DESTIGMATISING MENTAL ILLNESS?

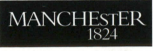

Manchester University Press

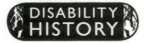

Series editors
Dr Julie Anderson, Professor Walton Schalick, III

This new series published by Manchester University Press responds to the growing interest in disability as a discipline worthy of historical research. The series has a broad international historical remit, encompassing issues that include class, race, gender, age, war, medical treatment, professionalisation, environments, work, institutions and cultural and social aspects of disablement including representations of disabled people in literature, film, art and the media.

Already published
Deafness, community and culture in Britain: leisure and cohesion, 1945-1995
Martin Atherton
Framing the moron: the social construction of feeble-mindedness in the American eugenics era
Gerald V. O'Brien
Worth saving: disabled children during the Second World War
Sue Wheatcroft

DESTIGMATISING MENTAL ILLNESS?

PROFESSIONAL POLITICS AND PUBLIC EDUCATION IN BRITAIN, 1870–1970

Vicky Long

Manchester University Press

Manchester and New York

distributed in the United States exclusively by Palgrave Macmillan

The right of Vicky Long to be identified as the author of this work has been asserted by her in accordance with the Copyright, Designs and Patents Act 1988.

Published by Manchester University Press
Oxford Road, Manchester M13 9NR, UK
and Room 400, 175 Fifth Avenue, New York, NY 10010, USA
www.manchesteruniversitypress.co.uk

Distributed in the United States exclusively by
Palgrave Macmillan, 175 Fifth Avenue, New York,
NY 10010, USA

Distributed in Canada exclusively by
UBC Press, University of British Columbia, 2029 West Mall,
Vancouver, BC, Canada V6T 1Z2

British Library Cataloguing-in-Publication Data
A catalogue record for this book is available from the British Library

Library of Congress Cataloging-in-Publication Data applied for

ISBN   978 0 7190 8581 9   hardback

First published 2014

The publisher has no responsibility for the persistence or accuracy of URLs for any external or third-party internet websites referred to in this book, and does not guarantee that any content on such websites is, or will remain, accurate or appropriate.

Typeset in 10/12pt Arno Pro by
Servis Filmsetting Ltd, Stockport, Cheshire
Printed in Great Britain by
TJ International Ltd, Padstow

For Terry and James Long

Contents

List of figures

Series editors' foreword

You know a subject has achieved maturity when a book series is dedicated to it. In the case of disability, while it has co-existed with human beings for centuries the study of disability's history is still quite young.

In setting up this series, we chose to encourage multi-methodologic history rather than a purely traditional historical approach, as researchers in disability history come from a wide variety of disciplinary backgrounds. Equally 'disability' history is a diverse topic which benefits from a variety of approaches in order to appreciate its multi-dimensional characteristics.

A test for the team of authors and editors who bring you this series is typical of most series, but disability also brings other consequential challenges. At this time disability is highly contested as a social category in both developing and developed contexts. Inclusion, philosophy, money, education, visibility, sexuality, identity and exclusion are but a handful of the social categories in play. With this degree of politicisation, language is necessarily a cardinal focus.

In an effort to support the plurality of historical voices, the editors have elected to give fair rein to language. Language is historically contingent, and can appear offensive to our contemporary sensitivities. The authors and editors believe that the use of terminology that accurately reflects the historical period of any book in the series will assist readers in their understanding of the history of disability in time and place.

Finally, disability offers the cultural, social and intellectual historian a new 'take' on the world we know. We see disability history as one of a few nascent fields with the potential to reposition our understanding of the flow of cultures, society, institutions, ideas and lived experience. Conceptualisations of 'society' since the early modern period have heavily stressed principles of autonomy, rationality and the subjectivity of the individual agent. Consequently we are frequently oblivious to the historical contingency of the present with respect to those elements. Disability disturbs those foundational features of 'the modern'. Studying disability history helps us resituate our policies, our beliefs and our experiences.

Julie Anderson
Walton O. Schalick, III

Preface

On a visit to London in 2009, I caught sight of a poster on the Underground produced by the campaign Time to Change. Titled, 'Is your mind made up about mental illness?' the poster sought to dispel nine 'myths' about mental illness with nine 'facts'. Drawing my partner's attention to the poster, I complained that some of the 'facts' which the poster conveyed – for example the statement that 'mental health problems affect one in four people' – would do little to ease the discrimination experienced by people with enduring mental distress. However, the black and white presentation of the issue precluded debate: either, it inferred, you agree with us, or you're bigoted. Understandably, my partner was puzzled that I would question a campaign for which the objectives appeared so self-evidently right. Who, after all, would not want to end mental health discrimination?

By this time, however, I'd begun to identify connections between the surge of current campaigns which sought to destigmatise mental illness, and a seemingly obscure piece of historical research that I'd undertaken some years earlier as a PhD student, which analysed the efforts made by healthcare professionals and charitable groups in the period between 1870 and 1970 to educate the public and tackle the stigma of mental illness. The conclusions I drew concerned me.

Current campaigns assert that stigma emanates from interpersonal interactions. They seek to change the behaviour of the public by replacing public misapprehensions with professional knowledge regarding the truth about mental illness. Such campaigns contend that a false divide exists between those who have mental health problems and those who do not; we are all, they imply, liable to experience mental health discrimination. Bracketing together all psychiatric diagnostic labels under the umbrella term mental illness, these campaigns stress that mental illness is very common and can be treated effectively. The healthcare workers and charitable groups whose earlier efforts to grapple with the stigma of mental illness had formed the basis for my doctoral research had likewise emphasised that many cases of mental disorder could be cured. They believed that if the public could be made aware of this, and of the scale of mental health problems, the stigma attached to mental illness and its treatment could be erased. Yet, as this book reveals, their efforts failed to convince, for most people were well aware that a brief episode of depression could not be equated with a diagnosis of schizophrenia. Moreover, such messages frequently compounded the stigma attached to chronic long-stay mental hospital patients. Could current campaigns have similar detrimental consequences for people who experience enduring mental health problems? My PhD research no longer seemed so irrelevant.

My research had revealed how political, economic and social factors had a profound impact upon the discrimination experienced by people then termed 'mental patients'. Worryingly, however, current campaigns seemingly pay little attention to the role of structural factors in generating the discrimination experienced by service users, focusing almost exclusively upon the role of public attitudes and behaviours. Indeed, charitable groups such as Mind appear to curiously dichotomise their activities. Thus, on the one hand Mind vehemently opposes welfare reform measures in Britain which (as Mind rightly observes) are having a deleterious impact upon service users, yet on the other it appears to unquestioningly support Time to Change, which tacitly sanctions many of the principles underlying welfare reform by asserting that mental illness is no barrier to employment, and that many people who suffer from mental health issues are very successful.

Rather than write yet another book which examines how public prejudice generates the stigma of mental illness, but in a historical context (a project which in any case would be methodologically flawed, as I'll elaborate in the introduction), I've turned my attention to professional bodies and voluntary groups which produced public education messages, and to the structural factors which shaped these messages. What follows is unapologetically a historical study of the efforts made by healthcare workers to educate the public and destigmatise mental illness in the period 1870 to 1970, and of the political, economic and social factors which constrained these endeavours. Anti-stigma campaigners, past and present, sometimes represent the problem as a black and white issue: the stigma of mental illness emanates from public ignorance, and can be cured by presenting the public with 'the truth'. In reality, the issue is far more complex than that, and this book has to reflect and engage with that complexity.

Yet history for me is as much about present concerns as it is about past debates, and I don't want to lose sight of the contemporary relevance of this research. Nor do I want to alienate service users, healthcare professionals or voluntary sector groups who have picked up this book because they want to know if past lessons can inform current efforts to challenge the discrimination experienced by people who suffer from mental disturbance. Therefore, the introduction to this book situates my historical research against the backdrop of current anti-stigma campaigns. For readers unfamiliar with the history of British mental health services over the period 1870 to 1870, I've provided a thumbnail sketch of the main developments in the introduction, and a timeline detailing key reports, pieces of legislation and the foundation of professional bodies and voluntary organisations, which can be found at the end of the book. The conclusion then critiques the limitations of current anti-stigma campaigns in light of my historical findings. Here, I've been inspired by a number of trenchant observations from service users who feel that current campaigns, rather than addressing the discrimination they experienced, risk compounding their problems.

Acknowledgements

Like many of my peers, I spent a number of years stuck at the postdoc stage (temporary contracts, hourly paid work, and unpaid work) before securing a permanent job. Without the generous support I have received from a number of institutions and individuals over those years, I doubt that I would ever have managed to turn my PhD into a book.

I am indebted to the Arts and Humanities Research Council, which funded my PhD within the Centre for the History of Medicine at the University of Warwick. Here, I was extremely fortunate to be supervised by Hilary Marland and Mathew Thomson, who subsequently managed my postdoctoral work at Warwick. I am very grateful for their intellectual and personal support over a number of years. I would also like to thank Jane Adams, Molly Rogers, Sheryl Roote, Brooke Whitelaw, Dan O'Connor, Sue Aspinall, Jonathan Toms, Julia Smith, Gauri Raj, Caroline Proctor, Stephen Soanes and Angela Davis for their support. Much of my research was undertaken at Warwick's Modern Records Centre, and I would like to thank Christine Woodland and her successor Helen Ford for all their assistance over the years. Colin Jones and Mark Jackson examined my thesis and provided constructive suggestions for rewriting.

After more than a decade at Warwick, I moved to a post within the Centre for the History of Science Technology and Medicine at Manchester (aka CHSTM / the Centre for Dog Studies). I'd like to thank Gill Mawson and friends from the postdoc corridor: Neil Pemberton, Elizabeth Toon, Emma Jones, Val Harrington, Stephanie Snow, Kat Foxhall and Mike Brown. In particular, I am grateful to Julie Anderson for all her support and friendship, and for encouraging me to write this book. Manchester was followed by a post at Northumbria University, where colleagues across the Humanities Department made me very welcome, especially Sasha Handley and Leigh Wetherall-Dickson, my collaborator in the Situating States of Mind research group. This book was finally completed at Glasgow Caledonian University, aided by a year largely free of teaching when I started. Here, I have enjoyed the support of colleagues in the History and Politics subject team, and from the Centre for the Social History of Health and Healthcare. In particular, I would like to thank Rhona Blincow for her friendship and assistance; colleagues from the reading group who commented on redrafts of the introduction and conclusion, and John Stewart, who very kindly read through a draft of the whole manuscript and gave me advice in the redrafting stage.

I am grateful to the archivists and librarians from the Wellcome Library, the BBC archives, the National Archives, the Lothian Health Services Archive and the Greater Glasgow Health Board Archive. Unison generously granted permission to reproduce material from the COHSE archive. Alisdair Cameron, team leader at Newcastle's Launchpad, kindly shared an article with me and bounced around ideas regarding Time to Change. Draft chapters from this book have been presented in seminars held at Glasgow Caledonian University, Manchester University, Northumbria University, Exeter University, Leicester De Montfort University and the London School of Hygiene and Tropical Medicine, as well as in conference papers for University College Dublin, the Situating States of Mind group (Northumbria), and the Medical Humanities Research Network Scotland (Glasgow University). I am grateful to everyone who gave me feedback at these events.

Emma Brennan and her colleagues at Manchester University Press have been professional, efficient, courteous and patient at every stage in the process. I am grateful to Walt Schalick, who co-edits the Disability History series with Julie Anderson; to the reviewers of the original proposal for their support for the project, and the reader of the manuscript for his/her constructive comments. Last, but certainly not least, I very gratefully acknowledge the support of friends and family over the years, especially Clare Hickman, who has bounced around ideas over the years as we've negotiated the postdoctoral minefield; my Dad, who spent years driving me up and down motorways as I moved progressively further away from Somerset, and my partner Sam, who, amongst other things, debated the merits of Time to Change with me, put up with the mounds of paper and post-it notes covered in incomprehensible scrawl in the lounge, and proofread the draft.

List of abbreviations

APSW	Association of Psychiatric Social Work
BBC	British Broadcasting Corporation
BJPSW	*British Journal of Psychiatric Social Work*
JMS	*Journal of Mental Science*
MACA	Mental After Care Association
NAMH	National Association for Mental Health
NHS	National Health Service
PRSC	Public Relations Sub-Committee of the Association of Psychiatric Social Work
PSW	psychiatric social worker
SANE	Schizophrenia: a National Emergency

Abbreviations used in the notes

BBC WAC	British Broadcasting Corporation Written Archives Centre
COHSE	Confederation of Health Service Employees
LHSA	Lothian Health Services Archive
MHIWU	Mental Hospital and Institutional Workers' Union
MRC	Modern Records Centre
NAWU	National Asylum Workers' Union
TNA	The National Archives, Kew

INTRODUCTION

This book examines the efforts made by British mental healthcare workers to destigmatise mental illness and its treatment. It covers the period 1870 to 1970, an era in which the polarisation of madness and sanity gave way to the belief that mental health and illness formed a continuum, and the asylum, which segregated the mad from the sane, began to be displaced by the policy of care in the community. In this introduction, I will commence by outlining the approach adopted within this book and the main lines of argument. I will explain why I have chosen to analyse the views of healthcare workers rather than public opinion, and I will outline the structure of this book. The rest of the introduction provides contextual information for readers approaching this study from different fields. For fellow historians of psychiatry and mental healthcare, I will situate the approach taken in this book within recent debates as to how histories of mental healthcare should be written. I will then provide an overview of the theoretical models which inform my approach. The concept of stigma is pivotal to this study. Yet, too often healthcare workers in the past – and anti-stigma campaigners today – draw upon a model of stigma which focuses upon public misconceptions and interpersonal interactions, overlooking structural factors which generated and perpetuated discrimination. Finally, for those readers with little or no prior knowledge of the history of mental healthcare, I will sketch out key pieces of legislation with affected the nature of psychiatric care in this era. Further details can be found in the timeline at the end of this book.

In 1993, Roy Porter and Mark Micale cogently argued that historians of psychiatry 'have told us a great many tales about the past, in the present, for present purposes'.[1] This observation by no means relates only to the history of psychiatry, for few historians would now contest that history is an interpretation of past events constructed by people whose contemporary preoccupations, consciously or unconsciously, influenced their choice of topic and interpretation.[2] However, few fields of historical inquiry better exemplify the truth of this observation than the history of psychiatry, for the subject matter, disciplinary boundaries and theoretical basis of psychiatry have long been, and continue to be, contested. In turn, these disputes inform histories of mental healthcare, imparting the multifarious contemporary preoccupations of their authors. Indeed, the appeal of history as a tool to legitimate current agendas is so alluring that its use is by no means confined to official histories of psychiatry. As we will see time and time again throughout this book, health-care workers, voluntary bodies and government officials frequently conjured a selective history of mental healthcare as a means of justifying their vision of reforming mental healthcare.

Nor is this book immune from contemporary concerns. Over the course of the 1990s, many of the traditional psychiatric hospitals in Britain closed down as the model of community care gained ascendancy over institutional provision. Yet the incessant wave of public education campaigns launched in the past decade suggests that this transition failed to end the stigma attached to mental illness. As a fledgling PhD student in 2000, I wanted to understand why people who experienced mental distress continued to face widespread discrimination, via a historical analysis. I thus sought to trace how public attitudes towards mental illness changed, starting my research against the backdrop of the Royal College of Psychiatrists' five-year 'national anti-stigma' campaign, 'Changing Minds'.[3] Part way through, five mental health organisa-tions in Scotland launched 'See Me', an on-going campaign, fully funded by the Scottish government, which seeks to end the stigma attached to mental ill-health. In 2009, three major mental health organisations launched 'Time to Change'. Funded by the Department of Health, Time to Change is described as 'England's biggest ever attempt to end stigma and discrimination and improve well-being'.[4] These campaigns tend to follow similar patterns. See Me, for example, is highly typical in that it seeks to change public understanding, attitudes and behaviours so that the stigma associated with mental ill-health is eliminated. It emphasises the prevalence of mental illness by asserting that one in four people will experience mental health problems at some stage and believes that the media play a significant role in shaping public attitudes.[5]

As new campaigns rapidly spring up when a campaign concludes, it seems that campaigners struggle to secure their objectives. Disability rights cam-paigner Liz Sayce suggests that 'the messages that the mental health move-ment believes will change attitudes often simply do not look the same to those who are supposed to have their attitudes changed'.[6] She illustrated this point with a New Zealand campaign slogan, 'if you have or have had a mental illness you are in good company'. This slogan sought to normalise mental illness by emphasising its prevalence, a common strategy in destigmatisation campaigns. However, the message people took away from the campaign was that 'there were a lot of dangerous people with mental illness in the community':[7] the campaign thus fuelled the beliefs it had set out to dispel.

Indeed, despite the seemingly incessant launch of destigmatisation campaigns, it is hard to identify any significant movement towards greater public tolerance; a recent survey of attitudes towards people with mental illness in England and Scotland published in the *British Journal of Psychiatry* in 2009 suggests that opinions became less positive between 1994 and 2003.[8] A similar picture emerges in figures gathered by See Me, which reveal that the percentage of people surveyed who agreed with the statement 'the public should be better protected from people with mental health problems' dipped from 35 per cent in 2002 to under 25 per cent in 2004, only to climb back over the 30 per cent mark in 2006.[9] Nor can England's 'Time to Change' campaign claim, as yet, to have made any significant inroads. Publishing the findings of the Office of National Statistics' 2010 survey under the lukewarm title 'Public Attitudes Heading Slowly in the Right Direction', Time to Change noted that while, for example, 16 per cent of the people polled could 'correctly' state the proportion of people who would have a mental health problem at some point – a 3 per cent rise – the percentage of people who agreed with the statement that 'people with mental illness are less of a danger than most people suppose' had remained static at 59 per cent.[10] Beliefs that mental health service users pose a risk thus appear particularly entrenched. The authors of the *British Journal of Psychiatry* report argued that anti-stigma campaigns have been undermined by media coverage linking mental illness and violence, fuelled in part by the shift in government policy towards managing the risk posed to the public by people who experience mental disorder.[11]

Such views are often held by mental health professionals and campaigners who complain that negative representations of mental distress overshadow positive coverage. In its 'Changing Minds' campaign, the Royal College of Psychiatrists aimed to 'increase public and professional understanding of mental health problems and to reduce stigma and discrimination'.[12] The College explained that the campaign would reveal 'the damaging effects of negative attitudes to mental disorders, and provide information about what we know about them. We hope to challenge you to think in new ways about mental disorders, and banish some of the myths and prejudices surrounding them.' The campaign, the College hoped, would 'close the gap between what health care professionals and the public perceive as useful treatments'.[13] This campaign was underpinned by the supposition that public ignorance of mental disorders and treatment methods sparked prejudice; stigma could be alleviated if the College succeeded in imparting its knowledge to the public.

This book is still driven by my desire to understand whether history can help us understand why people who experience mental distress today continue to face widespread discrimination. However, my initial efforts to answer this question by examining changing public opinion rapidly slipped into conceptual and methodological mire as I realised that 'the public' and 'public opinion' were not the readily definable objects I had initially presumed them to be, but frustratingly opaque and intangible concepts. Yet while I slowly pieced together a theoretical framework through which to structure my research, the healthcare workers who had authored my primary source materials were evidently not so encumbered; their articles, unfettered by any similar theoretical considerations, blithely depicted the public and public opinion as constant, knowable categories. Indeed, as I amassed a growing number of articles in which healthcare workers, activists and sufferers of mental distress ostensibly discussed public views of mental illness, it dawned on me that these sources revealed little about what 'the public' thought. In other words, 'the public' which surfaced in healthcare workers' writing did not correlate with an external referent, for the term reflected a construct; a category imagined by healthcare workers. However, such constructions of 'the public' revealed a good deal about the preoccupations, concerns and professional aspirations of mental healthcare workers, who frequently constructed the category of 'the public' as a binary opposite to their own self-image as rational and knowledgeable, in part as a means of asserting their professional status.[14] Over the course of the nineteenth and early twentieth centuries, psychiatrists and other healthcare workers consistently depicted the public as a homogeneous entity which needed to be indoctrinated with the correct views to hold so as to raise the status of psychiatry and allied health workers, a task rendered virtually impossible by the malleable character of the public and its unfortunate predilection for sensationalist reporting.

Let us turn, for example, to a speech given by John Charles Bucknill to an audience of fellow psychiatrists in 1881, in which he informed his colleagues that there were two kinds of public opinion, 'the one morbid and irrational, the other sound and intelligent. The latter is based, indeed, upon the efforts made by scientific men themselves to create enlightened public opinion on this subject.'[15] These sentiments encapsulate beliefs frequently expressed about the public by mental healthcare workers well into the twentieth century. Bucknill sought to preclude discussion by claiming that psychiatric knowledge was indisputable fact rather than opinion, debarring lay people from participating in debate. The function of the public, as envisaged by Bucknill and his colleagues, was to provide unquestioning support to professional expertise. Unfortunately, in the view of nineteenth- and early twentieth-century psychiatrists, the public were rarely this obliging. Discussions in the *Journal of Mental Science* (hereafter *JMS*), the forerunner of the *British Journal of Psychiatry*, complained of public prejudice towards asylums, asylum patients and those who treated them. Thus James Crichton-Browne warned his colleagues that it was 'hopeless to attempt by any amount of inquiry to pacify half-cured lunatics, or crack-brained enthusiasts, to conciliate the irreconcilables who must have a grievance, or to tranquillise the busy-bodies'. 'Life', he decreed, 'is too short for the education of idiots'.[16] 'There is a class who are profoundly ignorant of the whole matter, and never saw a lunatic in their lives', claimed G. Fielding Blandford, 'yet who are entirely convinced that patients are still barbarously ill-treated in asylums'.[17] In an equally defensive vein, Dr Dawson insisted that 'progress has come entirely from within. It has not come from officious criticism on the part of busybodies who think they know better than the men who have studied the subject for a lifetime.'[18]

Psychiatrists recognised that their professional status was inexorably entwined with public perceptions of mental illness and concurred that the public should be educated to counter the stigma surrounding mental illness and its treatment. Thus Dr G. Douglas McRae believed that 'public ignorance is the stigma'. Complaining that the public were 'very strongly prejudiced against asylums and asylum treatment', he suggested that 'we ought to stand up more firmly for our asylums and get the public to understand what work we really do'. McRae believed that the status of the profession could be raised if attention was drawn to its success in treating mental illness. 'I do not think we ought to leave the public under the impression that the mental specialist is a man who deals with chronic dangerous lunatics', he warned his colleagues.[19] We can detect similar professional considerations surfacing in debates and discussions amongst other mental healthcare workers, as for example in 1929 when one mental nurse successfully persuaded colleagues that it was time to change the name of their trade union, arguing that 'if we as a Union alter our title and do away with the false stigma of the word "asylum", the public will more readily realise that our institutions are actually hospitals dealing with mental diseases . . . We shall be doing something to raise the status of the mental nursing profession and to teach the public that our profession is a real asset to the social services of the country.'[20]

In many respects, mental healthcare workers' views of the public corresponded with a vision of the public shared by health educators in the twentieth century. Thus, Elizabeth Toon has shown how cancer experts viewed the public as 'gullible and emotional'.[21] The role of the expert was thus to cure 'mass ignorance through the provision of scientific facts, which would then encourage sensible behaviour'.[22] Similarly, David Cantor has argued that the clinicians and scientists who dominated the Empire Rheumatism Council viewed the public as 'an empty vessel of ignorance into which scientific and medical expertise could be poured'.[23] Ignorance was not the only barrier which healthcare workers believed they had to surmount; many healthcare workers bemoaned the public's emotional volatility, easily manipulated by sensationalist propaganda and liable to vacillate between apathy and terror. Thus, members of the Empire Rheumatism Council feared that rheumatism lacked the emotional, dramatic appeal of other diseases, depicting the public as complacent, ignorant and easily distracted.[24] Conversely, healthcare workers seeking to educate the public about cancer viewed public fear of the disease as a barrier to early treatment, and promoted the message that cancer was curable.[25]

Mental healthcare workers also viewed public fear of mental illness as a barrier to early treatment, and thus sought to emphasise the ability of psychiatry to cure mental disorder in its early stages. In another crucial respect, however, the efforts of mental healthcare workers differed. Most health education sought to persuade the public to seek treatment and, increasingly in the postwar period, to take responsibility for their own health by adopting a healthy lifestyle.[26] However, many mental healthcare workers believed that the main objective of public education should be to counter the stigma and prejudice which they felt their profession and their patients laboured under. The goal of improving mental health co-existed alongside the desire for enhanced professional prestige and better resources for the mental health services.

If we want to understand why the shift from institutional care to community care failed to effect a transformation of attitudes towards people who suffered from mental disorder, we must shift our focus away from the nebulous realm of public opinion, and examine mental healthcare workers' efforts to challenge the stigma attached to mental illness. In this book, I will argue that representations of mental illness conveyed by healthcare professionals were by-products of professional aspirations, economic motivations and perceptions of the public, sensitive to shifting social and political currents. Via their professional groups, healthcare professionals generated discourses which in turn shaped media coverage and perpetuated the stigma of mental illness. Challenging the idea that discrimination stems from public ignorance and media depictions of violent madmen, I contend that the image of public ignorance which lies at the heart of anti-stigma campaigns has, in part, been constructed by healthcare professionals.

The structure of the book mirrors this reflexive shift from the role played by the public to agents in the field of mental health. It starts by considering the narratives produced by patients and psychiatrists for a public audience, examining whether the shared world of the asylum engendered a degree of parallel stigma. While many of these narratives ostensibly sought to change public attitudes, the disparate objectives of their authors hindered the goal of destigmatising mental illness. The book then examines how psychiatric nurses and psychiatric social workers (hereafter PSWs) attempted to secure the position of their occupation within the field of mental health. This chapter argues that we need to examine the relative power and professional status of different occupational groups, and to consider efforts to destigmatise mental illness within the context of the broader goals of that occupation. Many healthcare workers sought to enhance the image of their profession by drawing attention to the development of new treatment methods for acute mental disorder and the expansion of extra-mural services, as the third chapter demonstrates. This strategy, I argue, reinforced the stigma of chronic mental illness and the mental hospital. The fourth chapter contests the interpretation that mental illness was predominantly gendered as female in the twentieth century, contending that the image of the dangerous male lunatic underpinned the stigma of mental illness. It examines how the gender dynamic within the profession of psychiatric nursing ignited stigmatising images of patients at times of professional crisis, a strategy which also tarred the professional image of psychiatric nurses. Healthcare professionals also sought to change public attitudes towards mental illness and its treatment through other spheres, as the final two chapters demonstrate. The fifth chapter examines the capacity of voluntary groups to promote different representations of mental illness and innovative treatment approaches. In practice, however, charities' activities remained intimately linked to state provisions and professional aspirations. The book culminates in a chapter which analyses the influence exerted by healthcare professions on programming on mental health issues produced by the British Broadcasting Corporation (hereafter BBC). I conclude by critiquing the limitations of current anti-stigma campaigns, in light of my historical findings.[27]

To substantiate this analysis, I have drawn upon a range of sources which span statutory and voluntary services, private interest groups, individual perspectives, media representations and institutional sources. The archives and journals of the main trade unions and professional associations which represented mental healthcare workers in this era are integral to this analysis. I have also used records which allow me to chart the activities of healthcare workers in other domains, notably the archives of the first charity established to assist people with a history of mental illness, and the records of the BBC, a media outlet whose distinctive ethos of public education provided a platform for some healthcare workers to exert a powerful influence over programming on mental health issues. To provide more detailed analysis of practice and experience at given moments, these sources have been complemented by a selection of published memoirs and newspapers, articles and blog posts by service users, and archival records generated by asylums, psychiatrists and the Ministry of Health.

By examining how healthcare workers constructed an image of public attitudes towards mental disorder, I aim to critique the one-dimensional message at the heart of many contemporary campaigns: that public ignorance and prejudice produces the discrimination experienced by service users. Many current anti-stigma campaigns depict 'the public' as a monolithic entity and seek to impose a preordained set of unequivocal messages. This approach overlooks the broader structural factors which generate the discrimination experienced by mental health service users. It imposes generalised messages which do not correlate with people's diverse experiences of mental distress and its treatment, and fails to convince target audiences. Moreover, all too often such campaigns focus upon acute and minor mental health problems, but fail to address the discrimination experienced by people who suffer from severe and enduring mental distress. I do not mean to trivialise the distress which a short-lived episode of depression can induce, but it is misleading to suggest that a person with this experience would face the same level of discrimination encountered by a person who experienced recurrent episodes of mental disturbance.

'The story I want to tell is straightforward', explained historian Edward Shorter in the preface of his 1997 book, which he described as 'a new history of psychiatry, an overview that will tell the basic story'.[28] Shorter's approach makes for an eminently readable story which effectively conveys his interpretation. Unfortunately, however, the history of psychiatry is far from straightforward, for, as Porter and Micale pointed out, 'in no branch of the history of science or medicine has there been less interpretive consensus'.[29] Shorter outlined a chronological narrative which 'commences with psychiatrists who believed that the brain was the basis of mental illness . . . is then interrupted by half a century divorcing brain from mind . . . and . . . concludes in our own time with the renewed triumph of views stressing the primacy of the brain'.[30] While disingenuously promising to 'rescue the history of psychiatry from the sectarians who have made the subject a sandbox for their ideologies',[31] Shorter plotted his narrative to fashion a story which conveyed his view that mental illness has a biological basis, recounting how the linear development of biological psychiatry was briefly derailed by Freud, before rightfully gaining ascendancy.

Historical narratives, observed Hayden White, arise from the desire to impose a moral interpretation upon past events.[32] The work of postmodernist and post-structuralist scholars like White has done much to dispel the notion that historians can use their skills to fashion one truthful account of what happened in the past from the available historical sources, and reminds us that a chronological narrative risks imposing a misleading coherence upon past events. I aim, instead, to reveal the plurality of discourses generated by groups in the field of mental health; the nonlinear direction of policy and ideology; the multifarious meanings which can be ascribed to particular developments in the field of mental healthcare.

Historiography, healthcare professionals and the field of mental healthcare

I have written this book not to challenge or defend any particular line of historical interpretation but to examine the efforts made by healthcare professionals to destigmatise mental illness. However, as noted above, the history of mental healthcare is a contentious field; I thus wish to situate my approach within the historiographical debate, and to outline the theoretical models which inform my account. Revisionist work on the history of psychiatry, following in the wake of path-breaking accounts by Andrew Scull and Michel Foucault,[33] sought to destabilise earlier whiggish accounts, which Scull pithily dismissed as 'humanitarianism + science + government inspections = "the great nineteenth-century movement for a more humane and intelligent treatment of the insane"'.[34] Viewing the asylum as an instrument of social control which psychiatrists exploited as a mechanism for professional aggrandisement, revisionists pointed to the ways in which psychiatry perpetuated notions of social, gender and racial inequality. Such studies traced how therapeutic optimism gave way to pessimism as theories of degeneration reinforced policies of custodialism by the 1870s, transforming asylums into custodial rather than curative institutions.[35]

Recent post-revisionist historiography has sought to 'free itself from its anti-psychiatric genealogy';[36] to temper 'the overly ideologised and unconvincingly theorised approaches' said to characterise revisionist work.[37] Post-revisionist historians thus issue pleas to untangle the nuances inherent in mental healthcare; to undertake detailed empirical studies which might unseat the synthesising, sociologically influenced interpretations of the revisionists; to study the shades of grey between the black and white. Consequently, post-revisionist work situates psychiatrists' actions within a broader socio-political context, arguing that revisionists have overestimated psychiatrists' agency in engendering change. Such interpretations can be applied to analyses of institutional care. In a detailed study focused upon one Devon asylum, for example, Joseph Melling and Bill Forsythe sketched a politics of madness which encompassed government bodies, Poor Law unions, county councils, the courts and relatives of the insane. They asserted that the county asylum was not a kingdom in which the medical superintendent wielded unmediated power but a 'locus for social conflict',[38] contesting Andrew Scull's interpretation of the powers exerted by psychiatrists.

However, many post-revisionist historians seek to unseat the asylum as the primary object of historical enquiry, pointing out that even in the heyday of the asylum forms of care in the community persisted. This has been amply demonstrated by contributors to David Wright and Peter Bartlett's 1999 edited collection, who explored the persistence of boarding out and care within the home.[39] Such studies were fostered by post-revisionists' interest in the role played by families in the care of the mentally disturbed, and a growing scepticism in the powers hitherto ascribed to psychiatrists. Thus, David Wright has drawn historians' attention to the role played by families in securing the discharge of their relatives from asylums and providing care in the nineteenth century,[40] while Akihito Suzuki similarly sought to problematise the idea that doctors controlled the care of the mentally ill by examining the persistence of home care.[41] Louise Westwood has demonstrated that forms of non-institutional care continued to be pioneered in the first half of the twentieth century, particularly for cases labelled as borderline or mentally defective.[42] Furthermore, the ways in which psychiatric and psychological knowledge filtered beyond the walls of the asylum to permeate diverse fields of social life, a trend which historians had ascribed to psychiatrists' professionalising ambitions, are now attributed to a broader range of social agents. Thus, in a case study of social therapy for sex offenders in West Germany, Greg Eghigian asserted that psychiatrists' professional jurisdiction was circumscribed by other bodies, such as social service agencies and courts.[43]

In many respects, this book furthers, rather than challenging, the interpretations of post-revisionists as regards the role of psychiatry in the history of mental healthcare. Considering the views and actions of psychiatrists alongside the role of other healthcare workers, voluntary groups and patients, it reflects the broadening scope of the historiography on the history of mental distress. Rather than portray healthcare professionals as omnipotent agents of change, I analyse how intra-professional politics, embedded within a broader socio-political context, shaped and constrained the ways in which healthcare workers represented mental illness. In so doing, I seek to complicate the question 'why did healthcare workers not do more to destigmatise mental illness?' by illuminating the factors which constrained healthcare workers' agency. Thus, this book explores the complex goals and strategies of each group (of which destigmatising mental illness was but one); it considers the broader socio-political context in which they sought to enact these goals; it analyses the inequalities certain groups laboured under.

However, while this book focuses on discourses which transcended the asylum or mental hospital as opposed to institutional practice per se, I feel compelled to express my misgivings about any attempt to erase or decentre the asylum in histories of nineteenth- and twentieth-century mental healthcare. After all, post-revisionist work which has explored the asylum has demonstrated how it served as a locus for struggle,[44] or a site of reform through which extra-mural provisions connected.[45] Volker Hess and Benoît Majerus insist that historians of twentieth-century psychiatry cannot use the problems encountered by old and chronically ill patients in the wake of deinstitutionalisation as an excuse to overlook the fact that 'in the second half of the twentieth century, in almost every European state, psychiatry detached itself from the model of care in institutions'.[46] I do not disagree with this statement, but feel that it would be equally disingenuous to use extra-mural developments as a justification for overlooking the history of chronically ill patients, particularly because (as this book will demonstrate) the experiences of, and provisions for, long-stay patients have historically been overlooked by healthcare professionals keen to emphasise the more promising sectors of their work.

The drawn-out process of hospital closure, which has hitherto largely been neglected by historians, surely deserves our attention and may help us understand why the shift to community care did not significantly lessen the discrimination experienced by mental health service users. Peter Barham's work provides some clues in this respect, suggesting that the 'place' of the asylum was relocated in the 1980s and 1990s to new extra-mural spaces such as the rehabilitation or day centre, helping to perpetuate the identity of the mental patient in the community care era.[47] Indeed, where changes in ideology did occur, they may not have benefited all service users. Ruminating on the transfer of mental health services from hospitals to the community, Barbara Taylor expressed her misgivings that the dependent care relationships she experienced while a patient in Friern Hospital in the 1980s had since been displaced. Observing that 'outpatient services which do not fit into the new recovery model, such as rehabilitation services and day centres, are disappearing everywhere',[48] Taylor characterised contemporary mental healthcare as 'individuated and disconnected from any communal body . . . the much-touted independence of the community-based user thus often equals a life of lonely isolation'.[49]

Three theoretical concepts loosely underpin this book, although as the objective has been to utilise theory to analyse the processes under discussion, rather than to use the processes under discussion as a means of elaborating theory, these ideas inform the work implicitly rather than explicitly. Firstly, following Nancy Fraser, I seek to give due consideration to the contribution made by private interest groups (such as professional bodies and trades unions) to debates on mental illness; to explore whether such groups offered arenas in which their members could formulate counter-discourses, and whether the participation of such groups enabled a more inclusive, and thus more democratic, debate to take place.[50] Secondly, to understand and analyse inequalities of power between different groups, and to nuance interpretations of healthcare workers' roles in destigmatising – or stigmatising – mental illness, I turn to Chris Nottingham's concept of the insecure professional.[51] Thirdly, I have drawn upon Pierre Bourdieu's work to further my analysis of the interconnections and interrelationships between different groups, viewing mental healthcare as a field.[52] The groups and individuals involved in mental healthcare shared a perceptual scheme which imposed a hierarchical order, classifying objects and agents within the field. Thus, for example, oppositions between treatment and care served to divide the field and to privilege the former over the latter. Yet the boundaries and classifications within mental healthcare which served to privilege certain groups over others were constantly contested. We can discern such struggles if we explore attempts made to change the title of a profession, to appropriate new words to describe work practices, to 'don the most flattering of the available insignia . . . or inventing new labels'.[53] The field of mental healthcare conveys the multi-directional nature of change which took place, while acknowledging that not all groups had equal capacity to effect change.

'Medicine in the twentieth century', remarked Gerry Larkin, 'is characterised by its ever-growing workforce and by an increase in the number and type of health worker'.[54] This observation certainly characterises the field of mental healthcare, where the number of occupations involved in the provision of care proliferated over the course of the century, each seeking to carve out a distinctive niche. However, the near-absence of occupational groups whose functions emanated from the delivery of 'technologies of investigation and measurement' alerts us to one of the more idiosyncratic characteristics of twentieth-century psychiatry: the limited impact of scientific practices, relative to other fields of medicine.[55] Within the field of mental healthcare, which bordered on to and overlapped with general healthcare, welfare and employment, the power of respective occupations and groups to influence government policy, media coverage, public opinion and other occupational groups was distributed unevenly. Many of the groups formed a specialist branch of a broader health-care occupation and sought to defend the credentials of their specialism within that occupation. Moreover, tensions existed within each occupational group which reflected differences in the sites in which practitioners worked, the patient groups they worked with, their perspectives on the nature of mental illness and suitable treatment methods, and the balance of gender within the profession.

Amongst the mental healthcare occupations, psychiatry was the most influential and held the most professional status. Nevertheless, at the start of the century it remained a 'Cinderella' speciality, lacking the professional status, therapeutic techniques and popular image enjoyed by other branches of medicine.[56] Moreover, as the field of mental healthcare expanded over the course of the twentieth century, divisions emerged within the profession between psychiatrists based within asylums and those practising in community services. Tensions also developed between those psychiatrists who believed that mental illnesses had biological causes and were best treated in general hospitals with standardised medical interventions, and those psychiatrists who believed that mental illnesses were influenced by the patient's social context and could be alleviated by psychosocial interventions.

Within the increasingly overcrowded asylums, patients had more contact with asylum attendants or nurses. Throughout the first half of the twentieth century, this group of workers, through their trade union, contested whether their claims for pay and status should be grounded in their ability to provide skilled nursing care to sick patients or their ability to manage dangerous inmates, a debate which often pitted men and women within the profession into conflict with one another, and into conflict with the feminised profession of general nursing. In the second half of the century, the Royal College of Nursing offered another vehicle through which the interests of nurses could be expressed.

In the emergent field of social work, the psychiatric social work profession – rooted in the mental hygiene movement – grounded its claims to professional status on specialised training. Aspiring to lead the way in terms of professional knowledge and status within the social work profession as a whole, this female-dominated occupation, via its Association, also sought to assert its professional superiority over psychiatric nursing. Psychiatric social workers came into conflict with mental welfare officers, who managed the certification of patients and stressed the value of practical experience and risk management over qualifications.

Within the voluntary sector, the National Association for Mental Health (hereafter NAMH) dominated. This body, which operated in England and Wales, was formed in 1937 from the amalgamation of the Central Association for Mental Welfare, the National Council for Mental Hygiene and the Child Guidance Council. The Mental After Care Association (hereafter MACA), which chose not to merge with the other groups in 1937, also remained active. The Scottish Association of Mental Welfare was established in 1923. It amalgamated with the Scottish Child Guidance Council to form the Scottish Association for Mental Hygiene in 1938, and subsequently changed its name to the Scottish Association for Mental Health in 1949. These groups, whose viability was dependent upon financial support, had to convince the public that they offered an important and distinctive function not provided by the state. Over the course of the century, the rationale of these organisations shifted dramatically in response to changing state provision and broader social currents. They also offered another forum in which mental health professions could air their views on mental illness and its treatment. Although the service user movement did not begin to coalesce until the early 1970s, some former patients were able to express their views on mental illness and its treatment earlier in the century by writing memoirs and newspaper articles, by contributing to hospital papers and by giving evidence to government committees. Here again, it would be misleading to suggest that all patients or former patients shared the same objectives in writing, and many accounts authored by former patients do not situate the writer as belonging to a larger community of patients and ex-patients. There were of course other professions and organisations involved in the field of mental healthcare which this brief sketch does not do justice to, such as occupational therapists, disablement resettlement officers and clinical psychologists.

The proliferation of occupational groups in the field of mental healthcare led to a plurality of discourses on the nature of mental distress and how it might most effectively be treated. Broadly, we can divide understandings of and responses to mental distress into social and psychoanalytic approaches or biomedical and physical approaches. This in turn prompted debate as to whether mental distress was best conceptualised as maladjustment or illness, whether it had a social or biological cause and how and where it should be treated. Consequently, while all groups working within the field of mental health agreed that the public should be educated to alleviate the stigma attached to mental illness – a message that, as we have seen, underpinned the Royal College of Psychiatrists' 'Changing Minds' campaign – there was no consensus as to what message they wanted to impart.

Stigma and discrimination

Groups or individuals working in the field of mental healthcare tended to complain of the public's ignorance regarding mental health issues, and of the irrational and morbid views which the public consequently held regarding mental illness and mental healthcare. Public ignorance, they argued, was the source of the stigma of mental illness. Similar assumptions guide many contemporary anti-stigma campaigns: a more informed public would behave in a more enlightened manner towards mental health service users, and the stigma of mental illness would cease. This approach views interpersonal interactions as the site in which discrimination is exercised, a conceptualisation of stigma elaborated at length by the sociologist Erving Goffman in his influential 1963 account, *Stigma: Notes on the Management of a Spoiled Identity*.[57] Goffman's conceptualisation of stigma offers a useful starting point for considering the impact of stigma upon affected individuals and their relationship with others who labour under the same stigma. However, as recent critics of Goffman's work have argued, this model of stigma pays insufficient attention to broader structural forces which generate discrimination. Efforts to destigmatise mental illness which focus solely on interpersonal interactions can thus only partially ease the discrimination experienced by mental health service users.

Goffman defined stigma as a discrediting attribute which differentiates the individual. However, Goffman believed that no attribute was intrinsically discrediting. Stigma, he argued, arose in a fluid interpersonal context. It did not involve 'a set of concrete individuals who can be separated into two piles, the stigmatized and the normal'.[58] Thus, he noted how individuals whose attributes marked them out as deviants would nonetheless employ normal strategies to conceal these undesirable attributes and frequently succeeded in passing as normal. Indeed, 'he who is stigmatized in one regard nicely exhibits all the normal prejudices held towards those who are stigmatized in another regard'.[59] Conversely, hitherto 'normal' individuals might find that attributes acquired through ageing could discredit them.

What are the consequences of stigma? 'We believe', wrote Goffman, 'that the person with a stigma is not quite human':

> On this assumption we exercise varieties of discrimination, through which we effectively, if often unthinkingly, reduce his life chances. We construct a stigma theory, an ideology to explain his inferiority and account for the danger he represents . . . We use specific stigma terms . . . in our daily discourse as a source of metaphor and imagery, typically without giving thought to the original meaning. We tend to impute a wide range of imperfections on the basis of the original one.[60]

The impact of discrimination upon lived experience is mediated by individuals' sense of identity. If 'protected by identity beliefs of his own', Goffman argued, the stigmatised individual could feel 'that he is a fully fledged normal human being, and that we are the ones who are not quite human', yet, by and large, 'the stigmatized individual tends to hold the same beliefs about his identity that we do'.[61] As a consequence, many stigmatised individuals exhibit a degree of ambivalence regarding their identity. This undermines the capacity of those sharing the same stigmatising label to support each other; instead, individuals vacillate between a desire to affiliate and a desire to sever any connection with those sharing the same stigmatising label. Those who acquire a stigmatising label part-way through their lives may be reluctant to accept their new status, while some may stratify others in their group 'according to the degree to which their stigma is apparent and obtrusive', taking up 'in regard to those who are more evidently stigmatized than himself the attitudes the normals take to him'.[62] This ambivalence of identity, Goffman argued, is evident in the humour of the stigmatised in which 'cartoons, jokes and folk tales display unseriously the weaknesses of a stereotypical member of the category, even while this half-hero is made to guilelessly outwit a normal of imposing status'.[63] Stigmatised individuals who sought to challenge the discrimination they experienced could find their efforts backfiring, for 'in drawing attention to the situation of his own kind he is in some respects consolidating a public image of his differentness as a real thing and of his fellow-stigmatized as constituting a real group'.[64]

Although Goffman stressed the fluid and interpersonal nature of stigma, other scholars and campaigners felt that the term *attribute* embodied stigma within the individual, neglecting the actions of those who discriminated against the stigmatised individual. On these grounds, Liz Sayce critiqued Goffman's model for its focus on 'individual self-perception and micro-level interpersonal interactions'. Sayce believed that the concepts of discrimination and oppression more effectively drew attention to structural forces which fuelled the social and economic exclusion experienced by service users.[65] Similarly, Bruce Link and Jo Phelan argued that Goffman's conceptualisation overlooked structural factors. They argued that stigmatised individuals were divided into separate categories to accomplish a 'them' and 'us' dichotomy; labelling an individual as 'a schizophrenic', for example, defined that individual solely in reference to the condition they have been diagnosed with.[66] Stigma existed where discrimination was experienced as a consequence of such categorisation, and in situations where the social, political and economic climate facilitated the labelling, categorisation and discrimination of stigmatised individuals. By way of illustration, Link and Phelan described how stigmatised conditions such as schizophrenia attracted less funding for research and treatment, and how healthcare workers seeking advancement were attracted to more prestigious areas. Stigma thus generated a series of structural factors which affected the lived experiences of stigmatised individuals, independently of the discrimination they encountered from individuals on the basis of the stereotype of schizophrenia.[67] Power relations are intrinsic to this definition of stigma; without power potentially stigmatising beliefs will not generate discriminatory consequences, while the relative power of stigmatised individuals will determine their capacity to resist stigmatisation.[68]

In interpersonal contexts, interactions with non-stigmatised people pose a number of challenges for the stigmatised individual. When the stigmatising label is either clearly visible or public knowledge, the stigmatised individual may feel exposed, and resent the labelling, and lack of privacy. S/he might feel frustrated when basic skills are praised as major accomplishments. 'I don't want to be a schizophrenic "doing well"', complained Ben, when interviewed for a study by Peter Barham and Robert Hayward in the 1980s. '"Isn't he good, even though he's had a mental illness?"'[69] At the same, the stigmatised individual is aware that minor lapses from exemplary behaviour, for example displaying irritation or emotion, are likely to be attributed to their stigmatising label. Given these frustrations, individuals may well seek to conceal their stigmatising label, yet this strategy leaves open the possibility that their stigmatising label will be revealed. For this reason, some may choose to distance themselves from others to avoid having to divulge information. Those who do succeed in passing may encounter derogatory remarks made about those who share the same stigmatising label.

Goffman argued that the stigmatised individual can expect support from representative groups. These lobby to ameliorate the stigma attached to the stigmatising label, for example by trying to persuade the public to use a softer social label for the category in question. While some representative groups include members of the stigmatised group they claim to represent, and some indeed are led primarily by such individuals, others are dominated by people who claim to campaign on behalf of the stigmatised group. Goffman notes that these differences in the membership and leadership can engender tensions between groups.[70] It would however be helpful to qualify his argument that stigmatised individuals are 'likely' to support agencies and agents who represent them. Support is dependent upon how the group seeks to represent the category it claims to serve, and how effectively it meets the disparate needs of individuals perceived to belong to that category. By no means all individuals who experience mental distress would, for example, unconditionally support Schizophrenia: a National Emergency, hereafter SANE, the charity established by journalist Marjory Wallace in 1986.[71]

The stigmatised individual, Goffman argued, could also expect support from 'the wise': people who do not share their stigmatising label, but who have an intimate knowledge of life with this attribute, either because they work in an institution that caters for individuals so labelled, or because they are related to a stigmatised individual. Goffman argued that the wise are sympathetic to the plight of the stigmatised group, who in return extend courtesy member-ship of their group to the wise. However, as this book will demonstrate, the relationship between mental healthcare workers and their patients was far more complex.

Goffman described how stigma 'spread out in waves, but of diminishing intensity',[72] tainting those close to stigmatised individuals. This observation can be used to analyse the strategies adopted by those working in the field of mental health. Pointing to the shared experiences of people with learning disabilities and those employed to care for them, whilst acknowledging the 'profound differences' in the histories of the two groups, Duncan Mitchell has in this vein argued that learning disability nurses shared the stigma of the people they cared for. In turn, Mitchell argued, this shaped the strategies of this occupational group and its professional status.[73]

The place of madness and mental illness

Healthcare professionals' debates about the nature of mental illness and its treatment were shaped by, and in turn shaped, the provisions established to deliver mental healthcare. For those with little or no prior knowledge of the history of British mental healthcare services, it is thus helpful to have a brief overview of the main developments which affected care in this era. Further details of the legislation regulating mental healthcare in Britain throughout the period 1870 to 1970 can be found in the time line at the end of the book.

In the eighteenth century, insanity was interpreted through a blend of religious, medical and social explanations. Consequently, provisions for those afflicted could be characterised by their plurality, encompassing care within the family home, boarding patients out and the establishment of public asylums and private madhouses (the latter operated on a for-profit basis by both medical practitioners and lay people).[74] Treatment within an asylum became the primary course of action in the nineteenth century, when a series of legal measures culminated in the Lunatics Act of 1845.[75] This was portrayed as a humanitarian measure which provided patients with potentially curative treatment, while seeking to prevent abuses such as wrongful confinement and poor asylum conditions. The Act required all counties to build an asylum for pauper lunatics, who were admitted via a process of certification, and established the Lunacy Commission, which inspected all asylums.[76] From the outset, the county asylums were thus Poor Law institutions,[77] a connection severed when the 1929 Local Government Act abolished the Boards of Guardians.

In the twentieth century, the boundaries between mental health and illness became more ambiguous. Thus, the interwar mental hygiene movement sought to promote good mental health and prevent the onset of mental illness. Efforts were made to provide treatment to incipient cases of mental disorder via the 1930 Mental Treatment Act. This allowed people to seek treatment of their own volition or to be admitted as temporary patients without undergoing the process of certification, and made provision for the establishment of out-patient treatment. The Act also sought to alleviate the stigma of mental illness by substituting the phrase 'mental hospital' for the word 'asylum'. Attempts to align mental health services with general health services gathered pace after the Second World War, when mental hospitals were nominally incorporated within the new National Health Service (hereafter NHS). In 1959, the Mental Health Act empowered local authorities to establish community mental health services provisions. The trend towards community-based provisions accelerated two years later when the Minister of Health announced plans to close down the psychiatric hospitals.

In deploying the term 'mental illness' in this study, I am adhering to one of the more commonly held terms used in the twentieth century. However, I am not utilising this term for this reason alone. The shift in terminology from madness to lunacy, insanity and mental illness – while by no means a linear process – reflects subtle shifts in how mental disturbance was understood. The term *mental illness* conveyed a belief that mental distress and disturbance emanated from an illness with a probable physiological cause and also served to bracket together individuals with a diverse range of experiences. Healthcare professionals predominantly talked in terms of mental illness when they discussed the stigma they believed attached to their profession and their patients in the public mind. In saying this, I do not seek to deny the reality of mental distress – I simply contend that 'mental illness' is, to paraphrase Lindsay Prior, a name for a theory, rather than a name for a thing.[78] I thus view 'mental illness' as a time-bound concept, generated to reflect and perpetuate a certain view of what mental distress is, which this book interrogates as an object of analysis as it explores the consequences of centring anti-stigma campaigns and debates on this concept. Sidestepping debates as to the extent to which mental illnesses are socially constructed or natural kinds, arguably a false dichotomy in any case,[79] one might observe that even those who adhere to the view that mental illnesses are natural kinds – biological entities observable in different historical eras – would acknowledge that 'mental illness' is a label which refers to a number of conditions. The 'mentally ill' are thus a heterogeneous cohort of individuals experiencing different fates. This book explores the consequences of collapsing the plural – mental illnesses – into the singular – mental illness.

Notes

1 R. Porter and M. S. Micale, 'Introduction: reflections on psychiatry and its histories', in M. S. Micale and R. Porter (eds), *Discovering the History of Psychiatry* (New York and Oxford, 1994), pp. 3–36; p. 26.

2 See, for example, the classic text on historiography: E. H. Carr, *What Is History?* (1961; Harmondsworth, 1990), pp. 24, 30, 134. For a now classic postmodernist take on the same matter, see K. Jenkins, *Rethinking History* (1991; Abingdon, 2009), p. 31.

3 Royal College of Psychiatrists, 'Changing Minds', www.rcpsych.ac.uk/campaigns/previouscampaigns/changingminds.aspx, 2008. The campaign ran from 1998 to 2003.

4 'Time to Change' was launched by Mental Health Media, Mind and Rethink; since its launch, Mental Health Media has merged with Mind, and Rethink has rebranded itself as Rethink Mental Illness. See www.time-to-change.org.uk/, consulted 9 June 2009.

5 See www.seemescotland.org, consulted 6 January 2012. 'See Me' was launched in 2002 and is ongoing (as of 2013).

6 L. Sayce, *From Psychiatric Patient to Citizen: Overcoming Discrimination and Social Exclusion* (Houndmills, 2000), p. 207.

7 Ibid., p. 208.

8 N. Mehta, A. Kassam, M. Leese, G. Butler and G. Thornicroft, 'Public attitudes towards people with mental illness in England and Scotland, 1994–2003', *British Journal of Psychiatry*, 194 (2009), 278–84.

9 See Me, 'Changing public attitudes', www.seemescotland.org.uk/about/-whatwedo/changingpublicattitudes, consulted 8 March 2011.

10 J. Tudor, 'Public attitudes slowly heading in the right direction', www.time-to-change.org.uk/news/public-attitudes-heading-slowly-right-direction, consulted 31 March 2010.

11 Mehta, Kassam, Leese, Butler and Thornicroft, 'Public attitudes'.

12 Royal College of Psychiatrists, 'Changing Minds: history of the campaign', www.rcpsych.ac.uk/default.aspx?page=1424, 2006.

13 Royal College of Psychiatrists, 'Mental disorders: overcoming prejudice', www.rcpsych.ac.uk/campaigns/changingminds/whatisstigma/mentaldisorderschallenging.aspx, last updated 11 September 2003.

14 The same point is made by David Cantor in his study of how the Empire Research Council represented the public: see D. Cantor, 'Representing "the public": medicine, charity and emotion in twentieth-century Britain', in S. Sturdy (ed.),

Medicine, Health and the Public Sphere in Britain, 1600–2000 (London, 2002), pp. 145–68.

15 Anonymous, 'Occasional notes of the quarter: the annual meeting and dinner', *JMS*, 27 (1881–82), 401–2; 402.

16 J. Crichton-Brown, 'Presidential address', *JMS*, 24 (1878–79), 350–72; 351.

17 G. Fielding Blandford, 'The President's address', *JMS*, 23 (1877–78), 309–24; 320.

18 Anonymous, 'Annual general meeting of the MPA', *JMS*, 68 (1922), 423–58; 438.

19 Ibid., 434.

20 Mr Harris, *National Asylum Workers' Union Magazine* (hereafter *NAWU Magazine*), 18 (August, 1929), 11. This example is examined in further detail in Chapter 2.

21 E. Toon, '"Cancer as the general population knows it": knowledge, fear, and lay education in 1950s Britain', *Bulletin of the History of Medicine*, 81 (2007), 116–48; 118.

22 Ibid., 119.

23 Cantor, 'Representing "the public"', p. 145.

24 Ibid.

25 Toon, '"Cancer as the general population knows it"'.

26 See V. Berridge, 'Medicine, public health and the media in Britain from the nineteen-fifties to the nineteen-seventies', *Historical Research*, 82 (2009), 360–73, and V. Berridge, 'Medicine and the public: the 1962 Report of the Royal College of Physicians and the new public health', *Bulletin of the History of Medicine*, 81 (2007), 286–311.

27 This book does not seek to provide a sustained analysis of the impact of discrimination on the lived experiences of people diagnosed with a mental illness in this period, or of the efforts made by patients and service users to challenge the discrimination they experienced. These important questions merit a study in their own right.

28 E. Shorter, *A History of Psychiatry: From the Era of the Asylum to the Age of Prozac* (New York, 1997), p. vii.

29 Micale and Porter, *Discovering the History of Psychiatry*, p. 4.

30 Shorter, *A History of Psychiatry*, p. viii.

31 Ibid., p. viii.

32 H. White, *The Content of the Form: Narrative Discourse and Historical Representation* (Baltimore and London, 1987), pp. 14.

33 See, for example, A. T. Scull, *Museums of Madness: The Social Organization of Insanity in Nineteenth-Century England* (London, 1979); M. Foucault, *Madness and Civilization: A History of Insanity in the Age of Reason* (London, 1967).

34 A. Scull, *The Most Solitary of Afflictions: Madness and Society in Britain, 1700–1900* (New Haven and London, 1993), p. 3.

35 See Scull, *Museums of Madness* and *The Most Solitary of Afflictions*.

36 V. Hess and B. Majerus, 'Writing the history of psychiatry in the twentieth century', *History of Psychiatry*, 22 (2011), 139–45; 141.

37 J. Andrews and A. Digby, 'Introduction', in Andrews and Digby (eds), *Sex and Seclusion, Class and Custody: Perspectives on Gender and Class in the History of British and Irish Psychiatry* (Amsterdam and New York, 2004), pp. 7–44; p. 13.

38 J. Melling and B. Forsythe, *The Politics of Madness: The State, Insanity and Society in England, 1845–1914* (Abingdon, 2006), p. 6.

39 P. Bartlett and D. Wright (eds), *Outside the Walls of the Asylum: The History of Care in the Community, 1750–2000* (London and New Brunswick, 1999).

40 D. Wright, 'The discharge of pauper lunatics from county asylums in mid-Victorian England: the case of Buckinghamshire', in J. Melling and B. Forsythe (eds), *Insanity, Institutions and Society 1800–1914: A Social History of Madness in Comparative Perspective* (Abingdon, 1999), pp. 93–112.

41 D. Wright, 'The discharge of pauper lunatics'; A. Suzuki, *Madness at Home: The Psychiatrist, the Patient, and the Family in England, 1820–1860* (Berkley and Los Angeles, 2006).

42 L. Westwood, 'Avoiding the Asylum: Pioneering Work in Mental Health Care, 1890–1939' (DPhil thesis, Sussex University, 1999).

43 G. Eghigian, 'Deinstitutionalizing the history of contemporary psychiatry', *History of Psychiatry*, 22 (2011), 201–14.

44 Melling and Forsythe, *The Politics of Madness*.

45 See S. Soanes, 'Rest and Restitution: Mental Convalescence and the English Public Mental Hospital, 1919–1939' (PhD Thesis, University of Warwick, 2011); S. Soanes, 'Reforming asylums, reforming public attitudes: J. R. Lord and Montagu Lomax's representations of mental hospitals and the community, 1921–1931', *Family and Community History*, 12 (2009), 117–29.

46 Hess and Majerus, 'Writing the history of psychiatry', p. 140.

47 See P. Barham and R. Hayward, *Relocating Madness: From the Mental Patient to the Person* (London, 1995).

48 B. Taylor, 'The demise of the asylum in late twentieth-century Britain: a personal history', *Transactions of the Royal Historical Society*, 21 (2011), 193–215; 214 and 200, footnote 26.

49 Ibid., 215.

50 J. Habermas, *The Structural Transformation of the Public Sphere*, trans. T. Burger (1962; Cambridge, 1999). I drew heavily upon Nancy Fraser's reinterpretation of Habermas's work in my PhD thesis, reworking her notion of a 'counter-public sphere' to outline the idea of 'sub-public spheres': parallel discursive arenas which enabled members of subordinated social groups to constitute their own alternative publics. See N. Fraser, 'Rethinking the public sphere: a contribution to the critique of actually existing democracy', in C. Calhoun (ed.), *Habermas and the Public Sphere* (1992; Cambridge, Mass., 1999), pp. 109–42, and V. Long, 'Changing Public Representations of Mental illness in Britain, 1870–1970' (PhD dissertation, University of Warwick, 2004).

51 C. Nottingham, 'The rise of the insecure professionals', *International Review of Social History*, 52 (2007), 445–75.

52 I draw here primarily from P. Bourdieu, *Distinction: A Social Critique of the Judgement of Taste* (1979; translation by Richard Nice 1984: Abingdon, 2005), esp. pp. 466–84.

53 Ibid., p. 481.

54 G. Larkin, 'Health workers', in R. Cooter and J. Pickstone (eds), *Companion to Medicine in the Twentieth Century* (London, 2003), pp. 531–42; p. 531.

55 Ibid., p. 534. An exception here is the development of psychopharmacology – scientists from academic and industrial backgrounds and clinicians who were involved in the development of new drug therapies in psychiatry. See E. M. Tansey, '"They used to call it psychiatry": aspects of the development and impact of psychopharmacology', in M. Gijswijt-Hofstra and R. Porter (eds), *Cultures of Psychiatry and Mental Health Care in Postwar Britain and the Netherlands* (Amsterdam, 1998), pp. 79–101.

56 On the insecure professional status of psychiatry, see A. Scull, C. MacKenzie and N. Hervey, *Masters of Bedlam: The Transformation of the Mad-Doctoring Trade* (Chichester, 1996); T. Turner '"Not worth powder and shot": the public profile of the Medico-Psychological Association, c. 1851–1914', in G. E. Berrios and H. Freeman (eds), *150 Years of British Psychiatry, 1841–1991* (London, 1991), pp. 3–16.

57 E. Goffman, *Stigma: Notes on the Management of a Spoiled Identity* (1963; Harmondsworth, 1968).

58 Ibid., p. 136.

59 Ibid., p. 164.

60 Ibid., pp. 15–16.

61 Ibid., p. 17.

62 Ibid., pp. 130–1.

63 Ibid., p. 132.

64 Ibid., p. 139.

65 Sayce, *From Psychiatric Patient to Person*, pp. 14–15.

66 B. G. Link and J. C. Phelan, 'Conceptualizing stigma', *Annual Review of Sociology*, 27 (2001), 363–84; 372.

67 Ibid., p. 373.

68 Ibid., p. 376.

69 Barham and Hayward, *Relocating Madness*, p. 155.

70 Goffman, *Stigma*, p. 36.

71 SANE is discussed in Chapter 4.

72 Goffman, *Stigma*, p. 43.

73 D. Mitchell, 'Parallel stigma? Nurses and people with learning disabilities', *British Journal of Learning Disabilities*, 28 (2000), 78–81.

74 See, for example, R. Porter, *Mind-Forg'd Manacles: A History of Madness in England from the Restoration to the Regency* (Cambridge, Mass., 1987); W. Parry-Jones, *The Trade in Lunacy: A Study of Private Madhouses in England in the Eighteenth and Nineteenth Centuries* (London, 1972); R. A. Houston, ' "Not simple boarding":

care of the mentally incapacitated in Scotland during the long nineteenth century', in Bartlett and Wright (eds), *Outside the Walls of the Asylum*, pp. 19–44; A. Ingram (ed.), *Voices of Madness: Four Pamphlets* (Stroud, 1997); M. MacDonald, *Mystical Bedlam: Madness, Anxiety, and Healing in Seventeenth-Century England* (Cambridge, 1981).

75 This Act covered England and Wales; similar legislation was passed in Scotland in 1857.

76 For a thorough account of lunacy legislation in the nineteenth century, Kathleen Jones's work is particularly helpful. See K. Jones, *Asylums and After. A Revised History of the Mental Health Services: From the Early 18th Century to the 1990s* (London, 1993).

77 See P. Bartlett, 'The asylum and the Poor Law: the productive alliance', in Melling and Forsythe (eds), *Insanity, Institutions and Society*, pp. 48–67.

78 See L. Prior, *The Social Organization of Mental Illness* (London, 1993), p. 7. Prior, in turn, was borrowing from psychiatrist John Wing in his choice of phrasing.

79 For a discussion of this debate and an attempt to surmount this dichotomy, see I. Hacking, *The Social Construction of What?* (1999; Cambridge, Mass., 2000), pp. 100–24.

PSYCHIATRISTS AND THEIR PATIENTS: MIRRORED NARRATIVES OF SANITY AND MADNESS

Roy Porter, whose work was pivotal in establishing the significance of patient perspectives to the history of madness, observed that psychiatrists and their patients often said 'intriguingly comparable things about agency and action, rights and responsibility, reason and nonsense, although applying them in fundamentally reversed ways'.[1] Porter's observation informs my examination of the efforts made by psychiatrists and patients to address the public and challenge the stigma attached to mental illness and its treatment. Analysing a selection of psychiatrist and patient accounts, this chapter considers how the shared world of the asylum and mutual experiences of discrimination created parallels. It draws upon Erving Goffman's analysis of stigma to consider the difficulties facing patients and former patients who sought to challenge the stigma of mental illness, and to shed light on the strategies adopted by writers. Goffman argued that those who worked in institutions catering for stigmatised individuals empathised with their plight and were in turn accorded honorary membership of the stigmatised group.[2] However, the frequently adversarial nature of the relationship between psychiatrists and patients hindered collaborative efforts to tackle the stigma attached to mental illness and its treatment.

Indeed, even if we confine our analysis to either psychiatrists' narratives or patients' narratives, no consensus can be discerned. We can partly account for the disparate nature of these narratives by examining how understandings of mental illness, treatment regimes and the nature of the doctor–patient relationship at the time of writing shaped each account. Equally, it is important to consider the objectives of the author and the intended audience of the piece. Analysing books published by psychiatrists for public audiences in different eras, the chapter examines psychiatrists' perceptions of the public and the range of messages which they sought to impart. These accounts are compared to a selection of narratives authored by former patients, sampled to illustrate the disparate experiences of mental illness and its treatment described in such accounts over this period. Analysing an asylum newspaper published by and for the institution's patients and staff members, I will argue that the playful inversion of sanity and insanity which pervades the paper figuratively challenged the hierarchy of power within the asylum, but indicates a degree of self-alienation amongst asylum inmates.

Matters are different if we turn to examine accounts written by discharged patients who had been committed to an asylum against their will. These authors often sought to reassert control over their lives by denying that they had ever experienced mental disturbance. To emphasise this point, writers frequently set themselves apart from fellow patients. Insanity, in these accounts, was visibly inscribed upon the bodies of sufferers, identifiable through stereotypical postures and behaviours. Such an approach reveals a tendency amongst stigmatised individuals, as described by Goffman, to 'stratify his "own" according to the degree to which their stigma is apparent and obtrusive', and 'take up in regard to those who are more evidently stigmatized than himself the attitudes the normals take to him'.[3] Within the narratives of former patients, this attitude alternates uneasily with pleas to raise standards of care within asylums and change public attitudes towards mental illness, illustrating how writers oscillated between identifying with fellow sufferers and detaching themselves from the group.

The impact of changing treatment regimes upon patients' narratives is amply demonstrated if we turn to Allan Ingram's edited volume of seventeenth- and eighteenth-century pamphlets written by people deemed to have experienced madness at some stage in their lives. Only one of the writers, Hannah Allen, vividly detailed her experiences of mental disturbance.[4] Allen described how she fell into a deep melancholy following news of her husband's death, in which the Devil began to test her faith.[5] Her interpretation of her experience typified understandings in this era of mental disturbance, which tended to be identified through an individual's actions and behaviour, was often believed to stem from personal misfortunes and was interpreted through a combination of medical, religious and magical explanations.[6] While Allen's experience was mediated by a number of factors, including the willingness displayed by her family network to care for her when she was disturbed, chronology plays no small part. Allen was the only one of the four authors to write in the seventeenth century, a period in which mental disturbance was rarely subject to institutional confinement and care. She was thus able to write about her experiences of madness without fearing the loss of her liberty.

By 1739, when Alexander Cruden wrote, madness was increasingly perceived as a public problem, for which one solution was the private madhouse.

Those who chose to write about their madness thus ran the risk of being confined against their will. Cruden and the two later eighteenth-century authors whose accounts featured in Ingram's edited volume denied that they had ever been mad, and used their narratives to complain of the treatment they had received in madhouses.[7] Moreover, perhaps by the mid-eighteenth century, people were less inclined to listen to the narratives of the mad. Foucault argued that the practice of confinement was inspired by a desire to separate reason from unreason. Communication with the mentally ill ceased, and their physical segregation from the community in asylums was matched by a disregard for their attempts at communication. 'As for a common language', he wrote, 'there is no such thing':

> The constitution of madness as a mental illness, at the end of the eighteenth century, affords the evidence of a broken dialogue . . . and thrusts into oblivion all those stammered, imperfect words without fixed syntax in which the exchange between madness and reason was made. The language of psychiatry, which is a monologue of reason about madness, has been established on the basis of such a silence.[8]

Consequently stories told by those diagnosed with a mental illness about their experiences have traditionally been excluded from the psychiatric record, an approach replicated by some historians of psychiatry.[9] For most of the period under study, psychiatry spoke on behalf of patients, adopting a biomedical approach in which patients' speech could be usefully interpreted only as a symptom of underlying disorder. Jonathan Andrews and Andrew Scull, in their examination of John Monro's 1766 casebook, illustrate how this transition affected the encounter between patient and practitioner. While Monro sought to engage his patients in conversation in order to discover any events or behaviour that might have precipitated their disturbance, Andrews and Scull found that he 'was not disposed to place much credence in the stories he heard from what were, for him, evidently suspect sources'.[10] Reworking Mary Douglas's observation, Roy Porter argued that, by the nineteenth century, madness involved 'sound out of place'.[11] The content of patients' speech was believed to have no meaning.

The creation of a nationwide network of asylums under the terms of the Lunatics Act of 1845 in turn forged a community of mental patients with a shared experience of confinement and shaped the development of the emergent psychiatric profession. In 1841, asylum superintendents established the Association of Medical Officers of Asylums for the Insane, the forerunner of the Royal College of Psychiatrists.[12] Twelve years later, the Association established the *Asylum Journal of Mental Science* (hereafter the *JMS*; it dropped

Asylum from the title in 1859), envisaged as a forum for debate and the exchange of ideas amongst a dispersed profession, and a means of communicating the profession's ideas to a wider audience: to 'make an otherwise clapperless bell articulate'.[13] In practice, debate often took second place to a didactic defence of psychiatric practice.

It would overstate matters to suggest that psychiatrists laboured under the same degree of discrimination experienced by their patients. Nevertheless, throughout the nineteenth century psychiatry remained a fledgling profession whose claims to be the rightful custodian of the mad frequently came under fire. Well into the twentieth century it was a 'Cinderella' speciality, lacking the professional status, therapeutic techniques and popular image enjoyed by other branches of medicine. Assessing the position of psychiatry in Britain in the early to mid-twentieth century, Hugh Freeman was of the opinion that 'frankly speaking, the standard of doctors working in mental hospitals then was generally low'. Most doctors working in this field, he noted, 'simply picked up their working knowledge in mental hospitals on the old apprenticeship system'. The diploma in psychiatry lacked the prestige of comparable specialist qualifications in medicine, while the Royal College of Physicians sought to usurp the Royal Medico-Psychological Association's position as the body which represented the interests of psychiatrists to the government.[14]

Press coverage of psychiatrists and asylums in the late nineteenth century veered paradoxically between attacking psychiatrists for failing to lock up dangerous lunatics and recounting how unscrupulous psychiatrists colluded with relatives to wrongfully confine sane citizens for monetary gain.[15] Nor could doctors practising in other fields of medicine be relied upon to support their besieged colleagues working within asylums. The *JMS* bitterly attacked *The Lancet*'s reports on the care of the insane, claiming that the coverage 'combining real ignorance and popular prejudice with a lofty affectation of knowledge in its hostile criticism in a way we never remember to have seen exhibited towards any other department of the profession'.[16] In 1871, the *JMS* turned its attention to the *British Medical Journal*, deriding one recent article as 'inspired by the sensationalist spirit of the worst sort of writing in the daily press'. Psychiatrists belonging to the British Medical Association protested that the article would 'make the separation between the speciality and the general body of the profession still greater than it is at present, and strengthening popular prejudices which are injurious to the true interests of the insane and of the medical profession'.[17]

We will return to the troubled relationship between psychiatrists and other doctors, and the ways in which the asylum mediated this relationship, in Chapter 3. At this point, it is pertinent to note that the growth of asylums, to which patients were generally admitted against their will and from which they could be discharged only at the behest of the asylum superintendent or at the request of their families, fundamentally reconfigured the relationship between patients and their doctors. While the dismissive attitude adopted by other doctors and the legal profession's claims to define mental illness circumscribed the power and credibility of psychiatrists in the public domain, they nevertheless retained the upper hand in the clinical encounter within the asylum. This balance of power persisted well into the twentieth century, as the psychiatrist R. D. Laing explained to the documentary maker Peter Robinson in 1971: 'if you are interviewing a patient in a mental hospital ward and you have a key in your pocket to get out and the patient hasn't, the gulf in power, in position, is enormous'.[18]

Psychiatric patients – many certified and brought to the asylum against their will – often did not view themselves as suffering from an illness. Consequently, the ensuing clinical encounter between patient and practitioner was rarely characterised by a mutual wish to identify what was wrong with the patient and how it should be cured. Instead, the psychiatrist would diagnose the patient – often described as 'lacking insight' into their condition – while the patient could either not respond or challenge the psychiatrist's judgement or seek to convince the psychiatrist that they were well. The asylum, which had thrown together the fates of the psychiatric profession and the psychiatric patient, thus frequently constructed an adversarial relationship between the two parties. While patients and psychiatrists both shared in and deplored the stigma attached to the asylum, it was rare for them to speak together when trying to redress perceived public misapprehensions.

If psychiatrists had reconstituted madness as the loss of reason and abandoned dialogue with their patients, one might expect each group to be saying very different things, or as Foucault put it, to lack a 'common language'.[19] However, the discourses of psychiatry and of the mad reflected the difficulties of living with stigma and the shared heritage of the asylum, and frequently converged.[20] Although psychiatry was keen to proclaim itself as a scientific discipline based on truth and observation, some asylum inmates argued that psychiatric practice was simply the realisation of unproven theories. Porter's study of patient narratives revealed that some thought psychiatry itself mad, rendering others 'the victims of its own delusions, by conjuring up its own fantasy world of the mad'.[21]

Shared world of the asylum

It is to the narratives which emerged within the asylum that we now turn, drawing upon the *Morningside Mirror*, a newspaper established by the Royal

Edinburgh Asylum in 1845. This was by no means the only asylum newspaper established in the nineteenth century, but such papers were more common amongst Scottish asylums. Moreover, the records of the Royal Edinburgh Asylum have attracted a good deal of historical research, allowing us to contextualise the function of the paper within the asylum regime. The *Mirror* offered some asylum inhabitants a forum in which to forge a different identity for themselves than that of mental patient, a place to discuss literary genius, exotic locations and historical events; to escape the humdrum routine of asylum life. Thus, the *Mirror* carried frequent reports of the activities of the Asylum Literary Club where staff and patient members took turns to present papers, temporarily levelling the hierarchy within the hospital. Lauding the talent of the Club, an 1885 poem enthusiastically proclaimed the superiority of the Club to local schools and colleges:

> Hurrah! Hurrah! For the R.E.A.
> And the Literary Club so grand;
> Where will you find, my shrewd wise men,
> A better in all the land.

> The Morningside College is nothing to us,
> Nor Merchiston's ancient renown
> Our C. and our K., and our S. and our T.
> Could beat all the town and the gown.[22]

Indeed, the *Mirror* did more than simply defend the intellectual abilities of the asylum's inhabitants. Contributors frequently promoted the idea that mental illness was a positive attribute and that those within the asylum were superior to the sane outside, ideas given credence by psychiatrists who sometimes argued that creativity and insanity were linked. Henry Maudsley, for example, argued that people with a predisposition to mental illness should not be prevented from marrying on the grounds that originality and 'certain forms of genius' had 'sprung from families in which there has been some predisposition to insanity'.[23] However, articles proclaiming the virtues of asylum patients within the *Mirror* were usually written in a humorous tone and frequently contained a degree of self-mockery. It is thus worth considering Goffman's interpretation that such accounts stemmed from the stigmatised individual's sense of ambivalence regarding his or her identity. In the jokes made by stigmatised groups, Goffman argued, we are often presented with half-heroes who display the stereotypical weaknesses attributed to individuals labouring under this stigma, yet who nevertheless manage to 'guilelessly outwit a normal of imposing stature'.[24] Such stories, Goffman suggested, are indicative of self-alienation.[25]

We can discern a degree of self-mockery in the response printed by the *Mirror* to a letter sent in 1878 from an Alabama asylum, which complained that the *Mirror* devoted too much space to articles on Tennyson while overlooking basic details such as how many patients were in the asylum and how they were supported. Here, hyperbole created an exaggerated picture of the asylum residents' literary skills:

> Fancy anyone preferring to know how we are 'supported' to reading that most brilliant article of ours on the poet laureate, – a production, we have no hesitation of saying, unequalled as a criticism for its ingenuity and perspicuity. Tennyson's real meaning was unknown until that critique appeared. The poet has himself acknowledged this . . . As regards the commonplace into which his mind seems set on, we beg to inform him that . . . more Kings, Emperors, gods of the first class; lords, authors, prophets, artists, inventors, and great men of whom the world was not worthy; live here than anywhere else in creation.[26]

Mockery was however by no means reserved for the asylum's patients. Coverage of sporting activities, in particular curling, the dominant sporting pastime within the asylum in the nineteenth century, offered plenty of scope to ridicule the asylum staff. 'Just watch that "tall wise-looking man", who yesterday might have been seen in all the glory of official headship of his department striding along with his wand of office in his hands, a terror to all evil-doers', began one report of an 1879 curling match, which poked fun at Dr Thomas Clouston, Superintendent of the Asylum from 1873 to 1911:

> It cannot be that the uncanny looking mortal whom we see today on the ice is the same. He is unkempt and strange. He wields a monstrous broom, with which he now frantically sweeps the clean ice, already as smooth as glass . . . and if you have any doubt that the man is clean crazy and beside himself, just listen for a little to him. No patient in the padded cell was ever so incoherent.[27]

As this description suggests, curling, like the Literary Club, acted as a levelling force by providing a space in which the asylum population could come together on an equal footing. Doctors were frequently defeated by patients in matches and the asylum team often triumphed over local teams. The excerpt typifies how the *Mirror* depicted the distinctions between madness and sanity as permeable; the comedy in this excerpt stems from attaching the attributes of insanity to the psychiatrist. Contributors frequently held up the *Mirror* as a mirror on sanity and insanity, reflecting commonly held beliefs about madness, only in reverse.

This is neatly exemplified in a series of annual columns authored by an anonymous contributor between 1898 and 1900. Describing the antics of the Secret Society of Certified Lunatics, the stories contested the nature of mental illness and the purpose of the asylum. These columns commenced by reversing the comedic devise used above, attaching the attributes of rationality to the patients. According to the author, discussion amongst the patients prompted by the opening of the parliamentary session led to a consensus that 'affairs in our little community were fast going to the dogs, and that the only way to set them right was the parliamentary one of full discussion'.[28] Using the occasion of the attendants' ball, the patients chose to debate 'were the doctors themselves *simple* or *dangerous* lunatics?'

In the course of this discussion, Mr A. stated his belief that psychiatrists' trappings of knowledge – their professional association and knowledge of Latin – marked them out as dangerous lunatics. Mr E concurred, supporting his contention on the grounds that the doctors 'had stopped his grog, a mean thing to do'. Mr F. also cited the doctors' desire to spoil the patients' fun as proof of their dangerousness. He recounted how he had taken a knife from the pocket of the trousers of one attendant and had used it 'for his own amusement' to rip up a sofa and two chairs, before an attendant had stumbled upon the scene, 'deprived him of the toy he had found and stopped his liberty'. 'Could there be stronger proof of dangerous lunacy than that?', asked Mr F. Conversely, Mr G. claimed that the doctors were not dangerous but simple lunatics, informing his fellow patients that 'he himself had only that morning called Dr C [undoubtedly Clouston] a d—d to his face. The doctor simply laughed and passed on . . . that conduct was more compatible with a simple type of lunacy than a dangerous one. If the doctor had called him a d—d fool he would have knocked him down.'[29] The meeting drew to a close when one patient, Mr J., ended the reversal of given knowledge about mental illness, suggesting that 'before they discussed the question of whether the doctors were simple or dangerous lunatics, they must first settle whether they were lunatics at all . . . For himself, he did not think they were lunatics, but very sensible and well-informed persons indeed'. 'It was evident to all of us', wrote the narrator, 'that his mind was unhinged'.[30]

Stifled by the presence of the treacherous Mr J., who had had the temerity to suggest that the doctors were not insane, the *Mirror* described how the Society was revived a year later following his discharge. 'How we laughed when we heard of it!', reported the narrator. 'Anyone who had read the account of our last year's proceedings could see that he was the only insane person present. That he should be discharged while we other perfectly sane persons were kept, afforded strong support for both sides in our celebrated debate, "are the doctors themselves simple or dangerous lunatics?"'[31] The patients used their meeting, again held on the night of the attendants' ball, to debate the question, 'what is insanity?' The first speaker decided it was 'merely a matter of opinion. A doctor thought his patient was insane, the patient thought the doctor was insane. Who was to decide?' To which Mr B. reflected on the imbalance of power between patient and psychiatrist, remarking that 'although it was difficult to say who should decide, there was no doubt about who did decide'. Mr C. questioned the existence of insanity itself, claiming the whole thing was 'humbug'.[32] However, to deny the existence of insanity was to deny that doctors were lunatics, as Mr D. pointed out. It was Mr E. who resolved the issue:

> There was lunacy, dangerous lunacy, but it was all outside . . . For himself, he felt glad and proud to be where he was. To be considered different from the rest of the world when all admitted that the world was mad was surely to prove conclusively the sanity of all the members of our little society. It might not be the opinion of the doctors, but the doctors belonged to the world, and *ergo* were themselves mad.[33]

The final report of the Society appeared in 1900. According to the account, 'one of the certified who had enjoyed the privilege and enlightenment of our company for six months, and who it was now rumoured was about to leave us', suggested that as all the sanity was on the side of the certified, and all the insanity on the side of the uncertified, the duties and responsibilities of the two sections should be switched.[34] Agreeing that Dr Clouston should be the first subject of the experiment, the patients again waited until the night of the attendants' ball before phoning the hall keeper and asking that the doctor be sent up to the ward. Once the doctor entered the ward, the patients pounced upon him and removed his keys. The narrator asked, '"What is all this about. Is this the new patient?" Chorus "Yes sir, it's the new patient, and a precious rough one he is, he nearly beat us."' Although the patients had attacked Clouston, when in the role of 'attendants', they attributed the violence to the 'patient', reflecting patient complaints of brutal attendants. Clouston was then put through a mock admissions procedure:

> When he entered the sitting room I asked what his name was. One of our members informed me that his name was John Jones; that he had just been sent in as a dangerous lunatic; that he had spent the greater part of his life in asylums; and that one of his funniest delusions was that he was Dr C—, the head of one of the largest asylums in the country.
>
> When this last delusion of poor Jones was mentioned great was the amusement of our company. Indeed so contagious is laughter, that poor Jones chimed in and laughed with the best of us.
>
> When the patient recovered, he said, resuming a grave tone 'you know very well who I am, and that I am Dr C—, and that you will smart for this stupid and cruel joke tomorrow.'[35]

The same idea underpinned a joke regarding an apocryphal admissions certificate for a patient that Dr Walter MaClay, Senior Commissioner of the
Board of Control in the 1950s, was fond of telling: 'This patient is arrogant,
overbearing, and suffers from delusions of grandeur. He thinks he is a medical
superintendent. In fact, he behaves just like a medical superintendent.'[36]

The admissions and treatment procedure which Clouston endured in the
story subverted medical discourse and practice by applying the treatment to
a nominally 'sane' subject in order to make him admit delusions. To coerce
Clouston into admitting that he was, indeed, John Jones, the patients twisted
his cravat, strangling him. They also pricked his rear with a pin and filled his
mouth with soap and water, until he renounced his 'delusion' that he was
head of an asylum. Medicalising the procedure, one patient took his pulse and
temperature, pronouncing them to be too high. The narrator wanted to shave
Clouston's head in order to 'draw the inflammation from the brain', but, under
protest from Clouston and the other patients, only a cold shower was given.
'Then informing him that the first stages of the cure were passed through, and
that what he required was a good night's rest, we pushed him into the strong
room and locked him up.'[37]

Within the *Mirror*, writers playfully subverted hierarchies of madness and
sanity, casting the psychiatrists as irrational and the patients as rational. The
asylum is depicted as a cosy, safe and informal environment, the tone is good
humoured, if somewhat disrespectful, and the paper illustrates that psychiatrists and patients drew on a common language when addressing one another.
However, the comical exaggeration of the virtues of the insane lends some
credence to Goffman's contention that such humour masked self-alienation;
while those admitted to the asylum may have found a degree of acceptance
amongst fellow patients, it seems plausible that many found it hard to accept
an identity which they might previously have viewed disdainfully.

Moreover, the paper masks the real balance of power within the asylum –
the *Mirror* was printed because the doctors permitted it to be printed. It is
clear from an examination of patients' letters retained by Thomas Clouston
that many held a deep resentment for the man they believed was responsible
for their unjust incarceration.[38] While it is tempting to believe that a ward of
patients kidnapped their doctor, this scenario seems implausible. The story
closely follows the genre of comedy identified by Goffman whereby half-
heroes displaying the stereotypical attributes assigned to their stigmatised
category outmanoeuvre a normal individual.[39] By providing patients with a
controlled outlet for their frustrations, the *Mirror* may well have quelled discontent and unrest. Indeed, it is impossible to rule out the idea that a member
of staff, perhaps even Clouston himself, wrote the articles on the Secret Society

of Certified Lunatics: rather than being given a taste of his own medicine, perhaps it was the doctor who had the last laugh?

Psychiatrists writing for the public

Psychiatrists recognised that their professional status was inexorably entwined with public perceptions of mental illness and concurred that the public should be educated to counter the stigma surrounding mental illness and its treatment. Acting on these concerns, a number of psychiatrists attempted to correct perceived misapprehensions by writing books for a popular audience. However, such works were shaped by the perception that public education should be a didactic process. Thomas Clouston's *The Hygiene of the Mind*,[40] for example, claimed to draw on incontestable fact rather than opinion and thus sought to preclude the possibility of debate and contestation by a lay readership.[41]

While any qualitative analysis must of necessity be selective, it is instructive to commence by examining the work of one of the most prolific writers for a public audience. James Crichton-Browne served as medical superintendent at Newcastle and Wakefield asylums before his appointment as Lord Chancellor's Visitor in Lunacy in 1875. His work included *The Doctor Remembers, The Doctor's Second Thoughts, From the Doctor's Notebook, Stray Leaves From a Physician's Portfolio* and a book on the Scottish poet Robert Burns.[42] However, as Michael Neve and Trevor Turner have noted, Crichton-Browne was 'surprisingly unforthcoming' about his own profession in his popular books.[43] Thus in his collection of essays, *Stray Leaves*, Crichton-Browne dealt briefly with dreamy mental states and brain rest before examining the work of the Brontës, Shakespeare, Burns and Sir Walter Scott. These topics would not have been out of place within the *Morningside Mirror*, illustrating how both patients and psychiatrists sought to bolster their image through recourse to literature and the arts. Meanwhile, *A Doctor Remembers* was not an autobiography of Crichton-Browne's experiences as a psychiatrist, but a compilation of his reminiscences of famous men and incidents from the Victorian era.

Crichton-Browne seemed motivated to write by his concern that his hobbies and extracurricular interests were saved for posterity, 'rescued from the oblivion of bygone magazines'.[44] 'Most physicians', he claimed, 'are peripatetics and stroll from time to time from the professional Lyceum into the shady walks that branch out of it in so many directions'.[45] If judged by his popular writing, Crichton-Browne would appear to have spent very little time in the professional lyceum at all. Educating the public to lessen the stigma of mental illness does not appear to have been Chrichton-Browne's goal, perhaps

because he believed it to be a futile exercise. 'Life is too short for the education of idiots', he informed his audience on the occasion of his presidential
speech to the Medico-Psychological Association in 1878.[46] Analysing Henry
Maudsley's *Physiology and Pathology of the Mind*,[47] Helen Small observed that
Maudsley privileged fictional examples of insanity over scientific learning on
the subject. 'The repeated emphasis on medicine as a creative art', argued
Small, 'indicates considerable social ambition on the part of a man who culti-
vated an extensive aristocratic clientele, and who fought to protect the gentility
of his profession'.[48] Similarly, Crichton-Browne's free-ranging popular writ-
ings could be construed as an attempt to depict psychiatry as a gentleman's
occupation, requiring literary and social attributes as well as scientific knowledge; or indeed as an attempt by Crichton-Browne to camouflage his area of
specialism, an interpretation supported by Crichton-Browne's decision to title
himself as 'doctor' or 'physician' in his books.

Another doctor writing for the public in the 1920s had no hesitation in
placing before the public gaze what went on within asylum walls. Dr Montagu
Lomax's 1921 exposé, *The Experiences of an Asylum Doctor with Suggestions for
Asylum and Lunacy Law Reform*, offered a distinctly critical view of asylum care
which in turn inspired a Ministry of Health investigation. Most psychiatrists
argued that the problems facing psychiatric patients emanated from public
ignorance of the nature of mental illness and its treatment, and believed such
issues could be resolved if the public would let themselves be educated by
psychiatrists. Conversely, Lomax believed that the problems facing psychiatric
patients emanated from mismanagement within the system of asylum care
and that, once the public were acquainted with this mismanagement, they
could force psychiatry to reform. That Lomax had no particular allegiance to
the psychiatric profession doubtless informed his interpretation. Lomax was a
retired general practitioner who temporarily assumed the role of a psychiatrist
by entering asylum service during the First World War; while he indicated his
authority to address the topic by styling himself an asylum doctor in the title
of his book, he had no interest in raising the professional status of psychiatry. He, was, as Stephen Soanes has observed, 'detached from the system he
sought to expose'.[49] Consequently, Lomax aimed to familiarise readers with
what he saw as the prison-like conditions within asylums, following in the vein
of other doctors who had published critical pieces on psychiatric practice.
The insane, Lomax argued, were not 'dangerous wild beasts' but intelligent
people with feelings who were painfully aware of their pitiful surroundings.[50]
Characterising the therapeutic regime as comprising solely of the (frequently
punitive) administration of sedatives and purgatives, Lomax observed that
'merely to confine the insane is not to treat them, and certainly not to cure

them', insisting that 'many recoverable patients' were made 'permanently insane' by the present system.[51] Furthermore, Lomax averred that medical staff supplemented their diet by plundering the food supplies intended for the patients, and deduced that the growing death rate amongst asylum inmates during the First World War could be attributed to starvation.[52]

Lomax admitted that public knowledge of the nature of mental illness and its treatment was deficient.[53] However, he argued, the medical profession was equally ignorant as to the nature of mental illness, and consequently treated the matter with 'apathy and indifference'.[54] 'It is not enough for specialists and experts to be satisfied of the necessity for reform', he insisted, 'it is for the public itself to take the lead. But to do this the facts must be known.'[55] By itself, Lomax's book might not have had a significant impact. However, public feeling about asylum treatment had been stirred by the treatment of ex-service patients as pauper lunatics, and Lomax was able to tap into the emotion generated by this issue.[56] Once in the public domain, Lomax's ideas could be twisted in wholly new directions: one doctor, writing in the *Evening Standard*, praised Lomax for daring to give the public 'the naked truth' and expressed sympathy for the 'poor things' in the asylums before suggesting that 'there are many put in asylums who might as well be put in their graves . . . Why not painless extermination?'[57] Arguably Lomax's decision to configure patients as passive, voiceless objects of pity aided such an interpretation.

An investigation by the Ministry of Health dismissed many of Lomax's allegations and discovered in the process that Lomax had been responsible for prescribing 253 of 333 doses of the purgative croton oil between October 1917 and March 1918.[58] This might indicate that Lomax's book had a minimal impact upon mental healthcare. However, T. W. Harding has argued that Lomax's book prompted the Ministry of Health to review the work of the Board of the Control, and contributed towards the Ministry's decision to establish the Commission on Lunacy and Mental Disorder in 1924.[59]

In the postwar era, the development of new treatment methods and the integration of psychiatric services within the NHS encouraged psychiatrists to attempt to raise the status of their profession in the eyes of the public by stressing its affinity to general medicine. We can gauge the impact of these changes by comparing the two books published on the topic of psychiatry in Penguin's mass-market non-fiction Pelican series in the 1950s.[60] David Stafford-Clark, a participant in radio programmes on mental health issues, published *Psychiatry To-day* in 1952. By 1963, the book had sold over 130,000 copies and had been translated into several languages. Henry Yellowlees's popular psychiatry work, *To Define True Madness*, was first published a year after Stafford-Clark's book, and was subsequently issued as a revised edition by Penguin's Pelican series in 1955. Stafford-Clark did not distinguish between the general public and the psychiatrist in his writing, talking instead of 'normal people', 'we'. He was careful not to attack his readership by deriding their prejudices as foolish. However, by rationalising the fear which he believed mental illness provoked, he suggested that people with a mental illness were different from other people. 'Why do normal people find it so hard to accept and understand the mentally ill?' asked Stafford-Clark. 'A refusal or inability to accept some or all of the demands of reality is characteristic of such patients, and it is this above all that separates them from their fellow men'.[61] His book discussed normal behaviour, the causes of abnormal behaviour, and treatments. It also examined broader, more contentious issues, such as the place of psychiatry within general medicine and the wider applications of psychiatry.[62]

However, when Stafford-Clark began to address the social problems mental illness posed, the inclusive manner he had previously used to address his readers changed: 'In essence', he claimed, 'it is still the problem of an attitude of mind on the part of the public, who in turn must look for leadership to members of my own profession'.[63] In the last chapter, Stafford-Clark adopted a didactic tone, distinguishing between educated psychiatrists and an ignorant public, who needed 'to be taught the truth about psychiatry . . . they need to be helped to overcome the shame and fear which have dogged the whole concept of mental illness for centuries'.[64] If mental illness was stigmatised then, in Stafford-Clark's eyes, the fault lay with an ignorant public.

Henry Yellowlees eschewed Stafford-Clark's inclusive tone, claiming that twenty-seven years working within mental hospitals enabled him to speak authoritatively on the matter. He hoped to inform and enlighten the 'lay public', focusing on topics where he felt 'public feeling has rather outstripped public understanding'.[65] His book discussed depression, psychological theory, hypnosis and the relationship between law and medicine. Yellowlees devoted much attention to the public attitude towards psychiatry and what he described as the 'mutual misunderstandings' that existed between the psychiatrist and the layman.[66] While this term might imply equal blame for the state of affairs, Yellowlees largely held the public accountable, apportioning residual blame to media coverage of mental health issues for not only illustrating the misunderstandings between the public and psychiatry but doing 'much to maintain it'.[67]

Indeed, Yellowlees appears to have been more preoccupied by the low status of psychiatry than Stafford-Clark, grumbling that it served as 'the butt and laughing stock of a majority of both the medical profession and the general public'. Representations of the psychiatrist as 'an idiotic and incompetent figure of fun' in film and fiction had plumbed new depths, he complained.[68] Yellowlees depicted psychiatry as a profession beset on all sides, distinguishing between an elite 'public', composed of professionals, and the man-in-the-pub public, who copied their betters.

Yellowlees was very dismissive of the general public, even questioning 'whether anything can or should be done to put them in a position to grasp just the very rudiments of the subject'.[69] 'We cannot stop people talking about psychiatry: cannot we get them to talk sense about it?' he asked.[70] However, Yellowlees's condescending tone may well have alienated his potential readership. Distinguishing between physiology and pathology, Yellowlees commented that 'the reader who has grasped even this elementary point is entitled to feel that he has already progressed a good deal further than the average layman':[71] hardly effusive praise. The book promised to enable its reader to 'think and talk intelligently about psychiatry', but only 'if he will allow it to teach him to do so'.[72] Concerned about public disregard for the profession, Yellowlees sought to impose his views upon his readers as facts not opinions to be disputed, and displayed no interest in opening up a debate.

Former patients writing for the public

Books authored by psychiatrists were not the only source of public information on mental illness and its treatment, for the casual reader could also choose from biographical memoirs published by erstwhile patients. However, while such accounts provided a means for former patients to re-establish their identities as sane citizens in the first half of the twentieth century, writers struggled to document their experiences of mental disturbance, and consequently found it difficult to challenge stereotypical views of mental illness.

Many of these accounts critiqued the brutality and irrationality of psychiatry, a genre which stretched back to the eighteenth-century private madhouse, described by Roy Porter as 'aggressive works of self justification, which expose foes and vindicate the author's own actions'.[73] This assessment characterises two accounts authored prior to the introduction of the 1930 Mental Treatment Act: Marcia Hamilcar's 1910 autobiography, *Legally Dead: Experiences during Seventeen Weeks' Detention in a Private Lunatic Asylum*, and Rachel Grant-Smith's memoir, *The Experiences of an Asylum Patient*, published in 1922.[74] These memoirs followed a similar template: both authors wrote to defend their sanity, to protest against what they viewed as their wrongful certification and deprivation of liberty, and to lobby for a change in the law. Yet despite the authors' critical views of the treatment they received, both books were introduced by a doctor with experience of psychiatry. This added an authoritative air and gave the views expressed by Hamilcar and Grant-Smith more credence. Sidestepping the allegations raised by Hamilcar, Dr L. Forbes

Winslow took the opportunity when introducing her account to attack private nursing homes and asylums, to castigate the ignorance of general practitioners on the subject of lunacy, and to state his view that asylums were suitable only for the treatment of chronic cases – a view shared by a number of psychiatrists in this era, as we shall see in Chapter 3.[75] Grant-Smith's account was introduced by Montagu Lomax, who met the author after the publication of his own book. Lomax depicted Grant-Smith's account as a counterpart to his own exposé, a parallel consciously emphasised in the titles of the two books. 'Whereas, in my last book, I gave the reader the "Experiences of an Asylum Doctor"', wrote Lomax, 'I now stand aside and give him "The Experiences of an Asylum Patient", leaving him to judge how far the one set of experiences corroborates the other'.[76]

Both authors hoped to reveal how the deficiencies of the 1890 Lunacy Act imperilled personal liberty. Hamilcar, for example, stated that her experiences illustrated 'how the law facilitates the immuring of an obnoxious member of a family, or anyone, in an asylum, whilst it places almost insuperable obstacles in the way of his or her discharge'.[77] Similarly, Grant-Smith likened asylum care to a term in prison, averring it was 'monstrous' that she had 'been made to suffer twelve years' imprisonment, during which time I was deprived of any chance of appeal against my sentence'.[78] Both acknowledged that they had become distressed following difficult circumstances. Hamilcar related how she suffered a breakdown after undertaking extra work in order to counter her financial problems; 'my mind was out of joint', she acknowledged, 'and I was physically too exhausted to right it myself'.[79] Grant-Smith, meanwhile, described how her husband's death following a morphia overdose 'plunged me into a profound sense of grief . . . which I found very difficult to shake off'.[80]

Although Hamilcar and Grant-Smith admitted that they had been distressed, both insisted that they had been wrongfully certified owing to trickery and ill-treatment. Hamilcar claimed that her sisters placed her in a nursing home in which she was made into a lunatic through ill-treatment and the administration of drugs. After five weeks in the home, Hamilcar was certified as insane and sent to an asylum, where her account of what happened was disbelieved. 'So unfortunately true is it', wrote Hamilcar, 'that a patient suffering from the very mildest form of mental disease is at once condemned as incapable of making a true statement'.[81] Grant-Smith had voluntarily entered Cheadle Royal for what she believed would be a short rest cure. She protested at the underhand way in which she was certified by two doctors who interviewed her while she was under the influence of a sleeping draught, without giving any clue as to the purpose of the interview. Once certified, Grant-Smith spent more than twelve years as a patient at five different asylums before obtaining her release. She constantly protested her sanity, but recalled bitterly that 'once "ticketed" mad, it is well-nigh impossible to remove the impression'.[82] She reported the abuses she witnessed and experienced within the asylums. However, her accusations repeatedly fell on deaf ears, for 'once a person is labelled "mad", "lunatic", or "of unsound mind", then the prevailing attitude towards such alleged lunatic is that of "poor thing, still suffering from delusions!"'[83]

Both authors expressed their compassion for other patients, or, in Grant-Smith's words, 'fellow sufferers'.[84] Hamilcar pursued this theme more actively, devoting her first two chapters to her goal of raising public consciousness about the plight of the insane, and closing her account by echoing Clifford Beers's arguments for reform to protect the legal status of the mentally ill in America.[85] However, both authors carefully distanced themselves from their fellow patients, distinguishing between their state of inner turmoil and distress, and the visible insanity which surrounded them. Grief and mental distress, both writers inferred, was a wholly different matter from the stereotypical insanity performed around them. They depicted fellow patients as passive, voiceless objects of pity and horror; 'afflicted creatures',[86] who were 'dreadfully disfigured and most repulsive in appearance'.[87] Both were insistent that they had never been insane. Grant-Smith explained how she was driven to write in the hope of 'clearing my name of the undeserved stain of lunacy'.[88] That Grant-Smith sought to clear her name, yet wrote under a pseudonym, illustrates the conundrum facing former patients who sought to critique the system of asylum care while painfully aware of the stigma that they faced. Both accounts illustrated how the stigma attached to mental illness and the threat of compulsory detention deterred former patients from identifying with those who shared their stigmatising label.[89] Instead, Hamilcar and Grant-Smith sought to reclaim their identities at the expense of fellow patients, reinforcing the stereotype of the chronic lunatic with whom it was impossible to communicate and replicating the suppression and silence practised by psychiatrists. Other former patients whose lives had been disrupted by their committal to a psychiatric institution similarly reworked the story of what happened to them in a way that was acceptable to their self-image as they sought to reintegrate themselves back into the community.[90]

People who recounted their experiences of what they viewed as wrongful confinement appear to have focused specifically on this period in their lives. Those who admitted that they had experienced mental difficulties which justified hospital treatment sought to make their breakdown socially comprehensible, situating their experiences of mental distress within the events of their lives. *The Autobiography of David*, published in 1946 by Victor Gollancz, entwined details of the author's mental troubles with an account of his life and work. David traced the emergence of his difficulties to an experience of agoraphobia when aged thirteen. His first hospitalisation occurred while he was living in Canada.[91] Here, David entered Toronto hospital, where he was transferred from the general ward to a ward for nervous diseases. Failing to improve, David was moved to a mental hospital, which he depicted as a chaotic, prison-like environment with barred windows, in which both staff and patients could be violent. 'I saw a young boy of seventeen thrashed with an attendant's belt', David recalled, 'about a week later at tea one man stabbed another in the neck'.[92]

Following his discharge from the hospital, David was deported from Canada and went home, remaining in what he described as a state of 'acute neurasthenia'. In 1908, while undergoing what he referred to as a 'nervous turn', David exposed himself, was arrested for indecent conduct and sent to an asylum. Although he sought to offer readers insight into the social factors which had led to his breakdown, he made no attempt to explain why other patients in the asylum had become distressed and offered virtually no insight into fellow patients' states of mind. Instead, he ranked patients according to the obtrusiveness of their disturbance, drawing upon popular stereotypes to conjure their behaviour:

> From the congenital idiot slavering away in his chair – a terrible monstrosity unable to feed himself – to the highly-strung victim of some unhappy love affair, biting his nails in an anguish of melancholy. The general paralytic, the degenerate, the religious maniac, the feeble-minded, and the imbecile were my companions. I do not think of them with horror or antipathy now, though at the time it was not easy to repress repulsion . . . the frequent scenes of horror inside the institution were always a nightmare to me: patients at times snarling like dogs, warders fighting with maniacs, the contortions of epileptics; the continuous moaning of those afflicted by melancholy as they passed up and down, never at rest, wringing their hands; and the horrible laughter of the exalted as they proclaimed themselves to be emperors and kings.[93]

During this stay, he found solace talking to an attendant, explaining, 'I had an intense desire for "sane" company'.[94] Echoing Hamilcar, David claimed that his purpose in writing was to set forward his experiences in the hope that they might be of assistance to others, 'to the helpless insane especially, who could not speak for themselves'.[95] Like Hamilcar, however, David frequently depicted his fellow patients as repulsive, dehumanised objects, defined solely by their psychiatric classifications, with which it was impossible to communicate.

John Vincent's account likewise sought to make the author's experience of mental distress comprehensible within the context of his life story. Consequently, only twenty-one of the 115 pages of *Inside the Asylum*, published in 1948, referred to the time Vincent had spent in an asylum.[96] Vincent believed that the onset of what he described as 'long periods of black depression' had been slow and insidious, stemming from his childhood. He portrayed his father as cruel and unloving, 'a morose and ill-tempered man who was an object of fear to his family and wife', and his mother as weak and incompetent, 'a feeble reed upon which to lean in any difficulty'.[97] Moreover, the family adopted what he viewed as a Victorian attitude towards sex, 'something furtive, unclean and unspeakable'.[98]

Vincent took up work as a Methodist preacher and married, but found himself impotent. Ostracised during the Second World War for taking a stance as a conscientious objector, Vincent's depression increased. 'I knew I was seriously ill mentally', he wrote, recounting how he had entered the local mental hospital as a voluntary patient.[99] Vincent described how the nurses could talk, yet not communicate with the patients, giving a sense of the hierarchical power structures operating in the hospital that formalised interaction between nurses and patients.

> I suddenly became aware of a man standing beside my bed. He was wearing the blue suit of the male nurses . . . I said 'good morning'. He made no remark and continued to stand and stare at me . . . Then he sat on the edge of my bed and asked me questions . . . He seemed to be the symbol of authority, of all the authority I had ever known, of the authority against which I had been a rebel all my life.[100]

Upon entering the common room, Vincent found that the patients were more willing to communicate with him: 'one or two of them greeted me cheerfully', he wrote.[101] Identifying himself as suffering from a mental illness, Vincent was able to relate to his 'fellow patients' without distancing himself from them.[102] Echoing the kind of self-referential humour and mockery evident in some of the *Mirror* articles, Vincent described how 'most of us retained a vestige of humour and there were a few stock jokes about asylums, lunatics and kindred subjects which usually raised a laugh'.[103]

We may partially account for the different tone of Vincent's memoir by taking into consideration the impact of voluntary admissions, introduced under the 1930 Mental Treatment Act. Unlike earlier writers who recounted the disruption wrought on their lives by involuntary confinement, Vincent chose to enter an asylum and in his account he claimed to have retained some control over his treatment. Alongside drugs treatments, Vincent had an analytical interview with the doctor every two or three days, which he believed cured his impotence. Considering that there were four psychiatrists for a patient population of thirteen hundred, Vincent appears to have been a privileged patient and had an unusually good experience of the asylum. In this respect, Vincent's account illustrates the divergent fates of acute cases and long-stay patients, which we will turn to in Chapter 3.

Rather than emphasising the problems of the asylum, Vincent chose to stress the consequences of popular prejudice towards those who had received asylum care. 'What of those who do leave the asylum?', he asked. 'They will forever bear a stigma. They will be regarded with suspicion by work mates and even by loving relatives. Prospective employers will shake their heads as the gap in the record is explained . . . it is most urgently necessary that the public should be educated to understand and sympathise with mental disorders.'[104] In its emphasis upon dialogue with practitioners and fellow patients, and its desire to situate the origins of mental distress within familial problems, Vincent's narrative foreshadows many of the characteristic features of later narratives produced by both patients and practitioners, to which this chapter now turns.

Shared narrative of madness

Speaking on camera for Peter Robinson's 1971 documentary 'Asylum', the psychiatrist R. D. Laing recalled how in the late 1950s and early 1960s:

> A number of us who were working as psychiatrists in mental hospitals became increasingly dissatisfied with the setting of the mental hospital as a place to work. If I really wanted to get to the bottom of . . . what sanity is and madness is, who is sane, . . . if anyone and who is crazy if anyone and what that distinction is, I for one would have to come off my perch and level out on a man to man basis, when I met another human being who was in a position of being classified by other people as crazy, and on that man to man basis, on a level, then I would take my chances and he would take his when we met.[105]

As we shall see in Chapter 3, Laing's frustration with the therapeutic constraints of the 1950s mental hospital was far from unique. However, the way in which Laing portrayed mental disturbance and his critique of conventional psychiatric care demands analysis, for Laing, who commenced his career in a conventional psychiatric hospital, later became a high-profile critic of this treatment regime.[106] Laing worked for just over a year at Gartnavel Royal Medical Hospital in Glasgow in the early 1950s, when patient numbers were rising and there was a shortage of medical staff.[107] It was here that he led an experiment in which a small group of chronic schizophrenic patients spent time with the same nurses each day, as part of a broader programme of research undertaken into schizophrenia within the Hospital during this period.[108] Laing's experiences within Gartnavel provided much of the material for his first book, *The Divided Self*. Published in 1960 by specialist press Tavistock Publications for an audience of fellow psychiatrists, this book stated that Laing's objective was 'to make madness, and the process of going mad, comprehensible'.[109] The focus of the book was schizophrenia, a disorder that by the mid-1950s was assuming a prominent position within psychiatry as a 'test subject' to examine different strands of psychiatric and psychotherapeutic practice.[110]

For the subsequent republication by Pelican, Laing authored a new preface that pitched the work to a broader audience and helped establish the status of the text within the nascent anti-psychiatry movement. He now represented mental illness as transcendence over a repressive, one-dimensional society. In an overt a dig at William Sargant, whose book on brainwashing, *The Battle for the Mind*, had been published three years earlier,[111] Laing complained that psychiatry, instead of aiding this transcendence, was all too often 'a technique of brainwashing', the restraints of old having been replaced by 'the more subtle lobotomies and tranquillizers that place the bars of Bedlam and locked doors *inside* the patient'.[112] He linked his arguments to critiques of industrialisation, nuclear weaponry and racism. 'A man who says that Negroes are an inferior race may be widely respected', he wrote. 'A man who says his whiteness is a form of cancer is certifiable'.[113] Pitching the book to nominally sane readers, Laing argued that 'our "normal" "adjusted" state is too often an abdication of ecstasy, the betrayal of our true potentialities'. It was only those individuals with 'an insistent experience of other dimensions' who escaped 'the pervasive madness that we call normality'.[114] These kinds of statements have understandably led some writers to view Laing's work as part of the broader counter-culture, embraced by people seeking personal development.[115] While this is undoubtedly the case, we should not lose sight of the fact that Laing chose to examine a condition associated with chronic psychosis, and that his book focused on the inner workings of the minds of his patients.

Nick Crossley suggested that Laing was attempting to change the field of psychiatry from within when he wrote the book by drawing on philosophical theories and progressive ideas within psychiatry, such as the importance of the social environment.[116] In practice, the text falls somewhere between Laing's initial attempts to underplay the radicalism of the book when pitching it to fellow psychiatrists, and the rather excessive claims made for the text on its reissue, by which stage Laing had given up on transforming psychiatry from within.

In *The Divided Self,* Laing sought to reconfigure the relationship between psychiatrist and patient. Madness, he suggested, was not a discrete thing which was observed by the objective, detached practitioner. It was brought into being by interpersonal relations, and the depersonalising 'objective' approach adopted by psychiatrists helped produce the disturbed behaviour then read by the psychiatrist as indicative of underlying malfunction. Speech, Laing argued, should no longer be interpreted as a symptom of disease. Yet the uneven distribution of power between patient and psychiatrist within the clinical encounter skewed dialogue. Laing described how patients at the mercy of a seemingly omnipotent psychiatrist subverted and mocked psychiatric authority, echoing the subversive humour of the *Morningside Mirror.* 'We schizophrenics say a lot of stuff that is unimportant', one patient was quoted as saying, 'and then we mix important things in with all this to see if the doctor cares enough to see them and feel them'.[117] Laing illustrated this point by citing an example related to him by a patient diagnosed with schizophrenia:

> During a first meeting with a psychiatrist he conceived an intense contempt for him. He was terrified to reveal this contempt in case he was ordered to have a leucotomy and yet he desperately wanted to express it . . . The psychiatrist asked him if he heard a voice. The patient thought what a stupid question this was since he heard the psychiatrist's voice. He therefore answered that he did, and to subsequent questioning, that the voice was male. The next question was, 'What does the voice say to you?' To which he answered, 'You are a fool.' By playing at being mad, he had thus contrived to say what he thought of the psychiatrist with impunity.[118]

Despairing of the mental hospital as a site in which a constructive therapeutic relationship could be created, Laing sought an alternative therapeutic environment. He explained to Peter Robinson how 'several of us in London were able to set up places where, if we were psychiatrists, we could live as we want, and if we were patients, we could also live, and anyone who lived and who is now living in these places would get no encouragement for playing the part of psychiatrist or playing the part of patient'.[119]

This new model of therapy formed the basis for the 1971 account *Mary Barnes: Two Accounts of a Journey through Madness.*[120] Embodying Laing's call for dialogue between patient and practitioner, this book, co-authored by Joseph Berke and Mary Barnes, interwove their accounts of their relationship at the Kingsley Hall community, in which Berke supported Barnes on a journey into madness. Set up by Laing in 1965, Kingsley Hall evolved from Maxwell Jones's idea of the therapeutic community – an attempt to blur the rigid staff–patient relationship and give patients more of a say in running the hospital – and was envisaged as an alternative therapeutic environment to the mental hospital, one that might be liberating rather than repressive. In his account, Berke described why he had chosen to specialise in psychiatry:

> Here was one discipline where it was still fashionable to talk to the patient, or so it seemed. On closer examination it became obvious that the reverse was true. Both the interview and treatment situations were carefully structured to prevent any genuine exchange between patient and therapist . . . During my clinical years it became clear to me that most psychiatrists are not only not experts in communication, but are not at all interested in what their patients have to tell them.[121]

Berke explained that he never had any difficulties understanding what his schizophrenic patients were saying. Few of his colleagues, however, agreed that what schizophrenic patients did or said contained any meaning, 'other than signs or symptoms of a progressive, debilitating illness'.[122]

Berke had come across a copy of *The Divided Self* while a medical student and in 1963 visited Maxwell Jones and Laing. Two years later, Laing invited Berke, who had recently qualified, to participate in the founding of Kingsley Hall. Barnes had experienced a breakdown in 1953 and spent a year in a conventional mental hospital. She believed that her madness grew out of destructive familial relationships and entered Kingsley Hall after an acquaintance put her in touch with Laing. The book details Barnes's description of her stifling childhood, her breakdown and her regression to a state of childhood at Kingsley Hall in which she withdrew to her bed and insisted on being bottle-fed. It describes, from Barnes's perspective, how she came 'up' again, learning to channel her emotions through painting – initially with her own excrement until Berke brought her some paint – and how she reconnected her experiences to her deeply held Catholic faith. For Berke, Barnes embodied the thesis 'that psychosis is a potentially enriching experience if it is allowed to proceed full cycle through disintegration and reintegration, or death and rebirth'.[123]

While Berke shared Barnes's belief that regressing into childhood and madness would ultimately prove therapeutic, at certain points in his narrative he expressed his discomfort with the more unconventional aspects of this process – feeding a forty-year-old woman with a baby bottle, for example. 'One day', he recalled, Mary presented me with the ultimate test of my love for her':

> She covered herself in shit and waited to see what my reaction would be . . . When I, unsuspectingly, walked into the Games Room and was accosted by foul smelling Mary Barnes looking far worse than the creature from the black lagoon, I was terrified and nauseated. My first reaction was to escape and I stalked away as fast as I could. I knew that if I didn't turn around and face that poor, shit-covered creature, I would never be able to face her or anybody like her again.[124]

Berke also remained conflicted as to whether he was a fellow resident and Barnes's equal, or her doctor. Barnes frequently vented her anger by punching and kicking Berke, and, on one occasion, Berke punched her back. 'I noticed that blood was pouring out of Mary's nose and all over her face and gown', he recalled. 'I was horrified and thought, "What way is this for a doctor to treat his patient?" This first reaction on my part is an extremely interesting one, because I had tried so hard to avoid the role of doctor at Kingsley Hall.'[125] And yet, as Berke elaborated, 'clinging to my medical mannerisms was an expression of intense anxiety about being perceived as a . . . "schizophrenic" by other members of the community or visitors'. In a passage strongly evocative of the more subversive articles published in the Morningside Mirror, Berke wrote:

> I think that anxiety about being confused with the 'mentally ill' is why the staff at most mental hospitals rigidly conform to a strict standard of dress and demeanour, and resist attempts to deinstitutionalise their relationships with patients. It was terribly amusing when such personnel used to visit Kingsley Hall.
>
> As soon as they noticed that most residents dressed and talked alike, one could smell their anxiety reaching record heights as they struggled to divide us up into staff and patients. Nine times out of ten their observations about who was who were dead wrong. I can't count the number of times Mary was seen as the chief nursing sister,[126] or one of the 'psychiatrists' was seen as a 'schizophrenic' and spoken of as such. Great waves of embarrassment always broke across the face of a visitor after he learned that the 'poor crazy' he had chatted up was Dr Laing or Dr Berke or Dr Redler.[127]

Echoing Laing's belief that the speech and actions of his patients were no mere symptoms but a window into their difficulties, Berke insisted that Barnes's actions, 'which may seem quite bizarre to the uninformed observer, could be seen to have an inner logic and outer predictability once one took the trouble to know Mary, her story, her experience, her circle of friends and relatives'.[128] Yet Barnes and Berke did not agree as to the meaning of her experience. Barnes felt that her experience had purified her, explaining that 'it brings me nearer to God, to myself, helps me to a more conscious awareness of God, to a fuller participation in the sight of God'.[129] Berke, however, attributed Barnes's troubles and behaviour to sexual frustration and a desire to regress back to the womb.

Conclusion

This chapter commenced by noting how eighteenth-century narratives diverged from Hannah Allen's account of her distress. Yet we end with a narrative which in many ways echoes Allen's account. For Mary Barnes, her madness was a journey of religious enlightenment which served a higher purpose, and Barnes is remembered on her website as 'Nurse, Madwoman, Explorer of the Underworld, Celebrant of Death and Rebirth, Member of Kingsley Hall Community, Artist, Writer, Healer, Catholic mystic, Visionary'.[130] Other cyclical patterns can be discerned within stories told by those who have experienced mental distress, pointing to the significance of the context in which these authors wrote. Thus, distinctions between madness and sanity which had sharpened in the era of the asylum become permeable by the late 1960s as the locus of care began to shift once more from the asylum to the community, while notions of madness as socially produced, displaced in the era of the asylum by the dominance of biological models which situated disorder within the body of the individual sufferer, appeared once again resurgent.

One might object that the subversive narratives produced within the Royal Edinburgh Asylum bear comparison to the efforts made by the Kingsley Hall community to break down barriers between patient and practitioner. And so they do. Yet here again we need to consider the context: the authors of the subversive narratives published within the *Morningside Mirror* were writing for the asylum community, and madness formed the grist of the humour which permeated the paper. Conversely, memoirs authored by former patients were intended for public consumption. Illness narratives, observed Mike Bury, function as forums in which the private sphere of experience is connected to public forms of knowledge, reintegrating authors into their cultural world.[131] They articulate 'the links between body, self and society'.[132] While many illnesses isolate the sufferer from the wider community, mental breakdown, as Peter Barham and Robert Hayward have argued, 'typically wreaks havoc upon the agent's sense of his own biographical continuity . . . upon the narrative coherence of his life'.[133] 'It's just like being kidnapped', explained Sarah, one of Barham and Hayward's research participants, a description which poignantly evokes how hospitalisation ruptured her lived experience.[134]

Many of the stories written by former asylum patients can be read as attempts to reassert control over lives which had been disrupted by mental breakdown and involuntary hospitalisation. The ability of former patients to borrow and invert the rationale of psychiatrists demonstrates the instability of psychiatric authority in the public realm, yet the stigma of mental illness and fear of further involuntary confinement led many who chose to write to protest their sanity, or at least to proclaim that they had never been insane. Stereotypical views of insanity suggest that the condition can be discerned visually.[135] However, the invisibility of mental disturbance encouraged many to conceal their experiences and attempt to pass as normal,[136] or to claim that they had been erroneously admitted to an asylum by careless or unscrupulous psychiatrists, an anxiety widely articulated in the press.[137] Owing to the ambivalence which many erstwhile patients felt towards those labouring under the same stigma, protestations of sanity could, and frequently did, co-exist alongside pleas to improve conditions within mental hospitals and generate greater public tolerance of mental illness.

Indeed, many former patients sought to reintegrate themselves back into the community by distancing themselves from the 'otherness' of mental illness, perpetuating the image of erstwhile fellow patients as crazed beasts beyond reason and incapable of speaking for themselves. Even Clifford Beers, the poster boy of the mental hygiene movement who acknowledged in his account that he had been insane and campaigned to advance mental health, sought to distance himself from the mentally ill once he had been discharged. As Porter argued, Beers appeared to have distinguished between the 'deserving' and 'undeserving' mad, believing that his own disturbance had been a natural outcome of nursing his brother and that he himself had brought about his own cure through the exercise of will power and self-help.[138]

Psychiatrists also sought to educate the public and counter the stigma of mental illness, but their adversarial relationship with patients prevented a co-ordinated approach, despite psychiatrists' recognition that their fates were bound together. Moreover, psychiatrists focused on raising the status of their profession and tended to treat the public as an apathetic and homogeneous mass. Ignorant, resistant to the careful efforts of psychiatrists to educate them and yet strangely prone to sensationalist reporting, the public as envisaged by psychiatrists were not capable of participating in a debate about the care of the mentally ill, even if it was possible to gain their attention. Thus, while psychiatrists sometimes acknowledged that public opinion might be a helpful thing if it could stimulate the government to improve conditions of work and the prestige of psychiatry, they believed this opinion should be created by the absorption of knowledge passed from psychiatry to the public. These views were still being expressed in the popular psychiatry books of the 1950s. Another factor that inhibited psychiatrists from entering into a debate with the public was their view that psychiatric practice was firmly grounded not on opinion or belief but on incontestable scientific fact. A logical consequence of this belief was that the public, who were not privy to this specific expertise, were unqualified to contest psychiatric practice.

Psychiatrists, both collectively and individually, tended to exhibit more concern about press coverage that attacked the professional status of psychiatry rather than coverage that represented mental illness in a negative light. Although they argued that it was necessary to advance the prestige of psychiatry before the problems faced by people diagnosed with a mental illness could be addressed, psychiatrists were more concerned with the former issue. After all, psychiatrists rarely argued that it was necessary to destigmatise mental illness before the prestige of psychiatry could be enhanced. Thus even when they did seek to address the public, psychiatrists often sought to create more positive representations of psychiatry rather than of their patients.[139]

The dynamic changed somewhat in the 1960s with the rise of anti-psychiatry. Part of a broader cultural movement which challenged established norms and authorities,[140] anti-psychiatry also reflected the demise of Enlightenment ideals, evident, for example, in the rejection of the rational and an embrace of the irrational, or, indeed, the desire to accept one's individual potential rather than be, in the words of John Vincent, a 'cog in an industrial machine'.[141] In the 1960s, some psychiatrists such as R. D. Laing sought to facilitate this objective, proclaiming themselves agents of liberation. Openly acknowledging the fundamental instability of psychiatric authority, Laing and Berke sought to challenge distinctions of sanity and madness and to seek dialogue with patients such as Mary Barnes. What is particularly striking about these developments was the focus not on incipient or acute mental distress but on schizophrenia. This observation will be developed further in Chapter 3, which focuses on how psychiatrists depicted acute and chronic mental disorder. It is also noteworthy that Barnes's narrative, far from seeking to conceal her madness from her readers, focused upon it.

In 1972, a group of patients and supporters drew up a pamphlet entitled 'The Need for a Mental Patients' Union'.[142] Situating the plight of the mental patient within an oppressive capitalist system in which the psychiatrist was all too often an agent of the ruling classes, the pamphlet stressed the social and economic causes of mental distress and urged fellow patients to form a union to assert their rights. The emergence of the service user movement in the 1970s suggests that the stigma attached to mental distress had diminished, as people were able to campaign for greater rights without seeking to conceal their experiences of distress. However, the resurgence of bio-psychiatry and the displacement, once more, of madness for mental illness, heralded again the divergence of patient and practitioner narratives. Driven by a consumerist model of mental healthcare which seeks to individualise provision and foster autonomy,[143] mental healthcare workers attempt to foster an empathetic relationship with their patients while guarding against dependency. 'These emotional defences', explains Barbara Taylor, are 'meant to keep the craziness on the patient's side, well away from professional sanity'. 'How do you stay sane?' she asked one psychiatrist. 'I don't always', he admitted. 'I don't think I should.'[144]

Notes

1 R. Porter, *A Social History of Madness: Stories of the Insane* (London, 1999), p. 4. See also R. Porter, 'Hearing the mad. Communication and excommunication', in L. de Goei and J. Vijselaar (eds), *Proceedings of the First European Congress on the History of Psychiatry and Mental Health Care* (Amsterdam, 1993), pp. 338–52, and R. Porter (ed.), *The Faber Book of Madness* (London, 1991). Other influential works which focus on narratives of the mad include A. Ingram (ed.), *Voices of Madness: Four Pamphlets, 1683–1796* (Stroud, 1997); D. Paterson, *A Mad People's History of Madness* (Pittsburgh, 1982); G. A. Hornstein, *Agnes's Jacket: A Psychologist's Search for the Meanings of Madness* (2009; Ross-on-Wye, 2012). Hornstein has also compiled a bibliography of first-person narratives of madness, which she regularly updates. See G. Hornstein, 'Bibliography of first-person narratives of madness in English (5th edition)', last revised December 2011, http://www.gailhornstein.com/files/Bibliography_of_First_Person_Narratives_of_Madness_5th_edition.pdf.

2 E. Goffman, *Stigma: Notes on the Management of a Spoiled Identity* (1963; Harmondsworth, 1968), pp. 40–5.

3 Goffman, *Stigma*, pp. 130–1.

4 H. Allen, 'A narrative of God's gracious dealings with that choice Christian Mrs. Hannah Allen', in Ingram (ed.), *Voices of Madness*, pp. 1–22.

5 Allen, 'A Narrative of God's Gracious Dealings'.

6 See M. MacDonald, *Mystical Bedlam: Madness, Anxiety, and Healing in Seventeenth-Century England* (Cambridge, 1981), and R. Porter, *Mind Forg'd Manacles: A History of Madness in England from the Restoration to the Regency* (Cambridge, Mass. 1987).

7 A. Cruden, 'The London-citizen exceedingly injured' (1739), S. Bruckshaw, 'One more proof of the iniquitous abuse of private madhouses' (1774), and W. Belcher, 'Address to humanity: containing, a letter to Dr. Monro; a receipt to make a lunatic, and seize his estate; and a sketch of a true smiling hyena', (1796), in Ingram (ed.), *Voices of Madness*, pp. 23–74, 75–126, 127–36.

8 M. Foucault, *Madness and Civilisation: A History of Insanity in the Age of Reason* (London, 1967), pp. xii–xiii.

9 R. Porter, 'Psychiatry and its history: Hunter and Macalpine', in de Goei and Vijselaar (eds), *Proceedings of the First European Congress*, pp. 167–77.

10 J. Andrews and A. Scull, *Customers and Patrons of the Mad-Trade: The Management of Lunacy in Eighteenth-Century London with the Complete Text of John Monro's 1766 Case Book* (London, 2003), pp. 107–8.

11 Porter, 'Hearing the mad', p. 348.

12 Renamed the Medico-Psychological Association in 1865. See E. Renvoize, 'The Association of Medical Officers of Asylums and Hospitals for the Insane, the Medico-Psychological Association, and their presidents', in G. E. Berrios and H. Freeman (eds), *150 Years of British Psychiatry, 1841–1991* (London, 1991), pp. 29–78.

13 D. Hack Tuke, 'Presidential Address', *JMS*, 27 (1881–82), 305–42; 342.

14 H. Freeman, 'Psychiatry and the state in Britain' in M. Gijswijt-Hofstra, H. Oosterhuis, J. Vijselaar and H. Freeman (eds), *Psychiatric Cultures Compared: Psychiatry and Mental Health Care in the Twentieth Century* (Amsterdam, 2005), pp. 116–40; p. 126.

15 M. J. Clark, 'Law, liberty and psychiatry in Victorian Britain: an historical survey and commentary, c. 1840–1890', in de Goei and Vijselaar (eds), *Proceedings of the First European Congress*, pp. 187–93; P. McCandless, 'Liberty and lunacy: the Victorians and wrongful confinement', in A. Scull (ed.), *Madhouses, Mad-Doctors and Madmen: The Social History of Psychiatry in the Victorian Era* (Philadelphia, 1981), pp. 339–61.

16 Anonymous, reviewing J. Mortimer Granville's book, *The Care and Cure of the Insane. Being the Reports of the 'Lancet' Commission on Lunatic Asylums, 1875–76–77* in *JMS*, 23 (1877–78), 393–6; 393.

17 'Occasional notes of the quarter: a social blot', *JMS*, 17 (1871–72), 230–4.

18 'Asylum', directed by P. Robinson (1971).

19 Foucault, *Madness and Civilisation*, p. xii.

20 Porter, *A Social History of Madness*, p. 4.

21 Ibid., p. 23.

22 University of Edinburgh Centre for Research Collections, Lothian Health Services Archive (hereafter LHSA), LHB7/13/5, 'Our literary club', *Morningside Mirror*, XL (1885), 35.

23 H. Maudsley, 'Presidential address', *JMS*, 17 (1871), 311–32; 317. For more details on Maudsley's career, see A. Scull, C. MacKenzie and N. Hervey, *Masters of Bedlam: The Transformation of the Mad-Doctoring Trade* (Princeton, 1996), pp. 226–67. Links between madness and creativity continue to be advanced by modern commentators. See K. Redfield Jamison, *Touched With Fire: Manic Depressive Illness and the Artistic Temperament* (New York, 1994).

24 Goffman, *Stigma*, p. 132.

25 Ibid.

26 LHSA, LHB7/13/4, 'A capacious critic', *Morningside Mirror*, XXXIII (1878), 12.

27 LHSA, LHB7/13/4, *Morningside Mirror*, XXXIV (1879), 5.

28 LHSA, LHB7/13/6, 'A surprising movement', *Morningside Mirror*, LIII (April, 1898), 25–7; 25.

29 Ibid., 26.

30 Ibid., 27.

31 LHSA, LHB7/13/7, 'The surprising movement', *Morningside Mirror*, LIV (January, 1899), 1–3; 1.

32 Ibid., 1, 2.

33 Ibid., 2–3.

34 LHSA, LHB7/13/7, 'The surprising movement', *Morningside Mirror*, LV (February, 1900), 9–13; 9.

35 Ibid., 11, 12.

36 P. Nolan, *A History of Mental Health Nursing* (London, 1993), p. 97.

37 'The Surprising Movement' (1900), 12, 13.
38 See M. Barfoot and A. Beveridge, 'Madness at the crossroads: John Home's letters from the Royal Edinburgh Asylum, 1886–87', *Psychological Medicine*, 20 (1990), 263–84; A. Beveridge, 'Voices of the mad: patients' letters from the Royal Edinburgh Asylum, 1873–1908', *Psychological Medicine*, 27 (1997), 899–908; A. Beveridge, 'Life in the asylum: patients' letters from Morningside, 1873–1908', *History of Psychiatry*, 9 (1998), 431–69.
39 Goffman, *Stigma*, p. 132.
40 T. Clouston, *The Hygiene of the Mind* (London, 1906).
41 N. Crossley, 'Transforming the mental health field: the early history of the National Association of Mental Health', *Sociology of Health and Illness*, 20 (1998), 458–88. For an analysis of Clouston's book, see 466–8.
42 J. Crichton-Browne, *The Doctor Remembers* (1932; London, 1938); *The Doctor's Second Thoughts* (London, 1931); *From the Doctor's Notebook* (London, 1937); *Stray Leaves from a Physician's Portfolio* (London, 1938); *Burns, From a New Point of View* (London, 1926).
43 M. Neve and T. Turner, 'What the doctor thought and did: Sir James Crichton-Browne (1840–1938)', *Medical History*, 39 (1995), 399–432; 417.
44 Crichton-Browne, *Stray Leaves*, p. vii.
45 Ibid.
46 J. Crichton-Brown, 'Presidential address', *JMS*, 24 (1878–79), 350–72; 351.
47 H. Maudsley, *The Physiology and Pathology of the Mind* (London, 1867).
48 H. Small, '"In the guise of science": literature and the rhetoric of nineteenth-century English psychiatry', *History of the Human Sciences*, 7 (1994), 27–55; 45.
49 S. Soanes, 'Reforming asylums, reforming public attitudes: J. R. Lord and Montagu Lomax's representations of mental hospitals and the community, 1921–1931', *Family and Community History*, 12 (2009), 117–29; 120.
50 M. Lomax, *The Experiences of an Asylum Doctor with Suggestions for Asylum and Lunacy Law Reform* (London, 1921), p. 253.
51 Ibid., p. 39.
52 Ibid., p. 120.
53 Ibid., pp. 252–3.
54 Ibid., p. 34.
55 Ibid., 13–14.
56 P. Barham, *Forgotten Lunatics of the Great War* (London, 2004). Fiona Reid's recent study of the Ex-Services' Welfare Society suggests that although civilian asylum patients may have benefited in the short term, the distinctions between ex-servicemen and other sufferers of mental distress became entrenched once more by the mid-1920s. See F. Reid, 'Distinguishing between shell-shocked veterans and pauper lunatics: the Ex-Services' Welfare Society and mentally wounded veterans after the Great War', *War in History*, 14 (2007), 347–71.
57 LHSA, LHB7/12/7, A. Wilson, 'Critic of English asylums: a doctor's book on alleged evils and abuses: can our system be reformed? By Albert Wilson,

M.D.' *Evening Standard* (26 July 1921). Similar arguments were also used to support the 'euthanasia' of German psychiatric patients under the Nazi regime. See M. Burleigh, *Death and Deliverance: 'Euthanasia' in Germany 1900–1945* (Cambridge, 1994).

58 Ministry of Health, *Report of the Committee on Administration of Public Mental Hospitals*, Cmd. 1730 (London, 1922), p. 45.

59 T. W. Harding, '"Not worth powder and shot": a reappraisal of Montagu Lomax's contribution to mental health reform', *British Journal of Psychiatry*, 156 (1990), 180–7.

60 Penguin's Pelican series was launched in 1937. For an overview of the intellectual and political contribution made by Penguin publications, see N. Joicey, 'A paperback guide to progress: Penguin books 1935 – c. 1951', *Twentieth Century British History*, 4 (1993), 25–56.

61 D. Stafford-Clark, *Psychiatry To-day* (1952; London, 1963), pp. 11–12.

62 Ibid., p. 297.

63 Ibid., p. 268.

64 Ibid., p. 297.

65 H. Yellowlees, *To Define True Madness: Commensense Psychiatry for Lay People* (1953; Harmondsworth, 1955), p. ix, and inside cover.

66 Ibid., p. ix.

67 Ibid., p. 25.

68 Ibid., p. 1.

69 Ibid., p. 3.

70 Ibid., p. 4.

71 Ibid., pp. 7–8.

72 Ibid., p. 26.

73 Porter, *A Social History of Madness*, p. 36.

74 M. Hamilcar, *Legally Dead: Experiences during Seventeen Weeks' Detention in a Private Asylum with an Introduction by Dr. Forbes Winslow* (London, 1910); R. Grant-Smith, *The Experiences of an Asylum Patient with an Introduction and Notes by Montagu Lomax M.R.C.S.* (London, 1922).

75 Hamilcar, *Legally Dead*, pp. 7–15.

76 Grant-Smith, *The Experiences of an Asylum Patient*, p. 8.

77 Hamilcar, *Legally Dead*, p. 17.

78 Grant-Smith, *The Experiences of an Asylum Patient*, p. 62.

79 Hamilcar, *Legally Dead*, p. 89.

80 Grant-Smith, *The Experiences of an Asylum Patient*, p. 53.

81 Hamilcar, *Legally Dead*, p. 69.

82 Grant-Smith, *The Experiences of an Asylum Patient*, p. 62.

83 Ibid., p. 63.

84 Ibid., p. 51.

85 Hamilcar, *Legally Dead*; C. Beers, *A Mind that Found Itself: An Autobiography* (London, 1908).

86 Grant-Smith, *The Experiences of an Asylum Patient*, p. 65.

87 Hamilcar, *Legally Dead*, pp. 161–2.

88 Grant-Smith, *The Experiences of an Asylum Patient*, p. 50.

89 Goffman, *Stigma*, pp. 50–1; 130–2.

90 Anonymous, 'They said I was mad', *Forum and Century*, 100 (1938), 231–7.

91 Anonymous, *The Autobiography of David, edited by Ernest Raymond* (London, 1946), p. 55.

92 Ibid., p. 56.

93 Ibid., pp. 62–3.

94 Ibid., pp. 61, 62.

95 Ibid., p. 14.

96 J. Vincent, *Inside the Asylum* (London, 1948). See pp. 83–103 for Vincent's account of time spent in the asylum.

97 Ibid., pp. 26, 31.

98 Ibid., pp. 57–8.

99 Ibid., p. 73.

100 Ibid., p. 91.

101 Ibid., p. 91.

102 Ibid., p. 93.

103 Ibid., pp. 95–6.

104 Ibid., p. 18.

105 'Asylum' (1971).

106 For Laing's own account of his changing views, see R. D. Laing, *Wisdom, Madness and Folly: The Making of a Psychiatrist 1927–1957* (1985; London, 1986).

107 See A. Beveridge, *Portrait of the Psychiatrist as a Young Man: The Early Writing and Work of R. D. Laing, 1927–1960* (Oxford, 2011), pp. 202–3.

108 See J. Andrews, 'R. D. Laing in Scotland: facts and fictions of the "rumpus room" and interpersonal psychiatry', in M. Gijswijt-Hofstra and R. Porter (eds), *Cultures of Psychiatry and Mental Health Care in Postwar Britain and the Netherlands* (Amsterdam, 1998), pp. 121–40; Beveridge, *Portrait of a Psychiatrist*, pp. 203–23.

109 R. D. Laing, *The Divided Self: An Existential Study in Sanity and Madness* (1959; Harmondsworth, 1965), p. 9.

110 Cameron and J. L. A. Esterson, 'Psychotherapy with a schizophrenic woman', *Psychiatric Quarterly*, 32 (1958), 304–17. Cited in Andrews, 'R. D. Laing in Scotland', p. 134.

111 Laing made disparaging remarks about Sargant's work in his private papers. See Beveridge, *Portrait of a Psychiatrist*, pp. 46, 65.

112 Laing, *The Divided Self*, p. 12.

113 Ibid.

114 Laing, *The Divided Self*, p. 11.

115 C. Jones, 'Raising the anti: Jan Foudraine, Ronald Laing and anti-psychiatry', in Gijswijt-Hofstra and Porter (eds), *Cultures of Psychiatry*, pp. 283–94; N. Crossley,

'R. D. Laing and the British anti-psychiatry movement: a socio-historical analysis', *Social Science and Medicine*, 47 (1998), 877–89; 884–6.

116 Crossley, 'R. D. Laing'.

117 Laing, *The Divided Self*, p. 164.

118 Ibid.

119 'Asylum' (1971).

120 M. Barnes and J. Berke, *Two Accounts of a Journey through Madness* (London, 1971).

121 Ibid., pp. 84, 87.

122 Ibid., p. 85.

123 Ibid., p. 237.

124 Ibid., pp. 268–9.

125 Ibid., pp. 250–1.

126 Mary was a qualified nurse and had worked in this capacity earlier in her life, so it is perhaps unsurprising that she was mistaken as such by visitors.

127 Ibid., pp. 250–1.

128 Ibid., p. 376.

129 Ibid., p. 351.

130 http://mary-barnes.net/about.htm, consulted 17 February 2012.

131 M. Bury, 'Illness narratives: fact or fiction?', *Sociology of Health and Illness*, 23 (2001), 263–85; 268.

132 Ibid., 281.

133 P. Barham and R. Hayward, *Relocating Madness: From the Mental Patient to the Person* (London, 1995), p. 91.

134 Ibid., p. 97.

135 See S. L. Gilman, *Disease and Representation: Images of Illness from Madness to AIDS* (Ithaca and London, 1988); S. L. Gilman, *The Face of Madness: Hugh W. Diamond and the Origin of Psychiatric Photography* (New York, 1977); M. Jackson, 'Images of deviance: visual representations of mental defectives in early twentieth-century medical texts', *British Journal for the History of Science*, 28 (1995), 319–37; S. Cross, *Mediating Madness: Mental Distress and Cultural Representation* (Houndmills, 2010).

136 See Goffman, *Stigma*, pp. 92–113.

137 See Clark, 'Law, liberty and psychiatry', and McCandless, 'Liberty and lunacy'.

138 Porter, *A Social History of Madness*, pp. 195–6; p. 196.

139 I discuss this in more detail in my PhD thesis. See V. Long, 'Changing Public Representations of Mental Illness in Britain, 1870–1970' (PhD thesis, University of Warwick, 2004), chapter 1.

140 See Jones, 'Raising the anti'.

141 Vincent, *Inside the Asylum*, pp. 114–15.

142 E. Irwin, L. Mitchell, L. Durkin, B. Douieb, 'The need for a mental patients' union' (1972). Reproduced on the Survivors' History Group webpage: http://studymore.org.uk/mpu.htm#FishPamphlet.

143 See, for example, Helen Spandler's reflections on the ways in which indi-
vidualist ideologies have inhibited collectivism in mental healthcare, or Barbara
Taylor's reflections on the discouragement of dependency in mental healthcare:
H. Spandler, *Asylum to Action: Paddington Day Hospital, Therapeutic Communities
and Beyond* (London, 2006), pp. 138–9; B. Taylor, 'The demise of the asylum
in late twentieth-century Britain: a personal history', *Transactions of the Royal
Historical Society*, 21 (2011), 193–215.

144 Taylor, 'The demise of the asylum', 202.

2

INSECURE PROFESSIONALS
AND THE PUBLIC

The relationship between psychiatrists and their patients, explored in the previous chapter, dominated the historiography of madness and psychiatry for many years. Yet examining other occupational groups provides an insight into the complexities of mental healthcare politics, demonstrating the impact of the economic and political climate on professional strategies, and revealing the interconnected fates of different professional groups. Over the course of the nineteenth and twentieth centuries, a number of occupational groups emerged to provide care and treatment to mentally disordered patients. These occupational groups frequently held divergent views as to what mental illness was, where it should be treated and how it should be treated, which reflected the origins of the occupation. As systems of healthcare evolved, these groups had to adapt to find a new role.

This chapter traces the ways in which two such occupations – psychiatric nurses and PSWs – represented mental illness and elicited public support as they sought to establish a distinct role in the field of mental healthcare. Revealing the challenges facing insecure professional groups who tried to balance their interests with those of their patients, I argue that we need to examine the relative power and professional status of different occupational groups, and consider efforts to destigmatise mental illness within the context of the broader goals of that occupation. Psychiatric nursing developed from the work of asylum attendants, and the profession remained invested in the system of hospital care, supporting therapies which appeared to transform hospital practice and enhance nurses' skills, and resisting proposals to move care outside hospitals. Attendants established a trade union in 1910 as a vehicle through which to campaign for their interests and formulate a professional identity. PSWs emerged to liaise with families and to arrange care for individuals at the boundaries of institutions; consequently they sought to colonise the field of social and community care. This group of workers established a professional association in 1929 to defend their interests and promote their views.

This chapter traces the development of the two occupations, the background and training of these workers and the conditions under which they worked, outlining the formation of representative bodies and journals. It foregrounds many of the issues discussed in Chapter 4 by exploring the interaction of gender and professional identity. Psychiatric social work was a predominantly female occupation and its practitioners felt this inhibited their claims to professional status. In contrast, psychiatric nursing, which comprised a roughly equal number of men and women, struggled to attain the same status as other branches of nursing because nursing's professional image was linked to feminine attributes.

The emergence of psychiatric nursing and psychiatric social work and establishment of representative bodies

Over the past twenty years, much historical research has focussed on psychiatry. Yet, as Peter Nolan notes, until recently nurses have been 'allocated only a marginal role in the pages of history despite having had the most intimate therapeutic role in relation to the mentally ill'.[1] The occupation developed in response to the emergence and expansion of a nationwide network of asylums, within which attendants were employed to manage and care for patients. While the in-patient population of asylums expanded dramatically between 1870 and the 1950s, there was no corresponding rise in the number of doctors employed in the sector. Consequently, patients' contact with psychiatrists declined throughout the period under study, heightening the influence nursing personnel had over patients' day to day experiences. In contrast to the pattern of care emerging in general hospitals where nursing developed as a female profession, men were employed as attendants within asylums to care for male patients. The 1919 Nurses Registration Act officially re-designated attendants as mental nurses, although the continual slippage between the terminology of nurse and attendant, patient and inmate, and care and management indicates that perceptions of the work and these workers did not rapidly change.

Nolan's observation regarding historians' lack of interest in the role of nurses applies equally to PSWs. While psychiatric nursing had originated within the walls of the asylum, the origins of psychiatric social work can be found in the activities of earlier charitable organisations that worked with the mentally disordered and their families within community settings, often

seeking to remedy people's difficulties by providing solutions to their economic problems.[2] Another factor that influenced the development of psychiatric social work was the growing acceptance of psychological explanations
for people's behaviour, and the emergence of the mental hygiene movement,
which sought to prevent mental illness from occurring by tackling the underlying causes.[3] One aspect of this movement was expressed in the growing
interest in the 'problem' child, exemplified in the work of the educational
psychologist Cyril Burt who was employed in 1913 to investigate cases of
difficult children in London schools and to carry out treatment. This paved
the way for the development of child guidance clinics in which PSWs were to
play a significant role.[4] In the 1930s, more PSWs were employed by mental
hospitals than in child guidance clinics, although the disparity later evened out
as the child guidance service developed. Community care, the third main field
of psychiatric social work, developed at a slower place, only equalling the other
two fields of employment by 1969.[5] In 1962, the number of trained PSWs had
reached 1,202, of whom 136 were men.

In the 1890s, asylum superintendents established the Asylum Workers'
Association, the first representative body which claimed to represent the
interests of asylum attendants. Superintendents believed that the failure
of other professions to recognise attendants as trained nurses undermined
their efforts to secure recognition of asylums as hospitals in which skilled

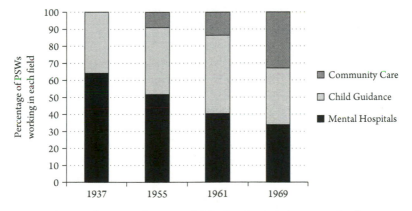

1 Distribution of PSWs in three main fields of work, 1937–69. Figures for the years
1937, 1955 and 1961 are drawn from data in Timms, *Psychiatric Social Work in
Britain*, pp. 69–70. The figures for the year 1969 are drawn from 'The Association of
Psychiatric Social Work Annual Report 1969', p. 17, MRC, University of Warwick,
APSW Archive, MSS.378/APSW/2/1/35.

medical personnel provided treatment to sick patients. The new Association idealised the professionalism of asylum attendants but overlooked the low wages and long hours that were endemic within the occupation.[6] Following the Association's failure to secure a non-contributory pension for asylum workers under the Asylum Officers' Superannuation Act of 1909, attendants from five asylums established the National Asylum Workers' Union (hereafter the Union) in 1910.[7] The fledgling Union capitalised on attendants' discontent with the Superannuation Act and the gulf between their salaries and those of medical superintendents, successfully attracting many former Asylum Workers' Association members to its ranks; by 1913, its membership stood at 7,900. Shulamit Ramon argued that attendants in the early years of the twentieth century focused on securing recognition as a protected group of workers, and 'did not attempt to achieve the status of a profession'.[8] Mick Carpenter echoed this view, asserting in his history of the Union it was 'created out of a hard-headed opposition to the pretensions of professionalism'. 'In place of the intangible benefits of status and prestige', he argued, 'the union had demanded better pay, shorter hours, and less irksome discipline'.[9] This orientation is evident if we examine the Union's objectives, which focused on working conditions rather than patient welfare:

> Objects – to obtain by legislation improvement of the status of asylum workers, reasonable hours of duty and of freedom, fair rates of wages, abolition of vexatious restrictions and other grievances, and a better regulation of the relations between employers and employed; and to assist members if wrongfully dismissed, and to provide legal aid when necessary, and to promote the welfare of asylum workers generally.[10]

The Union benefited from stable leadership for many years. Herbert Shaw, an attendant at the Wakefield Asylum, was appointed as Assistant General Secretary in 1911 after he was dismissed from his post for publicising the Union. Shaw served as editor of the Union's journal until his retirement in 1946. He focused his activities on his work for the Union, in contrast to George Gibson, who was elected as General Secretary in 1913 and retained this post until 1948. Gibson joined the Trades Unions Congress General Council in 1928 and served as Chairman in 1940. His activities were broadranging, and he served on the Overseas Settlement Board, the National Savings Committee, the Children's Overseas Reception Board, the Lancashire Industrial Development Council and the National Investment Council. For many members of the Union, Gibson's involvement with Winston Churchill in the United Europe campaign was the final straw; a motion was brought forward at the Union's 1947 conference seeking his resignation unless he withdrew from the campaign. Although the motion was defeated, Gibson retired from the post of General Secretary in 1947.

In the same year, Gibson was implicated by the Lynskey Tribunal of Inquiry for using his official powers to assist his friend Sidney Stanely to set up a business in expectation of personal gain. Gibson subsequently resigned from all his public posts, despite gaining little from the transaction: half a bottle of whisky, a dozen cigars, a suit (which he insisted he always intended to pay for) and three pounds of sausages.[11] His former colleagues at the Trades Unions Congress largely ignored Gibson's death in 1953, but Claude Bartlett, who served as President of the Union from 1926 to 1962, paid tribute to 'his vision and drive which enabled him to win such notable reforms for mental hospital and institution workers – and for patients too'.[12] Bartlett, who remained a mental charge nurse throughout his presidency, was a leading advocate of the amalgamation of health services trade unions which led to the Confederation of Health Service Employees. He took George Gibson's place on the Trades Unions Congress General Council in 1948 and was elected President in 1959. Bartlett also served as a member of the Royal Commission on Law relating to Mental Illness and Mental Deficiency, whose recommendations were incorporated into the Mental Health Act of 1959.

The Union's efforts to secure better wages and conditions for its members shaped its efforts to engage the public. Consequently, as the Union adapted to varying political and economic circumstances, the messages it sought to convey about mental illness and its treatment changed course. The first ten years of the Union marked a flurry of strikes and fluctuating membership.[13] Many asylum managements used a failed strike at Radcliffe in 1922 as an excuse to cut attendants' salaries, and membership fell from around 18,000 at the end of 1920 to 10,600 in 1926. By August 1930, when the Union renamed itself the Mental Hospital and Institutional Workers' Union, membership had increased to 12,488. These trends reflected national patterns, as overall trade union membership in Britain halved from 8.3 million in 1920 to 4.3 million by 1933.[14] During the 1930s, pay and hours only slowly improved as unemployment throughout the country remained high, but by 1942 the Union had 24,078 members. Four years later, the Union federated with the Hospitals and Welfare Services Union to form the Confederation of Health Service Employees, with a combined membership of 40,000. Unrest stirred again in the 1950s as recruitment to mental nursing declined and the Union struggled to negotiate better rates of pay and less overtime for mental nurses. In 1955, Union members picketed the Mental Health Exhibition, designed to tour the country, promoting the NHS. Health Minister Enoch Powell's plans to run down many of the mental hospitals in 1961 fuelled anxiety among many psychiatric nurses who feared losing their jobs.

The Association of Psychiatric Social Work (hereafter APSW) was formed in 1929 at the very inception of the British psychiatric social work profession with seventeen members. The new Association had no control over the training of PSWs but reinforced the importance of training by allowing only graduates of a specialised course to join. While the attendants' Union consciously rejected the ethos of professionalism, the founding members of the APSW hoped that their new Association would support their professionalising ambitions by publicising PSWs' expertise in the field of mental health and ensuring that training standards and working conditions were maintained. The first constitution of the APSW reflected these goals: the first object sought 'to contribute towards the general purposes of mental hygiene' through research and the sharing of experiences, while the second object aimed 'to raise and maintain professional standards, and to encourage the employment of fully trained workers at adequate salaries'.[15] The APSW offered a forum for the exchange and debate of ideas amongst its members through its national and local branch meetings, and its journal. The APSW also established a number of sub-committees that dealt with areas such as the management of its journal and other APSW publications; relations with other professions; training standards; salaries, and public relations.

The journals established by the APSW and the Union were intended primarily for the members of the respective organisations. The Union's publication, initially entitled *National Asylum Workers' Union Magazine* (hereafter referred to in the text as the journal) underwent radical changes in content, form and distribution over time.[16] Intended at first to cater for fewer than 8,000 mostly male asylum attendants, the journal initially adopted a socialist approach, fighting for its subscribers as members of the working class and attacking authority figures, especially superintendents, whom it depicted as over-paid and over-privileged. The journal portrayed membership of the rival Asylum Workers' Association as an act of class betrayal. As the working conditions of asylum staff slowly improved, the Union extended its horizons to encompass other issues, and the predicaments facing asylum patients came under closer scrutiny. In 1946, the journal began to incorporate the concerns of the former Hospitals and Welfare Services Union. By 1963, membership of the Union (and readership of the journal) stood at 67,000, reflecting for the first time a predominance of women members.

In 1947 the APSW Publications Sub-Committee established the *British Journal of Psychiatric Social Work* (hereafter *BJPSW*). The initial print run of 1,000 was cut to 600 copies in 1949 when it became clear that the APSW had a surfeit of unsold copies: membership of the APSW stood at only 398 by the end of 1948. From 1950, copies of the *BJPSW* were distributed to all subscribing members of the APSW. The remit of the *BJPSW* was initially to 'provide a vehicle for exchange of ideas regarding the methods of psychiatric social work. It will therefore be mainly of interest to a limited number of clinical workers.'[17] For historians, the *BJPSW* provides an insight into the professionalising aspirations of a nascent occupation; fragmentary perspectives from disparate locations, provided by authors for whom it is often impossible to ascertain even a first name. The APSW executive hoped that the issues discussed in the *BJPSW* would be debated in general meetings and branch meetings, linking the executive with its branch members.[18]

While the Union's journal functioned primarily as a vehicle for Union officials to outline policy and areas of concern to their members, and for members to share their views, contributions from Members of Parliament, doctors and pressure groups indicate that individuals outside of the Union were reading its publication. Nevertheless, as 'Onlooker' commented in 1934, while people with a vested interest in mental health issues could access a copy, 'as for the "general public", in so far as this refers to newspaper readers I do not think there is much scope for distribution.'[19] Similarly, 'A Satisfied Reader' ridiculed as a 'delusion' the idea that the journal could 'have an effect on public opinion outside the service'.[20] If anything, the ambitions of the *BJPSW* were even more limited; the editor Margaret Ashdown expressed the hope that it might help publicise the achievements of the APSW to related professions, serving as 'a whispering gallery, by means of which our voices, which some of us feel to be so feeble, can be made to carry to our professional neighbours, without fear or strain'.[21]

Insecure professionals and healthcare policy

As discussed in Chapter 1, psychiatry lacked the professional status, therapeutic techniques and popular image enjoyed by other branches of medicine. It remained, nevertheless, the most prestigious and well-established profession within the field of mental healthcare, and the difficulties its practitioners experienced in establishing their professional credentials were amplified in the fields of psychiatric nursing and psychiatric social work. Nurses and social workers belong to the group of occupations working in the fields of health, education and social welfare which Chris Nottingham has recently defined as 'insecure professionals'.[22] These professions, Nottingham argued, struggled to secure wage levels which placed them within the ranks of the middle classes because their claims to professional status on the grounds of unique professional skills and knowledge, verified through qualifications, were vigorously challenged. Viewed as agents of the state and entrusted with the task of resolving problem cases which transgressed social, educational or medical boundaries, insecure professionals were expected to persuade clients to conform to social expectations. Unlike the established professions, insecure professional groups struggled to persuade the state that they offered a unique skill which entitled them to establish a monopoly in a particular field. Consequently, insecure professionals tended to work within a field dominated by an established profession, or were unable to define the remits of their field of work. Nottingham's work offers a helpful frame through which to explore the difficulties encountered by PSWs and psychiatric nurses as they sought to demarcate their area of expertise and sites of practice within the field of mental healthcare. For both groups, the perception that their interactions with patients or clients could be characterised as care or assistance rather than treatment hindered professional advancement.

Although nurses had far more contact with patients than psychiatrists, they by no means enjoyed unfettered power in the discharge of their duties. Hampered by their low professional status in relation to psychiatrists and other branches of nursing, and subject to the authoritarian rules and regulations of the asylum which compelled many to live at the institution and restricted free time, nurses occupied an uneasy intermediary position which at times bore closer comparison with the experiences of the patients they cared for than with the doctors they worked for. George Gibson, the Union's first General Secretary, became an asylum attendant in the first decade of the twentieth century. In his reminiscences, he recalled the 'monotony of asylum life', in which 'the long hours of duty, the necessary confinement together within four walls and the atmosphere all tended to develop a remoteness from everyday life'.[23] In the late nineteenth- and early twentieth-century asylum, attendants' duties included supervising patients working within the asylum and its grounds, in the airing courts and during sports and leisure activities; caring for patients confined to bed; feeding, dressing and bathing patients; applying dressings; cleaning wards; keeping a watch on suicidal, sick and incontinent patients at night and controlling difficult patients.[24] Observing that the recovery rate was low, the death rate high, and that treatment could be summarised as 'read the Bible and keep your bowels open', Gibson described the work as 'a monotonous grind, which had few compensations'.[25] The ability to control difficult behaviour or to make a contribution to the asylum's football team or band could be as useful as nursing abilities.

Gibson recounted how he had stumbled into his post after being fired from bar work, the latest in a string of short-lived jobs.[26] His experience was doubtless far from atypical: given the low wages, long working hours, strict discipline and low status of asylum attendants, it seems unlikely that many entrants to the field in the early years of the twentieth century were motivated by a sense of vocation. Ruminating on the calibre of senior nursing personnel in the 1960s, one nurse observed that most had entered the profession in the 1930s, 'when mines were closed down, ship-yards were empty, the business world was in the doldrums and great numbers of people were on the dole . . . They hadn't wanted to become nurses; they did so because they had to.'[27]

High staff turnover prevailed in the sector, and asylum superintendents recruited staff from Ireland in the first half of the twentieth century to make up the deficit.[28] During the course of the Second World War, a number of refugee nurses found employment in the sector.[29] These trends continued in the postwar era as hospitals recruited nurses from Commonwealth nations and British colonies, despite opposition from Union branches who claimed that raising the salaries of mental nurses would encourage local people to join the profession.[30] As Mick Carpenter has noted, overseas nurses were primarily employed in low-status areas of work within the NHS and were thus disproportionately represented within the mental health sector.[31] This created a vicious cycle whereby the low status of the occupation inhibited recruitment, prompting the recruitment of overseas personnel to fill the gap, further lowering the status of psychiatric nursing. In contrast to other branches of nursing, asylums tended to employ men to care for male patients. The diversity of this workforce created internal tensions and undermined the capacity of mental nurses to campaign effectively for change.[32]

Recognising that their own status was inexorably bound up with the image of asylum attendants, psychiatrists began to introduce training schemes within their asylums for attendants.[33] In 1884, the Medico-Psychological Association intervened, commissioning four of its members to author a handbook for attendants. Published the following year, the text covered both nursing of the sick and care of the insane, providing an overview of the functions of the body and mental disorders.[34] In 1889, attenders at the annual meeting of the Medico-Psychological Association agreed to appoint a committee to report on a national scheme for training attendants, culminating in an examination, and a register of attendants who had passed the exam;[35] the first exam took place in 1891. Despite these steps to professionalise the occupation, mental nursing was still viewed as a distinct, and inferior, branch of nursing. The anomalous employment of men, in part rationalised on the grounds that men were required because the job entailed control and management as much as nursing, created friction with the general nursing profession, which sought to distance itself from mental nurses in order to maintain its own professional status. The Nurses Registration Act of 1919 established the General Nursing Council to regulate nursing and a register of qualified nurses, which included mental nurses in a separate section. Following this legislation, the General Nursing Council established a parallel system of training for mental nurses, reluctant to allow the Medico-Psychological Association to control training. In 1925, the General Nursing Council announced that it would recognise only mental nurses who had undertaken its own training and, increasingly, promotion to senior positions within mental nursing was dependent upon obtaining state registered nurse status.[36] Men were admitted on a separate male register and were not admitted to the general register of nurses until 1949, when the Royal Medico-Psychological Association ceased to administer its own examination for mental nurses and the General Nursing Council agreed to admit holders of the Royal Medico-Psychological Association qualification to its register.[37] Men were not entitled to join the Royal College of Nursing until 1960.[38]

Professional training for social workers in psychiatric fields was pioneered in the United States and exported to Britain. Thus, the Boston Psychopathic Hospital first developed professional training for PSWs in 1914, while four years later the Smith College offered the first course for training in psychiatric social work.[39] PSWs became part of the team in the newly established and Commonwealth-funded child guidance clinics, which aimed to prevent juvenile delinquency. When the Commonwealth Fund agreed to finance child guidance clinics in Britain, it stressed the need to train social workers in a university setting. In 1929, the London School of Economics established the Mental Health Course to train social science graduates with some experience in social work in psychiatric social work. Outlining the influence American funders had on the shape of the British training programmes, John Stewart has argued that British PSWs consequently adopted the medicalised approach to social work which characterised the field in America.[40] By 1944, only 257 people had qualified as PSWs, and not all of these people were using their qualification to work as a PSW. Approved courses then started in Edinburgh (1945), Manchester (1947) and Liverpool (1954).

Training on the courses consisted of fieldwork placements in a mental hospital and a child guidance clinic, lectures, and demonstrations on topics such as psychology, social casework and psychiatry.[41] Comparing the syllabuses at London from 1932 and 1960, Noel Timms observed that psychoanalytical theory increasingly shaped the approaches adopted in casework.[42] Noting that students had only a year to complete the diploma, and that much of this time was spent undertaking practical work and placements as opposed to academic study, John Stewart has questioned how feasible it would have been for students to acquire any depth of knowledge in the broad range of topics covered.[43] From 1958, the APSW admitted students who had qualified through generic social work courses, provided they undertook an additional psychiatric placement.

PSWs employed by mental hospitals emphasised the value of the social histories they compiled, representing this task as their distinct professional contribution. These social histories gathered information on the patient's social background, hereditary conditions, their physical and intellectual development, experiences, a study of their personality before their illness developed and factors that led up to the present situation.[44] Taking a social history, PSWs argued, yielded vital information which could assist the psychiatrist. As Margaret Ashdown explained to an audience of psychologists and psychiatrists, it enabled the PSW to enter the patient's home where she could 'lift the patient's case out of the atmosphere of bewilderment and fear, blame and recrimination, so that he can be regarded as simply a sick person to be helped'.[45] PSWs also helped their clients to readjust following discharge from hospital by encouraging them to join social clubs and assisting in the search for employment.[46] As John Stewart has observed, those PSWs employed by child guidance clinics focused their attention 'on the child in its domestic setting and, thereby, on the parents'.[47] Believing that the mother might have caused her child's disorder through her faulty parenting skills, PSWs undertook casework interviews with the mothers of children referred to the clinic. These interviews were influenced by psychoanalytical ideas, namely that the behaviour of the mother could be understood only if unconscious motivation, often extending back to childhood, was taken into account.[48]

Shulamit Ramon has argued that PSWs were comfortable with their status as medical auxiliaries and followed the conceptual framework adopted by psychiatrists, an interpretation which seems convincing if we turn to publications produced by PSWs in the 1930s and 1940s.[49] Entering the field of mental healthcare in the 1930s when it was professionally dominated by psychiatry, the first PSWs to qualify tried to sell their skills to those who might employ or work alongside them. As Peggie Armstrong commented in the first issue of the *BJPSW*, 'social workers needed the help of psychiatrists long before psychiatrists were prepared to acknowledge that they needed lay assistance in the form of trained and skilled PSWs'.[50] A 1943 pamphlet produced by the APSW thus stressed how the PSW could act as an assistant to the busy psychiatrist.[51] However, the APSW fiercely resisted the suggestion made in the Cope Report of 1951 that PSWs should be registered as medical auxiliaries,[52] expressing anxieties as to the impact this designation would have on 'the status of PSWs as professional social case workers with their training based at a university'.[53] Ultimately, the Ministry of Health decided not to proceed with the registration of PSWs as medical auxiliaries, but professional rivalry lingered on. In 1956, the APSW attacked the British Medical Association for the evidence it had given to the Working Party on Social Workers, complaining that when 'doctors emphasise so much "a real sense of vocation" and so little the acquisition of skills, they are perpetuating in the social field a state of affairs which would not be accepted in their own profession'.[54]

PSWs sometimes emphasised their professional status by asserting their superiority over other insecure professional groups in the field of mental health. Thus, in an edited volume published by the APSW in 1969, one contributor acknowledged that 'there seems to be a real fear of the nurse muscling in on the social worker's job', but insisted, 'one can expect the nurse to assail the status of the social worker, and the latter to endeavour to maintain his position'.[55] While the APSW frequently endorsed collaboration, it tended to envisage co-operation as a one-sided process. PSWs argued, for example, that their postgraduate university qualification fitted them to train and supervise psychiatric nurses, health visitors, child care officers and staff working in the probation service. Indeed, while doctors depicted PSWs as medical auxiliaries, the APSW countered by arguing that PSWs' specialised expertise enabled them to elucidate doctors on certain issues; in 1955, for example, the APSW suggested that PSWs could advantageously contribute towards the training of medical undergraduates who 'learnt very little about social and psychological factors in health and illness'.[56]

Most of the mental health services provided by local authorities were undertaken by social workers, usually designated as mental welfare officers, who had not qualified as PSWs; these workers had often gained extensive experience as Poor Law relieving officers and as duly authorised officers, responsible for certifying patients. In their oral history work with mental welfare officers, Sheena Rolph, Dorothy Atkinson and Jan Warmsley found that most were male and that in 'certain local authorities, a "macho" culture was allowed to thrive'.[57] After the implementation of the National Health Services Act, the range of functions undertaken by mental welfare officers increasingly included the care and aftercare of people who had experienced mental illness. Given the shortage of qualified PSWs, the APSW often suggested that the work of mental welfare officers could be supervised by a PSW. This was not well received: in 1961, one mental welfare officer asserted the superior value of 'hard experience' over training in the field of mental healthcare, complaining about the 'growing tendency to over-stress the powers or capabilities of the PSW'. 'We are dealing with human beings', he insisted, 'not explaining ways and means of launching space ships'.[58]

While mental welfare officers stressed the value of experience, the APSW emphasised the value imparted by training and sought 'to encourage the employment of fully trained workers at adequate salaries'.[59] This proved extremely difficult to achieve, for the value of the PSW postgraduate qualification was not always recognised. In June 1950, for example, the APSW protested when an advertisement was placed for a PSW, or alternatively an untrained worker at a higher salary.[60] The ambiguous status of the profession raised difficulties when the APSW attempted to market psychiatric social work as a career to potential recruits. Sometimes the APSW emphasised the 'vocational' aspect of the work, stressing the moral probity and thus professional nature of PSWs. An article in 1959 claimed, 'PSWs have an intense vocational spirit – their training is long and arduous and depends upon specialised practical and theoretical courses at a university'.[61] Public relations advisers, whose advice was sought by the APSW, suggested getting in touch with a teacher training college and a working women's college, as students at these institutions 'already knew that they wanted to try some other more interesting occupation if possible and were prepared to suffer financial hardship to achieve it'. The advisers suggested that the APSW should 'write some slightly different articles with some emotional appeal relating to what we get out of psychiatric social work, as it is obvious that we must get something as it isn't financially rewarding'.[62]

A 1951 APSW career pamphlet emphasised the distinctive characteristics of the profession. 'The PSW is a social therapist', it explained, 'whose previous training and experience in social work combined with additional training in the field of psychological medicine, give her a special role to play in the investigation and treatment of patients, a role which is no less important than that of the psychiatrist or psychologist'. The pamphlet did not mention that PSWs were paid considerably less than either of the other professions (a factor that was believed to cause the low levels of male entrants into the profession), focusing instead on the 'interesting and satisfying' nature of the work.[63] However, emphasising the emotionally satisfying, vocational nature of the work undermined the APSW's attempts to improve status and pay for the occupation as a skilled profession. In 1965, Margaret Barnes wrote in to The Times in response to an article on psychiatric social work as a career:

> Your correspondent suggested that psychiatric social work calls for a 'selfless character and that such workers are not likely to rate money that highly'. This image of social work is out of date and PSWs, like the medical and nursing professions, wish to have their skills recognised by adequate and fair remuneration.[64]

Changes in healthcare policy profoundly affected the strategies adopted by both occupations. In the next chapter, we will see how some psychiatrists seized upon the formation of the NHS and the nominal incorporation of mental hospitals within the new service as a means of aligning psychiatry with general medicine and elevating the status of the profession.[65] For psychiatric nurses too, the ostensible integration of mental health services into the new NHS presented an opportunity to heal the longstanding rift with general nurses by emphasising the similarities between mental hospitals and general hospitals and the nature of nurses' roles within each. At an organisational level, the merger of the Union with the Health and Welfare Services Union to form the Confederation of Health Service Employees in 1946 facilitated these developments; now responsible for representing the interests of all health workers, the Union's journal played host to a broader range of health concerns.[66] Articles relating specifically to mental nursing now drew on the model of general nursing to approximate the work of nurses and the needs of patients in both sectors. Thus, in an essay competition launched by Union's journal shortly after the merger – 'What are the Prime Essentials in Successful Mental Nursing' –Mr Yarnell suggested that more general nursing training should be included in the training of mental nurses:

> I think this is very necessary, otherwise the real meaning of the word 'hospital' loses its significance. The mental health of the nation is an integral part of the health system of this country . . . The mind and body are so closely associated that general and mental trained nurses should be similarly associated.[67]

Rising patient numbers however hampered efforts to approximate mental nursing and mental hospitals to general nursing and general hospitals. As the resident in-patient population of mental hospitals peaked in 1954 leading to widespread overcrowding, the Union submitted a motion to the Trades Unions Congress which urged the Minister of Health 'to take immediate action to relieve the overcrowding of patients in mental hospital wards and to improve the mental nursing staff conditions and salaries with a view to making the service more attractive to students and retaining trained mental nurses'.[68]

In his presidential speech to the triennial delegate conference of 1959, the year in which he was elected President of the Trades Unions Congress,[69] Claude Bartlett expressed satisfaction at the large advances made by the Union in representing the interests of nurses as professionals:

> When I compare the conditions in our mental hospitals today with those obtaining before the advent of the NHS, I often wonder whether some of my trade union colleagues are not trying to break down barriers which have long since ceased to exist. It is a far cry from the lunatic attendant of less than fifty years ago to the fully trained and qualified psychiatric nurse of today. I am naturally proud to have played some part, small perhaps, in raising a once lowly and much stigmatised occupation into a skilled and honoured vocation.[70]

Yet not all the audience members who listened to Bartlett's address viewed their future prospects with such equanimity, for radical changes in the shape of mental health services were afoot which would dramatically affect both psychiatric nursing and psychiatric social work. The 1959 Mental Health Act, which enabled local authorities to provide a range of community-based services, followed in the wake of the 1957 report of the Royal Commission on the Law Relating to Mental Illness and Mental Deficiency; this had urged the relocation of mental healthcare from hospitals to community settings.[71] Bartlett had served on the Committee which produced this report and was keen to emphasise what he viewed as its progressive characteristics. For the profession of psychiatric nursing as a whole, which had emerged to provide care to patients within the asylum and which had not, at this stage, laid claim to the delivery of care in the community, the shift threatened to undermine working conditions and steadily obliterate the need for the profession entirely.

Concerned that other professionals might usurp their role in caring for patients in community settings, delegates passed a resolution on the Mental Health Bill which expressed concerns at inadequate funding for the proposed measures and their hope that mental nurses' skills would be utilised in community care. Aware that the Royal College of Nursing also claimed to represent the interests of psychiatric nurses – indeed the College issued a report on the impact of the 1959 Mental Health Act and its implications for the roles of psychiatric nurses the following year – the wording emphasised the Union's role as crusaders for psychiatric patients and as leaders of public opinion.[72] 'The Confederation membership', it claimed, 'has played an important part in seeking to improve the standard of nursing and other services to those mentally ill and have attempted through this organisation to make the general public mental health conscious'.[73]

However, Enoch Powell's decision to close mental hospitals incrementally appeared to cement this shift in policy. Announcing the proposed closure of 75,000 hospital beds over a period of fifteen years, Powell warned his audience – the 1961 annual meeting of the NAMH – that this task would not be easy. 'Hundreds of men and women', he explained, 'have given years, even lifetimes, to the service of a mental hospital':

> They have laboured devotedly, through years of scarcity and neglect, to render the conditions in them more tolerable, and of late they have seized with delight upon the new possibilities opening up, and the new resources available, for these old but somehow cherished institutions . . . It would be more than flesh and blood to expect them to take the initiative in planning their own abolition, to be the first to set the torch to the funeral pyre.[74]

For Powell, the obsolescence of the psychiatric hospital entailed the obsolescence of the personnel who staffed it. However, PSWs opposed nurses' attempts to move into the field of community work as hospitals faced closure. One PSW concluded that nurses' training was limited to the management of patients within hospital settings and that the PSW was in most instances better equipped to visit patients in the community.[75] Yet limiting psychiatric nurses' work to hospitals during a period when government policy was devoted to shutting hospitals down posed problems; as one lecturer in nursing studies observed, 'it seems unlikely that one can find intelligent highly motivated people of the right kind of personality to staff the hospital wards if they are barred from all work which carries more interest, more prestige and more career opportunities'.[76] We will explore the impact of this policy on the strategy adopted by the Union and the way in which it represented patients in Chapter 4.

The proposed closure of the mental hospitals and the expansion of community provisions did not appear to auger well for the future of psychiatric nursing; as Peter Nolan and Barry Hopper have observed, 'psychiatric hospitals and the psychiatric nursing profession were in crisis during the 1950s'.[77] The prospects seemed rosier for PSWs, however. Recognising the potentialities in the 1959 Mental Health Act to expand and improve the status of psychiatric social work, the APSW gave a guarded welcome to the legislation. 'The Bill could achieve little without the allocation of adequate finance and staff', proclaimed an article in the *Daily Telegraph*, citing the APSW. 'PSWs had a vital part to play. But there must be better recognition of their professional status.'[78] On this front, a report issued in the same year by a working party which had been appointed to inquire into the proper field of work and the recruitment and training of social workers in the local authorities' health and welfare services appeared to substantiate the professional status of PSWs. Chaired by Eileen Younghusband, the Report distinguished between simple problems and those which required skilled casework, asserting the need for an elite cadre of 'professionally trained and experienced social workers'.[79] Noting that only twenty-six qualified PSWs were employed full-time by local authorities, the Report expressed the belief that 325 PSWs would provide adequate coverage to the local authority health departments.[80] One disgruntled correspondent to the journal *Medical Officer* complained that five of the ten working party members were social workers and viewed the exercise as 'blatant empire building'.[81]

The publication of the Younghusband Report in 1959 and the imminent Mental Health Act should have opened the path to professional advancement for PSWS. However, the inability of the APSW to clarify the unique professional skills and role of the PSW fuelled destructive attacks on the profession, undermining its image. In a House of Lords debate on the Younghusband

Report in 1960, Lord Pakenham questioned the value of a trained PSW and expressed concerns that PSWs were meddlers: 'what generated so much heat', he suggested, 'was the question whether there was such a thing as a professionally qualified social worker as distinct from someone with good sense and a wealth of experience'.[82] Speaking in the same debate, Barbara Wootton criticised 'the growing practice of giving people in trouble "pseudo-psychology" instead of practical help'. 'Many social workers', she claimed, 'were encouraged, when faced with a simple practical economic problem, to search for some profound disturbance underneath'.

Wootton's comments echoed the critique of social work she had advanced a year earlier in her book *Social Science and Social Pathology*, in which she had ridiculed social workers' adoption of psychological and psychoanalytical interpretations.[83] Social workers, she argued, had 'succeeded in exchanging the garments of charity for a uniform borrowed from the practitioners of psychological medicine'.[84] In the process of undertaking this transition, Wootton scathingly remarked, social workers had constructed a 'fantastically pretentious facade', emphasising some aspects of social work 'out of all proportion to their real significance'.[85] The claims made on behalf of social casework in particular drew her ire. Citing some of the definitions of casework advanced by social workers – many of which were American – Wootton insisted that only by marrying her client could the social worker hope to secure such ambitious and intimate objectives.[86] This was rather unfortunate for PSWs, who had long viewed casework as a professional activity which they had pioneered within the social work field and which consequently set them above other branches of the profession. Indeed, in a report of a training course organised by the APSW on 'The Boundaries of Casework', APSW Chairman Kay McDougall noted that 'psychiatric social work' and 'casework' tended to be used synonymously, and that the practice of casework could be viewed as constituting psychiatric social work.[87]

Wootton's diatribe also unravelled social workers' claims to be undertaking treatment. The social work literature, she noted, was 'richly strewn with references to "diagnosis", "therapy", "treatment" . . . caseworkers see themselves as a species of social doctor'.[88] It is noteworthy that the medicalised language used by PSWs to describe their work, which reflected the American origins of the profession, proved to be the very grounds on which Wootton challenged the professional status of social work.[89] She accused social workers of reducing 'moral and economic problems' to 'common psychiatric denominators',[90] misguidedly searching for a profound underlying psychological cause and blithely ignoring obvious environmental factors which had caused their clients' woes. Wootton castigated the language social workers used to describe their work as arrogant, defensive and preten-tious, favouring 'habitually misty vocabularies' over 'concrete language'.[91] 'Happily, it can be presumed that the lamentable arrogance of the language in which contemporary social workers describe their activities is not gener-ally matched by the work that they actually do', Wotton concluded, 'oth-erwise it is hardly credible that they would not get their faces constantly slapped'.[92] Having brutally dissected the professional aspirations of the social work profession, Wootton disingenuously expressed concerns at the 'considerable insecurity' of social workers' professional status, evidenced, in her view, by the proliferation of the words of 'profession' and 'professional' in the social work literature.[93] She insisted that the true value of the social worker lay not in any service she might herself provide, but in her ability to connect her client to another appropriate professional service. While Wootton's critique encompassed all social workers, it is noteworthy that the most disparaged aspects of the profession in her account – casework, the adoption of psychological explanations and medicalisation, reflected in use of the terns *diagnosis* and *treatment* – were those most strongly associated with psychiatric social work. Hitherto, PSWs had argued that it was pre-cisely these characteristics which set their specialism ahead of general social work in terms of professional status.

Admittedly, PSWs had long acknowledged that their inability to formulate an agreed definition of psychiatric social work obstructed their attempts to assert their professional superiority within the field of social work. Thus, in the second issue of the *BJPSW*, editor Margaret Ashdown observed that:

> We are . . . taking it for granted that there is something which distinguishes our work and makes it precious enough to justify us in claiming exemptions and privileges among other social workers . . . If we do this, we ought to be able to give an account of our speciality, yet it is doubtful whether we are able to formu-late it to our common satisfaction.[94]

At a meeting of the APSW's Public Relations Sub-Committee (PRSC) in 1959 Miss McClenan from the NAMH echoed Wootton when she accused the APSW of using 'a language so esoteric that the function of the PSW is incomprehensible to the ordinary lay mind. A clear but simple definition of what a PSW is and does has never, to her knowledge, been made public.'[95] Addressing a meeting of the APSW in the same year, the child psychiatrist Tom Ratcliffe also mirrored Wootton's criticisms, admonished his listen-ers for transcending their auxiliary role to provide interpretative analytical casework. There was a danger, he claimed, that the therapeutic approaches adopted by PSWs could become 'governed more by the training level – and dare we say the professional ambitions – of the therapist or caseworker, than by the level of therapy which is most appropriate to the client's needs and capacity'.[96] That these brutal indictments were delivered directly to the APSW by their supposed allies did not bode well: evidently, psychiatric social work was far from being comfortably entrenched as a recognised profession in command of a distinct set of skills and experience. A desire to confine PSWs to an auxiliary role in which they provided care but not treatment may have underpinned the hostility expressed in some quarters to interpretative as opposed to practical casework.[97] After all, PSWs sought to substantiate their claims to professional status by asserting that they provided skilled treatment – either through analytical casework or by providing psychiatric social treatment to individuals suffering from enduring mental health problems.[98]

Representing patients

The strategies adopted by members of both occupational groups to represent their interests and the broader context of healthcare policy in which these strategies were forged shaped the ways in which nurses and PSWs represented their patients. Given the initial focus of the Union on the pay and conditions of attendants, it is unsurprising that few early articles drew attention to the poor conditions in which the patients lived. When patients did feature in the journal, they tended to be represented as one of the dangerous and unpleasant features of asylum work, rationalising attendants' demands for higher wages. As we shall explore further in Chapter 4, representations of dangerous, violent and depraved male patients therefore predominated.

Very slowly, a few patients' voices infiltrated the journal. However, it was not until the formation of the Confederation of Health Service Employees and the broadening of the journal's remit to represent the interests of all health workers that a patient's account was cited with respect. Reviewing in 1946 *The Autobiography of David*, a memoir discussed in Chapter 1, the journal described how 'the anonymous author who triumphed over mental ill-health to become a staunch friend of this Union has gained an uncanny insight into the processes of mind derangement and he is generous in tribute to the powers of healing'.[99] In the 1946 August edition, the journal quoted 'David', giving qualified support to the care he had received, while arguing that the service would be better if only the government would improve the status and conditions of those who worked in mental hospitals: unsurprisingly, the Union writer chose to cite the most flattering paragraph referring to mental nurses in David's account:

Conditions can, and must, be greatly improved. The buildings, the staff (doctors have far too many patients to attend to, and so have the nursing staff), the living conditions of the nurses and their pay, provision for early treatment, money for reforms on an adequate scale – here is the ground on which we have to work and create the necessary reforms which will give the public, and particularly the patient, complete confidence in the services.[100]

The Union's decision to reproduce extracts from David's account within its journal demonstrated that a significant shift had taken place with regards to the patient. Formerly at the fringe of debates, deployed to highlight the pitfalls of asylum work, mental patients now assumed importance in their own right in the Union's discussions. Thus, in his opening speech at the 1928 annual conference, Claude Bartlett acknowledged that, while wages and conditions of work for members were the primary concern of the Union, it was also the duty of nurses to take responsibility for the welfare of their patients.[101] In addition to the usual motions relating to pay and conditions of service, delegates passed a motion pressing for an improvement of outdoor facilities for patient recreation. For Mick Carpenter, these developments marked the adoption of a 'user-centred and worker friendly approach' which persists today; a linear narrative which, as Chapter 4 will demonstrate, is difficult to substantiate.[102] Two years later, the journal once more aired David's views; in this instance, David praised a nurse who had rescued a mental patient from a dangerous situation. He reiterated the themes of patient–staff collaboration and the need for both 'a fuller understanding by the public of all the varied and difficult services rendered by the mental nursing staffs', and the effort 'to create a more humane public opinion towards insanity'.[103]

The Union's shift in strategy mirrored attempts by medical superintendents to redefine their field of work during the 1920s. As discussed in Chapter 3, this period witnessed a current of change in British psychiatric practice, with the establishment of out-patient clinics, reforms of the laws regarding hospital admission that enabled voluntary treatment, and reforms within hospitals themselves.[104] The Union formally enshrined its new concern for patient welfare at its 1935 annual conference, when a resolution was passed binding the Union 'to consider any matters relating to the care, treatment and general welfare of the patients in mental and other hospitals'.[105] In 1931 the Union started to report the activities of the MACA, whose work is discussed in Chapter 5. This charity dispensed paternalistic assistance to discharged patients, and its patient-centred, yet by no means radical or patient-led, approach appealed to the Union, which provided an annual subscription to the charity in 1931.

In its journal, the Union mirrored the view that the asylum had now become a mental hospital, where patients suffering from a curable disease would receive up-to-date treatment from skilled nursing professionals who supported the principle of voluntary admission enshrined in the 1930 Mental Treatment Act. This new conception, which focused less upon the mental nurse as the overworked and underpaid servant of the asylum authorities, required a new, more sympathetic representation of the mental patient. Early representations that depicted the mental patient as distinct from sane individuals gave way to the view that anyone could be susceptible to mental illness. Thus, Mr R. Bringloe, the runner-up in an essay competition in 1946, for 'What are the Prime Essentials in Successful Mental Nursing?', explained that 'the nurse must be able to place herself in the position of the patient, appreciate his predicament . . . Running counter to this is the attitude so easily developed of humouring a patient, based on the assumption that he is "mental".'[106] Bringloe's decision to gender the nurse as female indicates how the Union had begun to model mental nursing on the feminised model of general nursing as a means of professional advancement. Writing for the same competition, Mr F. Stamp urged nurses to empathise with their patients, challenging earlier rigid distinction between the sane and insane and representing patients as equals whose experiences were comprehensible:

> 'But for the grace of God, there go I', or words to that effect should be the outlook of a good nurse in a mental hospital because, as one well knows, the dividing line between sanity and insanity is a very narrow one. That depressed 'Monday morning' feeling, if magnified, gives one a slight impression of the tortures of the average melancholic . . . the average patient responds to kindness, when treated as an equal.[107]

Kathleen Woodroofe has argued that social workers in the 1920s and 1930s jettisoned their earlier concern with problems in the social environment that might impede individual adjustment. With the shift from an economic to a psychological approach to people's problems, 'it was assumed that if adjustment was not achieved the individual was to blame'.[108] Such attitudes can be discerned in the work of early PSWs, particularly in their discussion of working-class clients. In a case study prepared in 1932, the APSW explained that resolving the difficulties of R. D., a married man with children, would put an end to 'a distressing personal situation'. However, the APSW envisaged other tangible benefits from intervention, for 'R. D. seems essentially capable of contributing, as an intelligent and responsible citizen, to the community on which he has so long parasitically depended'.[109] Fifteen years later, the *BJPSW* printed similar ideas: 'we have to help the patient to assume social responsibilities for himself, his family and the community'.[110]

PSWs working in child guidance clinics sought to elevate their work with mothers as psychotherapeutic treatment, but a contradiction lay in the fact that it had been the child, and not the nominally healthy mother, who had been referred to the clinic with problems. One means of circumventing this unfortunate truth was to insist that children's problems usually stemmed from the mother's maladjustment. Thus Betty Joseph sought to collapse the boundary between child and mother, arguing 'that a mother and a young child are essentially emotionally one', and that consequently 'if one can alter, ever so little, the feeling in the mother, this fact will show itself in her child'.[111] Similarly, Margaret Tickler suggested that some mothers were 'regarded as patients in their own right'.[112] This approach enabled PSWs to conceptualise their work as treatment, but had the effect of pathologising mothers.

Insecure professional groups, argued Chris Nottingham, were tasked with the responsibility of persuading clients to conform to social norms.[113] This certainly characterised the approach taken by many PSWs in the 1940s and 1950s, who argued that the needs of their clients should not take precedence over societal demands. In 1950, E. L. Thomas argued that the PSW needed to avoid 'both an identification with the patient in his battles with authority and at the same time refrain from becoming a watchdog of the community'. The PSW's desire to facilitate a patient's optimal readjustment, Thomas warned, 'cannot be pursued to the point of jeopardising the welfare of others'.[114] However, attitudes began to change by the early 1960s. A careers pamphlet printed in 1960 adopted a more equitable approach, describing psychiatric social work as 'a branch of social case work which is concerned with helping disturbed people and society adapt themselves to one another'.[115] By 1963, the APSW appears to have inverted its original approach. Summarising discussion at the Association's annual conference, Chairman Irene Spackman observed that 'attention has been focused upon the responsibility of the social worker for influencing social policy. We have been reminded that casework is not a panacea for all social ills.'[116] A report of the conference in *New Editor* complained that people already disadvantaged by mental illness could not be expected to adapt to society if society failed to provide adequate resources.[117] In the original draft for this piece, PSW Jean Nursten reported how conference delegates felt that 'casework skills are misused and may be brought into disrepute when the aim is to adjust clients to situations which really require social action on a larger scale . . . social workers' responsibility lay in effecting change in the client *and* in society'.[118] While these changes may have been informed by the development of psychiatric social treatment,[119] they could also have served as a riposte to Barbara Wootton's searing criticisms. Wootton charged that the emphasis social workers placed on casework 'deflects attention away from the problems created by evil environments'.[120] Dependent upon psychiatric interpretation, social workers reduced 'moral and economic problems . . . to common psychiatric denominators'. 'Before we know where we are', Wotton warned, 'poverty no less than crime will rank as a form of mental disorder'.[121] Perhaps Wootton's diatribe had prompted some soul-searching amongst PSWs.

Educating the public

The increasing interest displayed by the Union in patient welfare from the late 1920s onwards went hand in hand with a desire to educate the public about mental illness and its treatment. Increasingly, the Union contested its inferior place within the professional hierarchy of mental health by presenting itself as a body which represented the interests of a skilled medical profession, appropriating new terminology to reflect its desired new image. This development was related to the introduction of new treatments and the 1930 Mental Treatment Act, which held out the promise of transforming psychiatry into a more esteemed branch of medicine. It was also connected to the uneasy relations between the Union and the general nursing profession following the establishment of the College of Nursing in 1916. Reflecting the middle-class background of its founders, the College, as its recent historians Susan McGann, Anne Crowther and Rona Dougall have described, adopted an 'unashamedly elitist' approach to nursing.[122] It explicitly eschewed a trade union approach in its Articles of Association, advocating in its place the advancement of nursing as a profession – a profession which excluded mental nurses and male nurses.[123] Following the Nurses Registration Act of 1919, the Union's Executive, via its journal, repeated called on all staff to obtain the Medico-Psychological Association Certificate so that mental nursing would be seen as a profession rather than an unskilled occupation only concerned with its financial rewards.[124] The growing interest displayed by the Union in establishing the professional credentials of its members can thus be viewed in part as a response to the explicit critique of trade unionism launched by the College, reflecting a desire to present the Union as a body equally concerned with professional advancement and working conditions. Consequently, the Union needed to depict its members – renamed mental nurses following the 1919 Act – as skilled medical professionals who delivered medical care within hospitals to sick patients. Images of attendants controlling violent asylum inmates began to fade from view, although this transition was a slow process.

Thus, at the Union's 1928 annual conference, where delegates debated motions concerning patient welfare, the Union endorsed the motion 'that this conference thinks it desirable for the general public to be enlightened in regard to public mental hospitals and the treatment therein'. Arguing for the motion, Mr Dixon argued that 'all the public know about mental hospitals is the worst side of them, and we think it would do much good if they were to come inside and look round'.[125] Like other healthcare workers, Union members depicted the public as an ignorant monolithic entity in need of enlightenment. In this vein, A. J. Goundry used the correspondence column in the journal in 1931 to express his concerns that the attitude of the 'general public' to mental nursing was outdated and ill-informed. 'The general public does not know enough of the more difficult type of nursing – mental nursing', he argued. 'As a matter of fact, a distorted view is often held.'[126]

In 1929 an unsuccessful attempt was made to change the title of the Union to the National Association of Mental Employees. The proposer argued that it would raise attendants' status. Asylums, he admitted, would 'still be asylums, but I think it gives us a higher standing if they are known as "mental hospitals"'. 'If we can get people to talk of us as "mental hospital workers"', he concluded, 'I think it will make things a bit better'.[127]

The proposal failed but nine years later a virtually identical suggestion succeeded. It raised the same concerns regarding public perceptions of the occupation, but voiced the belief that the change in name reflected an actual improvement in terms of treatment:

> If we as a Union alter our title and do away with the false stigma of the word 'asylum', the public will more readily realise that our institutions are actually hospitals dealing with mental diseases . . . We shall be doing something to raise the status of the mental nursing profession and to teach the public that our profession is a real asset to the social services of the country.[128]

Such concerns came to the fore following the formation of the Confederation of Health Service Employees, when the prospect of a national health service loomed on the horizon. Here again, the change in nomenclature was significant: the title of the new body had been decided upon in 1944 during the merger negotiations as those present felt 'there was an objection, maybe a "snobbish" one, to the word "Union"'.[129] If we turn back to the Union's 1946 essay competition, 'What are the Prime Essentials in Successful Mental Nursing?', we find that a desire to educate the public features prominently in contributions. Concerned that the stigma attached to mental illness and its treatment in the public mind would inhibit mental nurses' attempts to secure professional status, Mr G. Tiley claimed that 'there still exists a "fear" among the sane population of being contaminated by mental affliction and then being referred to as a "lunatic" in the "asylum"'.[130] Tiley's use of the word 'contami-

nation' evoked his anxiety that those unconnected with the mental health services believed that contact with patients somehow polluted nurses, a concern
that has been identified by Peter Nolan and Diane Gittins in their interviews
with former psychiatric nurses.[131] In her entry, Ward Sister Florence Marion
Harries-Jones complained that newspapers used outdated terms, which in her
view were derogatory and had failed to keep pace with developments within
mental healthcare:

> Unhappily, newspapers are only too prone to refer to a mental hospital as a
> lunatic asylum. The time is, however, now almost at hand when this old fash-
> ioned idea will be completely eradicated and mental nursing will be given the
> recognition it deserves for the skilled, highly trained and efficient profession
> which it has become.[132]

Four years later, the Union's National Executive Committee adopted a
resolution which expressed concern at 'the repeated use in the Press of the
words "Lunatic" and "Asylum" when reference is made to mental patients and
mental hospitals'.[133] One branch felt such a measure did not go far enough
and urged the Committee to secure the restyling of mental nurses as psychiatric nurses.[134]

While mental nurses were keen to improve the image of the mental hospitals in which they worked and to break down some of the barriers between
hospitals and the public,[135] PSWs were employed in a broader range of sites
and in roles which required them to liaise between their employers, their
clients and the community. Consequently, discussion of PSWs' potential
role as public educators began early in the profession's history. In 1936,
for example, Margaret Ashdown asked 'whether the PSW has not a special
responsibility to the community at large, as representing a certain attitude to
mental and nervous disorder'. Ashdown nonetheless cautioned her colleagues
to adopt a self-effacing approach, as in her view the PSW could most effectively
undertake this role 'if she does not carry a banner and is not too vocal'.[136] In
the second issue of the *BJPSW*, published in 1948, Pauline Shapiro expressed
her belief that the PSW had a dual function as a therapist to her patient and
an educationist to the community, responsible for conveying psychiatric concepts and attitudes. Mindful of the inauguration of the NHS, Shapiro stressed
the need for PSWs to accept their role as educationist 'at this time of new
legislation reflecting new social values and needs'.[137] Describing the problems
facing the mother of a child referred to a child guidance clinic, whose relatives
and friends, 'full of prejudice and the colourful propaganda of some recent
films, paint to her a grim picture of what will happen to her child once he gets
into the power of a psychiatrist', one PSW expressed concerns that treatment

objectives could be impaired if not accompanied by an attempt to change public opinion.[138]

While PSWs had from the inception of their profession expressed a belief that they were well placed to educate the public, this endeavour gained a new urgency following the transmission of the television series 'The Hurt Mind' on mental illness in 1956, which is discussed in detail in Chapter 6. In the wake of the series, the APSW established its PRSC, which noted in its inaugural meeting that, while 'The Hurt Mind' 'had been a much needed and excellent attempt at a difficult subject', 'the whole field of psychiatric social work was barely mentioned'.[139] Believing that it served as 'the public face of the Association',[140] the PRSC set out to monitor the press, radio, television and other publications in order to correct inaccuracies and provide constructive comment. Members also hoped to produce material publicising the profession and to get branches involved in collecting and replying to the press.[141] From the outset the PRSC concerned itself primarily with the profession of psychiatric social work; general issues regarding mental health and illness were further down, or even incidental, on its agenda.

Several factors constrained the PRSC's effectiveness. Virtually all the members serving on the Committee had full-time jobs as PSWs, and at one meeting members commented that people were being 'bludgeoned' into taking office because no one else would.[142] Indeed, minutes from the meetings suggest that serving on the PRSC could be a profoundly disheartening experience. As discussed earlier in this chapter, PSWs struggled to produce a definition of their work which substantiated their claim to professional status. While this posed difficulties for all PSWs, the burden laid heaviest on the PRSC, which believed that its first task was to produce 'a good definition of the functions of a PSW'.[143] PRSC members felt that the APSW executive looked to them to communicate to the public the role of the PSW and the viewpoint of the APSW, as 'it was felt that as a professional body it had a definite viewpoint to put across . . . even though there is within the Association a wide range of opinion on certain subjects'.[144] It did not help that psychiatric social work was, as one PSW observed, 'insuperably unpictorial. No uniforms, no badges, no exhibits, not even a photo could really demonstrate what we do, unless, as one of us gloomily observed, it were a photo of a woman on a wet day knocking at a door.'[145] When the PRSC attempted to create its first poster, members 'realised how hard the idea was to represent'.[146]

The PRSC believed they had to battle against widespread press and public ignorance and apathy about psychiatric social work, a view doubtless fuelled following high-profile attacks on social work led by Barbara Wootton. In his 1964 history of the profession, Noel Timms explained that his purpose in writing was 'to answer certain questions: who are PSWs? What do they do? Are they "half-baked" or adequately trained?'[147] He cited a pilot survey into public knowledge of, and attitudes towards, social work and the social services, in which 75 per cent of the sample interviewed had not heard of PSWs, while 80 per cent could not say what they did. Most of the remainder thought that PSWs were engaged in the actual treatment of mental patients, a view which Timms labelled as inaccurate, despite the claims of some PSWs to be undertaking treatment.[148]

The PRSC believed that ignorance of the functions of PSWs extended into, and perhaps emanated from, the press, and thus sent letters to the media to correct misrepresentations of PSWs and to attack omissions of PSWs' work. Mrs Finch, the chair of the PRSC, commented to the chair of the medical committee established to advise the BBC that 'it was felt to be misleading to show doctors functioning by themselves in programmes without any mention of other professional and technical staff'.[149] Finch however acknowledged the futility of this approach in a letter to the *Guardian* television critic Mary Crozier, expressing her view that 'it is impractical and even petty to keep writing letters of protest when, for instance, a PSW is shown on the BBC doing nothing more than getting into bed with a psychiatrist or removing a coat from her back to put it on that of a patient'.[150] Feeling powerless to stop misrepresentations of their occupation, the PRSC produced and circulated positive images of their work as a skilled profession to different audiences. They sought to persuade potential employers that a PSW could be a useful and productive member of the team and to reassure potential clients, especially mothers of children referred to child guidance clinics, that their work was helpful. PSWs also wanted to give the public a more informed – and positive – view of psychiatric social work, although their main objective was to boost recruitment to the profession.

PSWs' belief that the public knew little about their work impeded their efforts to share their ideas about mental illness with a broader public, and in practice many of their ruminations on the public do not appear to have escaped the confines of the *BJPSW*. 'Have we not a responsibility to play a more active role than hitherto in shaping public opinion on the needs and care of the mentally ill?' asked the PSW Elizabeth Irvine in 1958:

> If we are seldom consulted or mentioned by those who broadcast on mental health . . . may this not be because we ourselves have a certain diffidence about public expression . . . which seriously impedes the communication of our special knowledge and experience on topics of public importance. Much as we welcome copy for this journal, we must bear in mind that what is published here reaches only a very small and specialised public.[151]

Conclusion

Discussing the proliferation of emergent medical and paramedical occupations in the field of medicine as a whole over the course of the twentieth century, Gerry Larkin observed that 'there are no entirely "separate" histories of medical and paramedical occupations; they are all interconnected'.[152] By examining the paths followed by nurses and PSWs as they sought to delineate their occupational activities and secure improved working conditions and professional status, this chapter has revealed how decisions adopted by one occupational group were affected by the policies adopted by either another occupational group within the field of mental health or a related branch of the same occupation active in other fields of health and welfare. As Larkin argued, changes within medical practice, such as the adoption of new therapeutic approaches, reshaped the division of medical labour as occupational groups acquired new roles, changing the relationship and boundaries between occupational groups.[153] The political and economic climate in which these decisions were taken further complicates this picture.

This chapter has illustrated how attempts to secure professional status were often made by attacking other professional groups and more or less prestigious branches of the same profession. It has revealed the difficulties experienced by insecure professional groups in accessing and speaking to the public, demonstrating that one must understand imbalances of power in the field of mental health in order to evaluate the efforts made by different occupational groups to destigmatise mental illness. As the following chapter will demonstrate, a desire to enhance prestige within the field could lead some healthcare professionals to focus on particular patient groups and neglect others, a course of action which had profound ramifications for the ways in which healthcare professionals depicted mental illness and sought to destigmatise mental illness.

The occupations of mental nursing and psychiatric social work evolved at different historical moments in different institutional sites and reflected ideas regarding the nature of mental illness and its treatment which held currency at that time. Thus attendants emerged to care for and manage patients within asylums in the eighteenth and nineteenth centuries. Bound up intimately with the asylum, attendants initially rejected professionalisation, adopting in its place a trade union model in an effort to tackle the pervasive poor working conditions which characterised the occupation in the early years of the twentieth century. In so doing, they sought to secure improved rates of pay and greater freedom for their members by emphasising the disciplinary regime of the asylum and the unpleasantness of their patients. This strategy did not endear attendants to the professionalising feminised body of general nurses, who stressed the vocational nature of their work and refused to recognise attendants as nurses unless they achieved qualifications set by the General Nursing Council. However, as new treatment approaches and legislation encouraged psychiatrists to realign psychiatry and the asylum with general medicine and the hospital, the Union seized the opportunity to reposition itself as a body which campaigned both for nurses' working conditions and for patient welfare and professional status – a position which served to undermine the Royal College of Nursing's claim to be the only body which campaigned for nurses' professional interests.

It was in this interwar era that psychiatric social work emerged. Its roots were more complex, on the one hand stemming from the work undertaken by charitable workers in the nineteenth century and on the other embracing psychological understandings of mental disturbance formulated in the United States. Part of the flourishing mental health movement of the interwar years, this nascent, female-dominated profession was diffusely spread across different sites, where its practitioners initially sought to readjust individuals so as to enable them to function more adequately in society. Vacillating between psychiatry and social work, PSWs sought to secure professional advancement via their Association, which stressed the importance of appropriate training. Yet its dual medical and social orientation posed difficulties for the APSW as it struggled to identify exactly what PSWs did and why they deserved professional status. Thus in a letter to the television critic Mary Crozier in 1961, Mrs Finch of the PRSC agonised that 'we are accused of being in an ivory tower, we are inarticulate, our professional language is incomprehensible to ordinary people who say they simply do not know what we do that common kindness and neighbourliness cannot do'.[154] Indeed, while the APSW sought to outline the unique professional identity of the PSW, the Association's historian and practising PSW Noel Timms cited one American study which found that PSWs 'value psychiatry more than their own profession and many wish they were psychiatrists rather than social workers'.[155] Intriguingly, a resolution brought by one branch of the Union in 1951 which sought to enable mental nurses to train and qualify as PSWs suggests that at least some mental nurses, in turn, coveted the role of a PSW,[156] while, at the top of the professional hierarchy, many psychiatrists resented their relative inferiority to other branches of medicine and some sought to reinvent themselves as physicians.[157]

While PSWs' peripheral position within the field of mental healthcare – between professions and between institutions, the patient and the community – led them to develop unique insights into the nature of mental disturbance and its treatment,[158] it also inhibited their ability to convey these ideas to other groups. And while the APSW rejected the trade union route adopted by mental nurses, it had to tread a fine line between emphasising the vocational nature of psychiatric social work on the one hand, and claims for higher wages on the other. Representing psychiatric social work as an occupation requiring vocation suggested to some that PSWs were akin to voluntary workers and thus did not require the remuneration a qualified professional might expect.

The shift in government policy which led to the eventual abandonment of psychiatric hospitals and the adoption of the policy of community care was greeted differently by the two occupations. For psychiatric nursing, which had developed within the hospital, such a development threatened to destroy the profession. Its response to this challenge is studied in more detail in Chapter 4. At this stage, it suffices to say that the subsequent route adopted by psychiatric nurses severely stretches Mick Carpenter's interpretation that the Union progressively adopted patient welfare as a key aspect of its agenda,[159] and suggests that the flourishing of interest displayed by the Union in the professionalisation of mental nursing and patient welfare in the 1930s, 1940s and 1950s might be contingent upon the political set of circumstances in which the Union found itself. In short, narratives which seek to depict a linear path adopted by any one group of healthcare workers are bound to be rather reductionist. It is however worth emphasising that psychiatric nurses had long languished at the bottom of the heap of mental healthcare workers and the nursing profession at large in terms of prestige and working conditions. Frequently excluded from the more innovative and prestigious developments within mental healthcare,[160] nurses were thus driven to more extreme measures to ensure their professional survival.

For PSWs, the shift towards community care initially appeared to herald new prospects, yet the persistent difficulties experienced by the occupation in defining its role, ruthlessly dissected by Barbara Wootton and echoed by other critics, undermined the confidence of the profession. In 1970, the APSW and its 1,550 members were absorbed into the British Association of Social Workers and the specialised university training that had previously distinguished PSWs from their fellow social work colleagues was assimilated into the new generic training for all social work. For psychiatric nursing, the increasing rapprochement with general nursing served to enhance its professional status, while undercutting the claims of the Union to be the sole body representing the interests of psychiatric nurses. Within social work, the merger was marketed as a result of rising professional standards and training throughout social work as a whole which obviated the need for distinct specialities. However, not all PSWs viewed the absorption of their speciality with such equanimity. The APSW, recalled Elizabeth Irvine, 'constituted a small professional elite of well-qualified social workers who were deeply committed to the maintenance of high professional standards'. Its loss, she insisted, was 'keenly felt' amongst many of its members.[161]

Notes

1 P. Nolan, *A History of Mental Health Nursing* (London, 1993), p. 1.

2 For example, the MACA, examined in Chapter 5, deployed lady volunteers to visit its cases in their homes or places of work to check on the progress of their recipients and resolve any difficulties with their employers. The Central Association for Mental Welfare also engaged in work with the mentally disordered within the community. See L. Westwood, 'Avoiding the Asylum: Pioneering Work in Mental Health Care, 1890–1939' (DPhil thesis, Sussex University, 1999).

3 On the growing popularity of psychological thought, see M. Thomson, *Psychological Subjects: Identity, Culture and Health in Twentieth-Century Britain* (Oxford, 2006), and N. Rose, *Governing the Soul: The Shaping of the Private Self* (London, 1989). The role of the mental hygiene movement in the emergence of psychiatric work is discussed in K. Woodroofe, *From Charity to Social Work in the United States and England* (London, 1962), pp. 124–39.

4 A discussion of Burt's significance can be found in D. Thom, 'Wishes, anxieties, play and gestures: child guidance in inter-war England', in R. Cooter (ed.), *In the Name of the Child: Health and Welfare, 1880–1940* (London, 1992), pp. 200–19. On the history of child guidance, see J. Stewart, *Child Guidance in Britain, 1918– 1955: The Dangerous Age of Childhood* (London, 2013).

5 A thorough examination of the numbers of PSWs entering different fields of work and their geographical location can be found in N. Timms, *Psychiatric Social Work in Britain, 1939–1962* (London, 1964), pp. 66–89. Not all qualified PSWs went in to these three fields of work, and Timms should be consulted for details of other employment fields.

6 A survey conducted by the National Asylum Workers' Union (hereafter NAWU) of thirty-one mental hospitals in 1912 revealed attendants' working weeks to be in excess of seventy hours, in some cases more than eighty or ninety. See M. Carpenter, 'Asylum nursing before 1914: a chapter in the history of labour', in C. Davies (ed.), *Rewriting Nursing History* (London, 1980), pp. 123–46.

7 The name of this body changed several times. For clarity, it will be referred to throughout in the main text as the Union, although the footnotes will give full details.

8 S. Ramon, *Psychiatry in Britain: Meaning and Policy* (London, 1985), p. 85. Judging from her footnotes, Ramon appears to have based her conclusions upon the *Nursing Mirror*, a publication for the nursing profession in general, as opposed to asylum attendants.

9 M. Carpenter, *Working for Health: The History of the Confederation of Health Service Employees* (London, 1988), p. 98.

10 *NAWU Magazine*, 1 (October, 1912).

11 *Report of the Tribunal Appointed to Inquire into Allegations Reflecting on the Official Conduct of Ministers of the Crown and Other Public Servants* (1949), Cmd. 7617, p. 81; G. Gibson, edited by W. Gibson, *Reminiscences* (Eastbourne, 2004), pp. 68–78.

12 *Health Services Journal*, 6 (1953), 4.

13 For a history of mental nurses' trade union activities, see Carpenter, *Working for Health*.

14 D. F. MacDonald, *The State and the Trade Unions* (London, 1976), p. 97 and p. 113.

15 Modern Records Centre, University of Warwick (hereafter MRC), APSW Archive, MSS.378/APSW/2/1/1, 'The APSW report for the year 1936 (with foreword on the years 1930–5)', p. 5.

16 Renamed the *Mental Hospital and Institutional Workers' Union Journal* in 1931 and the *Health Services Journal* in 1946 following the formation of the Confederation of Health Services Employees (hereafter in notes COHSE). In notes, the appropriate publication is indicated by the terms *NAWU Magazine*, *MHIWU Journal* and *Health Services Journal*.

17 APSW Archive, MSS.378/APSW/2/1/9, 'APSW Annual Report 1946–47', typescript, p. 7,

18 M. Ashdown, 'Introduction', *BJPSW*, 1:1 (1947), 3–7; 6.

19 *MHIWU Journal*, 23 (January, 1934), 14.

20 Ibid., 15.

21 M. Ashdown, 'Editorial', *BJPSW*, 1:3 (1949), 3–6; 3.

22 C. Nottingham, 'The rise of the insecure professionals', *International Review of Social History*, 52 (2007), 445–75.

23 Gibson, *Reminiscences*, pp. 10, 9.

24 See Nolan, *A History of Mental Health Nursing*, pp. 56–60.

25 Gibson, *Reminiscences*, p. 12

26 Ibid., pp. 7–8.

27 M. Osbaldeston, 'Nobody wants to know', in B. Robb, *Sans Everything: A Case to Answer* (London, 1967), pp. 13–18; p. 17.

28 Nolan, *A History of Mental Health Nursing*, pp. 90, 110–11.

29 See J. Stewart, 'Angels or aliens? Refugee nurses in Britain, 1938 to 1942', *Medical History*, 47 (2003), 149–72; 156.

30 See P. Nolan and B. Hopper, 'Revisiting mental health nursing in the 1960s', *Journal of Mental Health*, 9 (2000), 563–73; 565. One nurse interviewed for this article who was recruited from Jamaica described how both staff and patients had frequently directed racist remarks at him.

31 Carpenter, *Working for Health*, pp. 284, 317.

32 On tensions between British nurses and those recruited overseas, see ibid., pp. 284–5, and Nolan, *A History of Mental Health Nursing*, pp. 110–11. On tensions between men and women within the mental nursing profession, see V. Long, '"Surely a nice job for a girl?" Stories of nursing, gender, violence and

mental illness in British asylums, 1914–1930', in P. Dale and A. Borsay (eds), *Nursing the Mentally Disordered: Struggles that Shaped the Working Lives of Paid Carers in Institutional and Community Settings from 1800 to the 1980s* (forthcoming).

33 Nolan, *A History of Mental Health Nursing*, p. 61.

34 Ibid., p. 63.

35 Ibid., pp. 65–8.

36 See Carpenter, *Working for Health*, pp. 99–100.

37 Ibid., pp. 260–3.

38 J. Hallam, *Nursing the Image: Media, Culture and Professional Identity* (London, 2000), p. 100.

39 For more information on the development of psychiatric social work training in America see E. Lunbeck, *The Psychiatric Persuasion: Knowledge, Gender and Power in Modern America* (Princeton, 1994), pp. 35–45.

40 J. Stewart, 'Psychiatric social work in inter-war Britain: child guidance, American ideas, American philanthropy', *Michael Quarterly*, 3 (2006), 78–91.

41 See Timms, *Psychiatric Social Work in Britain*, pp. 28–36.

42 Ibid., pp. 31–2.

43 J. Stewart, 'The scientific claims of British child guidance', *British Journal for the History of Science*, 42 (2009), 407–32; 425.

44 APSW Archive, MSS.378/16/4/1, M. Ashdown, 'The role of the PSW: an address delivered before the medical section of the British Psychological Society on February 26th 1936', undated printed pamphlet, p. 7.

45 Ibid., p. 8. I have gendered the PSW as female in this passage as there were no men employed as PSWs at this time.

46 For a detailed overview of PSWs' activities within mental hospitals, see Timms, *Psychiatric Social Work*, pp. 110–19.

47 J. Stewart, '"I thought you would want to come and see his home", child guidance and psychiatric social work in inter-war Britain', in M. Jackson (ed.), *Health and the Modern Home* (Abingdon, 2007), pp. 111–27; p. 115.

48 For a detailed overview of PSWs' work in child guidance clinics, see Timms, *Psychiatric Social Work*, pp. 90–109. For an analysis of child guidance, see Stewart, *Child Guidance in Britain*.

49 Ramon, *Psychiatry in Britain*, pp. 206–19.

50 P. Armstrong, 'Aspects of psychiatric social work in a mental hospital', *BJPSW*, 1:1 (1947), 36–44, 6.

51 APSW Archive, MSS.378/APSW/16/4/7, 'Psychiatric social work in mental hospitals', APSW pamphlet printed around 1943, p. 3.

52 *Report of the Committee on Medical Auxiliaries*, Cmd. 8188 (London, 1951).

53 APSW Archive, MSS.378/APSW/2/1/17, 'The APSW Annual Report 1951–52', p. 5.

54 M. A. Lane and H. E. Howarth, 'Social workers', *British Medical Journal*, 4983, supplement 2685 (1956), 5–6, 6.

55 T. Smith, 'The role of the psychiatric nurse in the community', in APSW, *New Developments in Psychiatry and the Implications for the Social Worker* (London, 1969), pp. 40–6; p. 40.

56 APSW archive, MSS.378/APSW/2/1/21, 'The APSW Annual Report 1955', p. 16.

57 For an account of the role played by mental welfare officers in the provision of community care services, see S. Rolph, D. Atkinson and J. Warmsley, '"A pair of stout shoes and an umbrella": the role of the mental welfare officer in delivering community care in East Anglia: 1946–1970', *British Journal of Social Work*, 33 (2003), 339–59; 355.

58 APSW Archive, MSS.378/APSW/P/14/4/59, K. Bain, 'Duties of PSWs', *Health and Social Services Journal*, 10 March 1961.

59 'The APSW Annual Report for the Year 1936', p. 5.

60 APSW Archive, MSS.378/APSW/2/1/15, 'APSW Chairman's Report 1950–51', typescript, p. 3.

61 APSW Archive, MSS.378/APSW/14/4/14, K. Sansacre, 'The sympathetic ear', untitled newspaper, June 1959, pp. 164–5; p. 165.

62 APSW Archive, MSS.378/APSW/15/3/47, letter to Mrs Colwell from Mrs B. Cautrey, 'Re meeting with our public relations advisors on 4 Feb.', 5 February 1960.

63 APSW Archive, MSS.378/APSW/16/4/9, C. Hay-Shaw (on behalf of the APSW), 'Training for psychiatric social work', undated pamphlet, c. 1951, pp. 2, 6.

64 APSW Archive, MSS.378/APSW/14/3/108, M. Barnes, letter to *The Times* in response to the article 'Open door to mental health', published 30 March 1965.

65 This is discussed in further detail in Chapter 4.

66 On the formation of the COHSE, see Carpenter, *Working for Health*, pp. 238–42.

67 *Health Services Journal* (June, 1946), 7.

68 In the event, this was raised under the general council report rather than as a resolution. MRC, COHSE Archives, MSS.292/CO/1/1/3, COHSE National Executive Committee minutes, 1–3 June 1954.

69 Bartlett was elected President of the Trades Unions Congress in 1959, serving as President in 1960.

70 *Health Services Journal*, 12 (July–August, 1959), 10.

71 *Report of the Royal Commission on the Law Relating to Mental Illness and Mental Deficiency*, Cmnd. 169 (1957).

72 The Royal College of Nursing often portrayed itself as the organisation that represented the views and interests of psychiatric nurses. See 'Changes urged in mental nursing', *The Times* (22 April, 1960), p. 20, which stated that the report 'contains the views of a representative group of mental and mental deficiency nurses'.

73 *Health Services Journal*, 12 (July–August, 1959), 49.

74 E. Powell, speech given to the NAMH (1961), text from http://studymore.org.uk/xpowell.htm.

75 Smith, 'The role of the psychiatric nurse', p. 40.
76 A. Altschul, 'The role of the psychiatric nurse in the community', in *New Developments in Psychiatry*, pp. 37–9; p. 39. Altschul fled Austria at the outbreak of the Second World War. She subsequently trained as a nurse, a psychiatric nurse and a tutor in England, emphasising the importance of the therapeutic relationship between patient and nurse in her work. See P. Nolan, 'Annie Altschul's legacy to 20th century British mental health nursing', *Journal of Psychiatric and Mental Health Nursing*, 6 (1999), 267–72.
77 Nolan and Hopper, 'Revisiting mental health nursing', 565.
78 APSW Archive, MSS.378/APSW/14/4/12 '"Revolution" in mental care: Bill welcomed', *Daily Telegraph and Morning Star* (23 March 1959).
79 Ministry of Health, *Report of the Working Party on Social Workers in Local Authority Health and Welfare Services* (London, 1959), pp. 7, 8.
80 Ibid., pp. 227–8.
81 APSW Archive, MSS.378/APSW/P/14/4/32, I. A. G. MacQueen, 'Surfeit of social workers', *Medical Officer* (29 May 1959).
82 'Distrust of psychiatry: House of Lords', *Daily Telegraph and Morning Post* (18 February 1960), p. 23.
83 B. Wootton, *Social Science and Social Pathology* (1959; London, 1963). For a recent account of Barbara Wootton's life and career see A. Oakley, *A Critical Woman: Barbara Wootton, Social Science and Public Policy in the Twentieth Century* (London, 2011).
84 Wootton, *Social Science*, p. 270.
85 Ibid., p. 271.
86 Ibid., p. 273.
87 K. F. McDougall, 'Chairman's introduction' in E. M. Goldberg, E. E. Irvine, A. B. Lloyd Davies and K. F. McDougall (eds), *The Boundaries of Casework: A Report on a Residential Refresher Course Held by the Association of Psychiatric Social Work* (London, 1959), p. 8.
88 Wootton, *Social Science*, p. 273.
89 Stewart, 'Psychiatric social work in inter-war Britain'.
90 Wootton, *Social Science*, p. 292.
91 Ibid., p. 287.
92 Ibid., p. 279.
93 Ibid., p. 287.
94 M. Ashdown, 'Editorial', *BJPSW*, 1:2 (1948), 3–9, 8.
95 APSW Archive, MSS.378/APSW/14/1:21, APSW PRSC Minutes, 10 July 1959.
96 T. A. Ratcliffe, 'Relationship therapy and casework', *BJPSW*, 5:1 (1959), 4–9; 4.
97 A. Scull, 'Somatic treatments and the historiography of psychiatry', *History of Psychiatry*, 5 (1994), 1–12.
98 On psychiatric social treatment, see V. Long, '"Often there is a good deal to be done, but socially rather than medically": the psychiatric social worker as social therapist, 1945–1970', *Medical History*, 55 (2011), 223–39.

99 E. Raymond (ed.), *The Autobiography of David* (London, 1946), reviewed in *Health Services Journal* (June, 1946), 1. There was no volume number for the 1946 *Journal*.

100 *Health Services Journal* (August, 1946), 2.

101 *NAWU Magazine*, 17 (August, 1928), 4.

102 M. Carpenter, *Normality Is Hard Work: Trade Unions and the Politics of Community Care* (London, 1994), p. 3.

103 *Health Services Journal*, 1 (September, 1948), 19.

104 These developments are summarised in K. Jones, *Asylums and After. A Revised History of the Mental Health Services: From the Early 18th Century to the 1990s* (London, 1993), pp. 126–35.

105 *MHIWU Journal*, 24 (August, 1935), 17.

106 *Health Services Journal* (August, 1946), 12.

107 *Health Services Journal* (June, 1946), 7.

108 Woodroofe, *From Charity to Social Work*, p. 132.

109 APSW Archive, MSS.378/APSW/16/4/3, 'Psychiatric social work and the family by the APSW. Part II illustrative material: a study in preparation for the second international conference on Social Work', p. 7. Produced for a conference held in 1932.

110 G. Hamilton, *Theory and Practice of Social Case Work* (London, 1940), quoted in Armstrong, 'Aspects of psychiatric social work', 44.

111 B. Joseph, 'A PSW in a maternity and child welfare centre', *BJPSW*, 1:2 (1948), 30–45; 34.

112 M. Tickler, 'Indications for successful work with parents in a child guidance clinic', *BJPSW*, 1:1 (1947), 80–4; 82.

113 Nottingham, 'The rise of the insecure professionals'.

114 E. L. Thomas and K. M. Lewis, 'Papers on the role of the PSW given to the AGM of the psychiatric session of the BMA in 1950', *BJPSW*, 1:4 (1950), 18–24; 22.

115 APSW Archive, MSS.378/APSW/16/4/14, 'A career as a psychiatric social worker', folded information sheet, printed 1960 or 1961.

116 APSW Archive, MSS.378/APSW/2/1/29, 'The APSW Annual Report 1963', p. 7.

117 APSW Archive, MSS.378/APSW/14/4/120, 'Social work: who's out of step?', unnamed, undated paper. Judging from the phrasing of this article, it appears to be the one sent by PSW Jean Nursten to the editor of *New Society* reporting on the APSW conference 'Psychiatric Social Work: Developments in Training and Practice', held in Manchester 8–13 September 1963, MSS.378/APSW/14/3/106a. Nursten entitled her piece 'A question of adjustment'.

118 Nursten, 'A question of adjustment'. Underlining in original text.

119 Long, '"Often there is a good deal to be done"'.

120 Wootton, *Social Science*, p. 286.

121 Ibid., p. 292.

122 S. McGann, A. Crowther and R. Dougall, *A History of the Royal College of Nursing 1916–90: A Voice for Nurses* (Manchester, 2009), p. 37.

123 For an account of the formation of the College, see ibid., pp. 5–17.

124 See for example *NAWU Magazine*, 9 (January, 1920), 3.

125 *NAWU Magazine*, 17 (August, 1928), 20

126 *MHIWU Journal*, 20 (March, 1931), 3.

127 *NAWU Magazine*, 9 (June, 1920), 5.

128 Mr Harris, *NAWU Magazine*, 18 (August, 1929), 11.

129 Minutes of joint meeting between the MHIWU and the Hospital and Welfare Services Union, 22 June 1944. Cited in Carpenter, *Working for Health*, p. 239.

130 *Health Services Journal* (June, 1946), 7.

131 D. Gittins, *Madness in Its Place: Narratives of Severalls Hospital, 1913–1997* (London, 1998), pp. 21–4, and Nolan, *A History of Mental Health Nursing*, pp. 109–10.

132 *Health Services Journal* (June, 1946), 7.

133 COHSE Archive, MSS.292/CO/1/1/2, National Executive Committee minutes, 8–9 May 1950.

134 COHSE Archive, MSS.292/CO/1/1/3, National Executive Committee minutes, 17–18 September 1950.

135 The psychiatrist J. R. Lord made similar arguments in publications in the 1920s. These are discussed in S. Soanes, 'Reforming asylums, reforming public attitudes: J. R. Lord and Montagu Lomax's representations of mental hospitals and the community, 1921–1931', *Family and Community History*, 12 (2009), 117–29.

136 Ashdown, 'The role of the PSW', p. 19.

137 P. C. Shapiro, 'Some "after-care" patients in rural areas', *BJPSW*, 1:2 (1948), 51–70; 70.

138 E. Brown, 'The preparation of parents for treatment in a child guidance clinic', *BJPSW*, 1:2 (1948), 46–50; 46.

139 APSW Archive, MSS.378/APSW/14/1/3, meeting of the APSW PRSC, 7 February 1957, p. 2. The making of 'The Hurt Mind' is discussed in detail in Chapter 6.

140 APSW Archive, MSS.378/APSW/14/1/31, APSW PRSC minutes, 21 February 1961, p. 3.

141 APSW Archive, MSS.378/APSW/14/1/1, from the APSW PRSC terms of reference.

142 APSW Archive, MSS.378/APSW/14/1/24, APSW PRSC minutes, 23 October 1959, p. 3.

143 APSW Archive, MSS.378/APSW/14/1/12, APSW PRSC minutes, 16 May 1958, p. 2.

144 APSW Archive, MSS.378/APSW/14/1/4, APSW PRSC minutes, 14 March 1957, p. 2.

145 R. Morrison, 'Reflections on an exhibition', *BJPSW*, 3:1 (1955), 32–5; 32.

146 APSW Archive, MSS.378/APSW/14/1/15, APSW PRSC minutes, 25 July 1958, p. 1.

147 Timms, *Psychiatric Social Work*, p. 1.

148   Ibid., pp. 7–8. On PSWs' claims to be undertaking treatment, see Long, '"Often there is a good deal to be done"'.

149   APSW Archive, MSS.378/APSW/14/1/35, APSW PRSC minutes, 29 September 1961.

150   APSW Archive, MSS.378/APSW/14/3/84, letter from Mrs Finch to M. Crozier, 12 October 1961.

151   E. E. Irvine, 'Editorial', *BJPSW*, 4 (1958), 3.

152   G. Larkin, 'Health workers', in R. Cooter and J. Pickstone (eds), *Companion to Medicine in the Twentieth Century* (London, 2003), pp. 531–42; p. 533.

153   Ibid., p. 541.

154   Letter from Mrs Finch to M. Crozier.

155   A. Zander et al., *Role Relations in the Mental Health Professions* (Amsterdam, 1957), p. 41, cited in Timms, *Psychiatric Social Work*, p. 93.

156   COHSE Archive, MSS.229/CO/1/1/3, COHSE National Executive Committee minutes 4–6 December 1951.

157   Psychiatrists' insecurities receive consideration in Chapters 1 and 3; for examples of psychiatrists who depicted themselves as physicians, see discussion of William Sargant, Thomas Clouston and James Crichton-Browne.

158   For more details on the therapeutic approaches adopted by PSWs, see V. Long, 'Changing Public Representations of Mental Illness in Britain, 1870–1970' (PhD Thesis, University of Warwick, 2004), pp. 142–60.

159   Carpenter, *Normality Is Hard Work*.

160   Shulamit Ramon made this point specifically in relation to mental nursing in the 1920s, but her observation remains applicable throughout much of the twentieth century. See Ramon, *Psychiatry in Britain*, p. 86.

161   E. Irvine, cited in E. Younghusband, *Social Work in Britain: 1950–1970. A Follow-Up Study Vol. 2* (London, 1978), p. 164.

3

CHALLENGING THE STIGMA OF MENTAL ILLNESS THROUGH NEW THERAPEUTIC APPROACHES

Perceptions of the asylum changed dramatically between 1837, when the alienist W. A. F. Browne painted a compelling picture of the therapeutic powers of the ideal asylum, 'a spacious building resembling the palace of a peer, airy, and elevated, and elegant',[1] and 1961, when Enoch Powell, then Minister of Health, unveiled plans to close Britain's psychiatric hospitals.[2] Like many other mental health reformers, Powell conjured a history of psychiatry which legitimated his objectives, representing mental hospitals as cumbersome relics of a bygone era, irrevocably tarnished by their Victorian heritage. Embarking upon a new course of mental healthcare, he implied, could be accomplished only by literally dynamiting the current system – and the past – out of existence. 'There they stand', he told his audience, 'isolated, majestic, imperious, brooded over by the gigantic water-tower and chimney combined, rising unmistakable and daunting out of the countryside – the asylums which our forefathers built with such immense solidity to express the notions of their day'.[3]

Juxtaposing these two quotations may suggest that a radical rupture had taken place, but this would be misleading. When Brown wrote in 1837, many alienists viewed the asylum as a vehicle for establishing their professional credentials. As Andrew Scull, Charlotte MacKenzie and Nicholas Hervey asserted on the first page of *Masters of Bedlam*, a volume of biographies of some of the most significant figures within psychiatry in nineteenth-century Britain, the birth of the asylum was 'intimately bound up with the emergence and consolidation of a newly self-conscious group of people laying claim to expertise in the treatment of mental disorder'.[4] Yet, as the biographies within this volume repeatedly demonstrate, a number of leading psychiatrists rapidly became disenchanted with the asylum. W. A. F. Browne, for example, helped mobilise support for a nationwide network of asylums with his portrayal of the utopian asylum in his 1837 book *What Asylums Were, Are and Ought to Be*. When he authored his final report as Superintendent of the Crichton Royal Asylum some twenty years later, Browne was considerably less sanguine regarding the therapeutic powers of the asylum system he had helped entrench. Comparing the asylum to the hospital, Browne found it to be wanting and pointed the finger of blame at the patients or 'inmates', who inconveniently refused to recover. 'An asylum', he asserted, 'is only in one sense a hospital'. In a hospital, he observed, 'the patients enter, depart, die', whereas in an asylum, 'the inmates, or about one-half of them, remain for life'.[5]

A similar disillusionment with the asylum can be detected in the career of John Charles Bucknill, Superintendent of Devon County Asylum, first editor of the *JMS* and President of the Association of Medical Officers of Asylums and Hospitals for the Insane from 1860 to 1861. This veteran alienist boarded out some of his asylum patients in local cottages and at Exmouth, the local coastal town, in part as a pragmatic response to overcrowding within the asylum, but also because he increasingly came to believe that the view that 'a lunatic is a lunatic and an asylum is the best place for him' was a 'stereotyped prejudice'.[6] In 1862, Bucknill left his position as superintendent of the Devon County Asylum to take a lucrative role as a Lord Chancellor's Visitor in which he advocated the merits of treating lunatics in a domestic setting as opposed to consigning them to an asylum.[7] Henry Maudsley, son-in-law of the renowned alienist John Conolly, commenced his career as a promising star in the Medico-Psychological Association. Following his election as President of the Association in 1871, Maudsley blithely informed his colleagues that asylums rarely cured patients and could exacerbate insanity.[8] Rapidly rejecting a career within a county asylum, Maudsley devoted his energies to private practice, penning numerous articles which delineated the broader social import of psychiatric knowledge. The Maudsley Hospital, founded out of a bequest in Maudsley's will, sought to offer an alternative to the asylum by providing treatment to early cases of mental disorder, often on an out-patient basis.

Browne, Bucknill and Maudsley were by no means isolated figures. Throughout the late nineteenth and twentieth centuries, a number of mental healthcare workers sought to alleviate the stigma attached to mental illness and its treatment and, in so doing, raise the status of their profession. If the asylum no longer enhanced the prestige of psychiatry, then it would either have to be reinvented as a hospital or be jettisoned, and the delivery of mental healthcare relocated to general hospitals. Asylum patients posed similar problems for practitioners aspiring to greater status. If they could not be cured in the asylum as had initially been promised by reformers, then new therapeutic methods would have to be found which presented psychiatry in a more appealing light, or more promising patients who responded to therapeutic measures would have to be identified. Such endeavours however need to be situated within the field of mental healthcare, which impeded healthcare workers' agency.[9] Constrained by the political, economic and social context in which they operated, healthcare workers were both agents of change and reactors to change; their efforts necessitated the involvement, and at times obstruction, of other groups of healthcare workers. Whilst change could emanate from any sector of the field, the relative power and status of different occupational groups shaped their capacity to effect change.

Tracing innovations in mental healthcare policy and practice in Britain from the late nineteenth century through to the 1970s, this chapter reflects upon the intimate relationship between understandings of mental illness, therapeutic models and the professional aspirations of occupational groups working within the field of mental healthcare. In so doing, it seeks to build upon an observation made by Mathew Thomson in his work on mental deficiency: that efforts to advance mental health and destigmatise some forms of mental distress served to reinforce the stigma and reduce the resources available to more severe and chronic cases.[10] When Thomson wrote in 1998, the history of learning disability was subsumed and overlooked within the literature on madness and he thus rightly sought to emphasise 'the distinction between the mentally ill and the mentally disabled . . . in histories of mental health care'.[11] As this historiographical neglect has now at least partially been addressed, it is perhaps time to query this distinction; to examine whether responses to patients diagnosed with chronic mental illness and patients diagnosed with mental disability converged, and to ask why this occurred.

This chapter explores the extent to which the asylum operated as a site of reform in which new treatment approaches were adopted, or whether new measures functioned to undermine the prestige and viability of the asylum. Equally, it asks whether reforms aimed to help acute cases of mental disorder, or whether they addressed the needs of long-stay patients. It commences by analysing attempts to identify incipient cases of mental disorder and provide treatment in general hospitals and community settings, and asks how these developments impacted upon long-stay mental hospital patients and individuals diagnosed as mentally defective. Analysis then turns to the expansion of biomedical treatments in the postwar period and the government's decision to relocate mental healthcare from psychiatric hospitals to general hospitals and community services. Proponents of biomedical approaches claimed that mental illnesses had a somatic aetiology and hoped to bridge the gap between psychiatry and general medicine with new physical treatments designed to alleviate psychological symptoms by inducing physiological change. Psychiatrists and PSWs who worked primarily with individuals who experienced enduring mental health problems expressed different views, however.

Incipient mental distress and the mental hygiene movement

As the careers of Browne, Bucknill and Maudsley demonstrate, it did not take long before a number of doctors began to question whether asylums offered suitable treatment for all cases. As asylum populations expanded and the anticipated cure rates failed to materialise, some doctors suggested that incipient cases of mental illness would be ill-served by removal to an overcrowded asylum. Moreover, they reasoned, insanity was more easily cured if caught at its onset, and individuals would be more willing to seek treatment at an early stage if certification and the asylum could be avoided. In 1896, the British Medical Association unsuccessfully lobbied for a new clause in the lunacy legislation governing England and Wales which would allow up to six months' treatment, without the need for certification and admittance to an asylum.[12] In a joint deputation to the Lord Chancellor from the British Medical Association and the Medico-Psychological Association, Dr Blandford argued that friends and family would do all they could to avoid the stigma of certification and thus only brought patients to the asylum when the case had become chronic, and 'the chance of recovery was past'.[13]

Six years later, Sir John Sibbald, a retired Commissioner in Lunacy for Scotland, suggested establishing wards in general hospitals for acute cases of mental disorder. This, in his view, would enable medical treatment to be provided at a stage when mental disorder was most amenable to cure, preventing patients from falling into 'incurable insanity' and 'relegation to an asylum'.[14] Sibbald rationalised his suggestion on the grounds that treatment methods for mental disorder increasingly resembled those adopted for the treatment of bodily disorder, referring to the use of bed rest, hydrotherapy, and the nursing of male patients in asylums by female nurses.[15] In a follow-up discussion Dr Thomas Clouston enthusiastically endorsed Sibbald's proposal, echoing the view that asylums were ill-suited to the treatment of early stages of mental disorder because 'unfortunate and cruel prejudices and repulsions' attached to the asylum deterred people from seeking treatment: a statement which attributed the stigma of mental illness to public ignorance.[16] Treating mental disorder in general hospitals, Clouston believed, would help educate the public that mental disease was like any other disease and was not shameful. To allow mental disturbance to exacerbate until an individual was certifiable, Clouston argued, 'seems a cruel neglect ... for the man so afflicted ... becomes incurable'.[17] This argument did not convince some audience members, who queried the wider ramifications of Sibbald's proposal. As Dr Yellowlees observed, 'this scheme almost seems to suggest that an asylum is a place by all means to be avoided'. 'Have we not been spending our lives in showing that asylums are merely hospitals for the insane?' he asked his colleagues.[18]

At this point let us turn to examine another protagonist in this debate: Thomas Clouston, the Physician Superintendent of the Royal Edinburgh Asylum figuratively locked up by his patients in Chapter 1. Clouston sought to enhance his professional standing through the campaign for mental hygiene. His 1906 work *The Hygiene of the Mind*[19] outlined how diet, education and lifestyle could prevent the development of mental disorder: the word asylum appears only on the title page in the book in reference to Clouston's various roles. The mental hygiene movement constituted an attempt to extend the field of psychiatric practice 'beyond the treatment of severe forms of mental illness in mental hospitals'.[20] Its proponents fostered the idea that mental health and illness formed a continuum and that more effort should be made to tackle incipient cases of mental distress in community settings. Emerging in the context of a growing interest in health promotion and preventive medicine, the movement began in the United States following the publication of Clifford Beer's widely read account of his experiences as an asylum patient in *A Mind that Found Itself*.[21] Within Britain, the mental hygiene movement influenced the establishment of new forms of non-institutional care pioneered in the first half of the twentieth century, particularly for acute or 'borderline' cases.[22] Equally, the nascent profession of psychiatric social work, examined in the previous chapter, was a product of and advocate for the mental hygiene movement.

It might be tempting to argue that mental health reformers in the early twentieth century bypassed the asylum to reach new groups. However, remodelling the asylum formed an integral part of reforming mental healthcare for some psychiatrists. For example, George M. Robertson, Clouston's successor at the Royal Edinburgh Asylum, sought to hospitalise the asylum by refashioning its purpose, structure and operations upon the template of the general hospital and replacing male attendants with female nurses.[23] Introducing a discussion on the diagnosis and treatment of borderline cases at an annual meeting of the British Medical Association in 1921, Robertson used the opportunity to plead for 'the emancipation of the mental hospital'. He urged a liberalisation of the legislation governing admissions, not to extend treatment outside mental hospitals but to allow patients to seek treatment at an early stage in 'our modern mental hospitals', before reaching a stage at which they were certifiable.[24]

Indeed, as Stephen Soanes has recently argued, the asylum could also be redeveloped so that its functions extended to encompass the provision of care for incipient and convalescent cases of mental disorder.[25] This approach was adopted by John R. Lord, a leading figure in the mental hygiene movement, who served as a member of the General Nursing Council, the Child Guidance Council and a founder member of the International Committee for Mental Hygiene. Lord was also a prominent member of the British psychiatric profession, elected President of the Royal Medico-Psychological Association in 1927 and serving as editor in chief for the *JMS* from 1911 until his death in 1931. In his publications Lord sought to elicit greater public support for mental hospitals, viewing hospitals as sites in which community psychiatric services could be based. Yet, as Soanes acknowledges, Lord's publications obscured the fates of long-stay patients, instead painting an 'idealised picture . . . based on a minority of recoverable patients'.[26]

Opening a nurses' home in 1928, the newly appointed Chairman of the Board of Control Sir Laurence Brock stated his belief that public attitudes had begun to change. Conjuring a version of the past which suited his purposes, Brock argued that present-day methods and curative treatment contrasted starkly with 'the cruelty and violence practised in asylums in the Victorian era', insisting that the innovations in treatment which had already been made were only an instalment of much greater advances which would be seen in the next few decades.[27] Brock's optimism characterised the aspirations of interwar mental health reformers, whose confidence was fuelled by the passing of the 1930 Mental Treatment Act. This legislation extended admittance procedures to allow for voluntary and out-patient hospital treatment and renamed asylums as mental hospitals, which many healthcare workers hoped would help counter public prejudice. In response, a number of hospitals constructed new admissions blocks to encourage people to seek hospital treatment of their own volition.

Studying healthcare workers' reports regarding these new facilities allows us to see how these developments, while potentially alleviating the stigma attached to incipient and borderline mental disorder, entrenched the stigma attached to long-stay patients. In 1930, for example, the mental nurses' Union (an organisation studied in the previous chapter) reported that Durham Mental Hospital was considering building an admission hospital where cases of a 'recovering type' could be received. They could then be discharged 'without coming into contact with permanent patients'.[28] A report from Derby Mental Hospital in the same year expressed the hope that many recoverable cases would go straight from the admission unit to convalescent villas without entering the main hospital at all, suggesting a similar fear of 'contagious' chronic patients.[29] These divisions between chronic and acute patients paral-

lel the increasingly distinct provision made for mentally defective patients in
'colonies' in the interwar years. Ruminating on practices of racial segregation
within British colonies, and the use of colonies as a solution for crime and
unemployment, Mark Jackson observed that the 'multiple connotations' of the
term colony 'neatly captured and reinforced the discriminatory politics of segregation'.[30] Advocates of the colony solution conjured an image of a homely,
village-like atmosphere. However, such ideals fell victim to economic considerations as local authorities were urged to spend less per capita on barracks-
like accommodation for mentally defective patients than on mental hospitals
or working-class housing, demonstrating in concrete terms the perceived
inferiority of mental defectives. As Mathew Thomson has argued, removing
mentally defective patients promised to improve the status of psychiatry by
alleviating 'the twin problems of overcrowding and low cure rates'.[31] Indeed,
desirous of enhancing the image of mental hospitals as curative, therapeutic
institutions following the passing of the 1930 Mental Treatment Act, the
Board of Control considered removing patients deemed to be suffering from
chronic and incurable mental illness to mental deficiency institutions.[32] These
proposals were never enacted, but they suggest that the distinctions drawn
between mental illness and mental deficiency could prove more permeable
than the boundaries between chronic and acute mental illness, for interwar
advocates of mental health reform tended to envisage a two-tier system of care
which privileged acute and minor cases of mental disturbance. Supporting
the Mental Treatment Bill in the House of Commons, the Minister of Health
Arthur Greenwood discussed the plight of 'the man broken down by overwork
or the woman suffering from puerperal mania', who 'ought to receive treatment different from that of the certified lunatic'.[33]

As Thomson argued, removing difficult cases in the interwar years could
enable the mental hospital to 'align itself with the curative model of general
medicine, whereas the defective colony assumed the role of institutional
"dumping ground"'.[34] This observation is equally illuminating if we wish to
consider why many healthcare workers sought to construct a dichotomous
relationship between chronic and acute cases of mental illness at different
points over the course of the nineteenth and twentieth centuries. While historians of the nineteenth-century asylum have drawn our attention to the ways in
which distinctions of class, gender, race, prognosis and diagnosis were embodied within asylum architecture,[35] further study of interwar mental health
reform, and of the building spree which created separate facilities for acute,
chronic and mentally defective patients – as if trying to disguise the very existence of long-stay patients – may well provide more insight into how distinctions between those perceived 'curable' and 'chronic' were enacted, dispelling

the notion that mental hospitals were monolithic entities which homogenised the fates of their inmates.

Reinforcing stigma: mental defectives

Examination of debates within the mental nurses' Union regarding the management of individuals diagnosed as mental defectives reveals that efforts to destigmatise mental illness were partial at best and illustrates how the line between mental deficiency and chronic mental illness could become blurred. In Thomson's authoritative analysis of policy relating to mental deficiency in this era, this Union played a pivotal role in halting the legalisation of sterilisation by bringing a resolution before the 1934 Trades Union Congress opposing such a move. The Union's General Secretary George Gibson was, Thomson argued, 'a lone voice in the trades union movement', whose actions 'made it clear that powerful groups within civil society would make sure that the Labour Party resisted any attempt to introduce sterilization'.[36] Gibson did indeed bring forward such a resolution, yet analysis of debates within the Union's journal leading up to this paints a rather murkier picture.

For those healthcare workers who sought to raise the status of psychiatry by depicting it as just another branch of medicine, mental deficiency posed problems. Education and training had evolved as the main forms of treatment for such patients and it proved difficult if not impossible to reconceptualise mental deficiency as an illness amenable to biomedical interventions in a hospital setting. Thus, while Laurence Brock had reflected on the potential of new treatment methods to transform perceptions of the mental health services when opening a nurses' home in 1928, his observations took on a more pensive character when he opened an extension to the Aston Hall Certified Institution for Mental Defectives in 1935. On this occasion, Brock discussed the 'grave problems' entailed by 'the aggregation of the socially inefficient, estimated at 300,000'.[37] As Brock was in contact with members of the Eugenics Society and was personally sympathetic to sterilisation, these sentiments were entirely in character.[38] Indeed, Brock had chaired the Departmental Committee on Sterilisation, which recommended legalising voluntary sterilisation for persons suffering from mental deficiency, mental disorder and transmissible physical disability.[39] Reporting Brock's speech, the *Mental Hospital and Institutional Workers' Union Journal* chose to accompany the story with an illustration from its regular cartoonist, 'Barlow'.

This full-page image depicted Brock's views with a figure whose featureless 'shadow', emblazoned with the number of mental defectives cited by Brock, fell menacingly over the country, emphasising the scale of the problem.

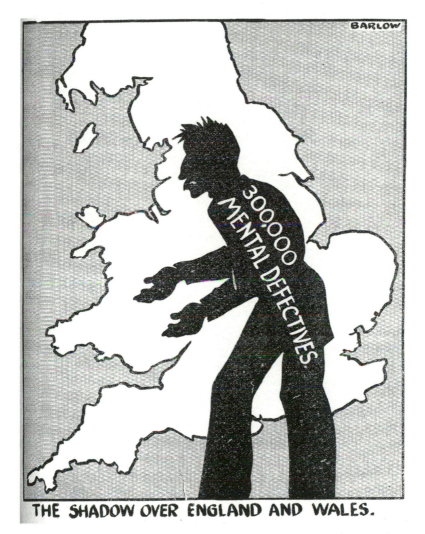

THE SHADOW OVER ENGLAND AND WALES.

2 Barlow, 'The Shadow over England and Wales', *MHIWU Journal*, 24 (July, 1935), 9.

Equating mental deficiency with physical deformity, the cartoon mirrored beliefs that mental defectives constituted a distinct and pathological race, arising from an atavistic reversion to a more primitive stage of human development. Difference was therefore embodied within and inscribed upon the defective, facilitating 'medical claims to diagnostic and managerial expertise'.[40] Conflating deficiency with criminality, pauperism and working-class immorality, proponents of these beliefs argued that mental deficiency lay at the root of many social ills, and viewed sterilisation as a biological solution.[41] By depicting the figure with palms outstretched this cartoon illustrates these concerns, recalling the view that mental defectives were socially inefficient and an economic drain on the normal population. Barlow's decision to represent the defective as featureless suggested that the attributes of mental deficiency overpowered the individuality of those diagnosed, while echoing concerns that mental defectives were difficult to identify, ascertain and segregate. By gendering the figure as male and not female, Barlow played to concerns that male defectives posed a danger to women and children, evoking earlier discussions amongst mental nurses in the Union regarding the danger posed by male asylum patients.

As the previous chapter demonstrated, the mental nurses' Union began to display an interest in patient welfare in the interwar years. Bolstered by the 1930 Mental Treatment Act which promised to usher in a new era of curative mental healthcare, the Union expressed concerns that negative media coverage could have a detrimental impact on public perceptions of mental illness and its treatment. However, this optimism did not encompass the field of mental deficiency. Within psychiatry, mental deficiency was a low-status field and those who specialised in the work rarely achieved much in terms of professional recognition or influence.[42] These difficulties translated into the field of mental nursing: in contrast to their counterparts in mental hospitals, fewer staff working in mental deficiency institutions held qualifications, pay rates were lower, the Union exerted less influence and working conditions were inferior.[43]

Between 1929, when an interdepartmental report on mental deficiency claimed that the mentally defective population was much larger than previously imagined,[44] and 1934, when another interdepartmental committee advocated the legalisation of voluntary sterilisation,[45] the Union's journal played host to pessimistic reports in which boards of guardians, county councils and the Board of Control ruminated glumly on the seemingly irresolvable social and medical problems posed by mentally defective people. While these reports were incorporated into the journal without editorial endorsement for the sentiments they expressed, their inclusion points to a sustained interest in the topic, and perhaps tacit approval for the opinions expressed. Drawing upon the pervasive correlation of mental deficiency with a parasitic residuum, organisations and individuals urging sterilisation depicted mental defectives as a distinct and rapidly expanding species which posed a menacing threat to society. Thus, West Riding County Council passed a resolution urging the government to sterilise mental defectives to 'stop the propagation of a species which, if continued, would in time be an enormous burden to the ratepayers';[46] the economic allure of sterilisation, which promised to reduce the number of people requiring costly institutional care, ensured that support for sterilisation amongst county councils transcended party political lines.[47] Meanwhile, Judge Henry McCardie, prone to delivering iconoclastic pronouncements on a range of social issues,[48] expressed his belief that 'unless steps were taken, either by greater measures of segregation or by sterilisation, the hideous process of multiplying the mentally unfit would go unchecked, and an army of mental defectives, which now numbers 400,000 would increase daily and almost hourly'.[49]

Thomson has argued that the Board of Control prioritised policy for mental illness at the expense of mental deficiency policy, generating an 'unnecessarily sharp division' between the two systems of care in which the 'incarceral' nature of mental deficiency institutions appeared even more anomalous than before.[50] While the Board acknowledged that sterilisation would not obviate the need for institutional provision, its members held a pessimistic view of the intrinsic nature of the mental defective. 'Many', the Board argued in its 1929 annual report, 'cannot resist criminal impulses'. 'Some have so little self-control that they are apt to . . . attack others and to commit crimes of violence . . . Many are sexually unrestrained or perverted, and are a constant danger to women and children.'[51] Portraying the condition as one characterised by a lack of social conformity and loss of self-control, rather than an illness, the Board's solution was to ascertain and institutionalise as many detectives as could be detected in the community, while accepting that cure was unlikely.[52]

When nurses began to write in to the journal in response to the coverage devoted to mental deficiency, debate focused on the merits of sterilisation. Ultimately the Union rejected sterilisation, yet the resolution of the debate can hardly be termed a resounding humanitarian triumph. The first nurse to comment on the sterilisation debate in the journal, Mr H. Noble, had previously contributed articles recommending improvements in hospital buildings so as to benefit patients. His interest appears to have been piqued by a letter sent from Dr Neil Montgomery of Storthes Hall Mental Hospital,[53] which argued against sterilisation on the grounds that mental defectives made an important contribution to the economy.[54] In response, Mr Noble claimed that the only output produced by the mentally deficient was 'trouble', and that 'when they have reproduced themselves ad infinitum they will be in the majority', a perspective which echoed the sentiments expressed in many of the reports which the Union's journal had chosen to reprint.[55] Some opponents of sterilisation, such as the Labour MP Dr Hyacinth Morgan, viewed it as a punitive measure which would be applied only to the working classes.[56] Dr Montgomery tapped into such anxieties when he countered Noble's views by alluding to the shared class backgrounds of nurses and their patients, stressing their interdependency. Noting that mental defectives produced 'a living, and a more or less congenial occupation for such people as Mr Noble (I presume) and myself', Montgomery argued that sterilisation 'is sure to be tried out first on the poor, who are less capable of resisting than the rest of us, especially if they happen to be pauper imbeciles'.[57]

If this was an attempt to sway Noble by echoing the narrative of class power frequently deployed by the Union's journal, it was unsuccessful. Noble grounded his argument on the basis of his personal experience, and his next letter suggested disillusionment with asylum work. 'I base my opinion solely on my observations during my service with mental cases', he wrote, a phrase which conflated mental illness and mental deficiency. Noble claimed that hereditary factors caused the difficulties experienced by many of his patients, and that a number of those discharged as cured later returned to the institution, 'very often after begetting another generation of mentally deficient'.[58]

Alec Flanaghan, a vocal member of the Union who frequently proposed resolutions at annual conferences, expressed misgivings that advocates of sterilisation had hijacked the Union journal as a vehicle for their views without protest. Flanaghan served as a member of the National Executive Committee for the Confederation of Health Service Employees from its formation in 1946 until his retirement in 1955.[59] He noted disapprovingly that hitherto mental nurses had been excluded from the debate, and implied that this state of affairs should cease. 'Articles under the heading "sterilisation" have appeared from time to time without causing the controversy one would expect', he commented. 'While we of the mental nursing profession look on, others are propagating their theories . . . Forces are massing beneath a banner whose motto is apparently "sterilisation first; realisation afterwards".' Criticising the scientific and ethical grounds for sterilisation, Flanaghan reiterated Montgomery's class concerns, asking whether 'this is not something like class legislation under a new name'.[60]

Flanaghan's letter triggered twenty responses from nine different nurses, four in favour of sterilisation and five opposed. H. C. Tusker reiterated the belief that mental deficiency was a biological condition which generated all manner of social problems; such patients, he insisted, were 'sexual perverts, and time after time they give birth to mentally defective children'. Querying why the state should be obliged to support such children, Tusker concluded that compulsory sterilisation was justified in such circumstances. He situated the problem of mental deficiency within the body of the individual, suggesting that the interests of the state ran counter to those of the mentally defective.[61] Conversely, E. Carnell echoed concerns that sterilisation could serve as a tool of class oppression which might be applied by the authorities to the unemployed.[62] Downplaying the role of biology, Carnell conflated mental deficiency with other forms of mental disorder which he argued emanated from social relations, rather than individualised failings. 'Mental disease', he insisted, 'is a product of a social condition, and can therefore only be explained by that condition. Insanity, like crime and prostitution, should be treated, not as an individual disease, but as a social relation.'[63]

At least one nurse stepped beyond the issue of sterilisation to contemplate killing those in their care. Writing in the column 'Things We Would Like to Know', the correspondent asked 'who will have the courage to recommend the lethal chamber for those suffering from hopeless insanity accompanied with physical disease?'[64] Intriguingly, this proposition referred to chronic mental illness, demonstrating that the line between chronic mental illness and mental deficiency blurred easily in the Union's journal. Despite the call for the 'courageous' to come forward, the writer masked his or her identity under the pseudonym 'Iconoclast', and phrased the issue as a question, rather than proclaim himself or herself in favour. No responses to this query appeared, although the journal printed a similar argument in 1934 when it reported a speech made by Professor J. A. Berry, the director of medical services at Stoke Park Colony in Bristol.[65] Under the guise of humanitarianism, Berry argued that some of those in his care should be killed:

> It was difficult for anyone who saw these human mental monstrosities almost every day to understand why society took such extraordinary pains to keep them alive. 'With complete absence of all human qualities or intelligence', he said, 'they have to be clothed, fed, housed and waited on hand and foot at the nation's expense, and one wonders why. Surely a kindly euthanasia is the only really kindly treatment for this pathetic side of mental deficiency.'[66]

The editor of the Union's journal conveyed his scathing disapproval of Berry's logic by titling the article '"Kindliness" of Euthanasia'.

The intervention of the Union's General Secretary George Gibson on the issue of sterilisation effectively closed the debate and provided an official policy statement from the Union. Ostensibly opposing sterilisation, Gibson nevertheless tacitly endorsed these perspectives, a paradox encapsulated by the title of his article: 'Sterilise the Unfit – When You Can Identify Them!' If it could be proved that a category of patients could be sterilised with no ill effects, Gibson would declare himself in favour. Indeed, like the proponents of sterilisation, Gibson in practice distinguished between the interests of society and the interests of the mentally defective, which he perceived to be in conflict. 'The test obviously must be the measure or degree of social benefit secured by sterilisation of a particular person or class of persons', he wrote. 'Segregation or detention during the reproductive period may be a better way in many cases . . . admittedly, society has a right to protect itself'.[67]

The debate regarding sterilisation was one of the few occasions where mental deficiency was discussed within the Union's journal, reflecting the low status of mental deficiency nursing in relation to mental nursing, as well as the comparatively low levels of unionisation amongst mental deficiency nurses. On one level, sterilisation could be viewed as a means of accomplishing the principles of mental hygiene by preventing future mental illness. Indeed, C. P. Blacker, a member of the Eugenics Society, portrayed sterilisation as a progressive medical right, comparing voluntary sterilisation to the introduction of voluntary treatment under the Mental Treatment Act.[68] Yet such a rights-based discourse was strikingly absent from the pages of the Union's journal, where proponents of sterilisation constructed a 'them' and 'us' dichotomy, depicting the mentally defective as a wholly alien species which jeopardised the well-being of society. Parallels can be drawn between these depictions of mentally defective patients as violent and sexually depraved, and the ways in which mental nurses represented male patients in the early years of the twentieth century, which are discussed in Chapter 4. Moreover, nurses advocating sterilisation did not confine their discussion to cases of mental deficiency.

Aware that to some extent they shared in their patients' stigma, nurses appear to have been torn between their desire to separate themselves from their patients and their desire to protect patients' interests – and by extension their own.[69] Thus while some nurses aligned their interests with society and against their patients, others articulated a duty of care to their patients, or alluded to a shared experience, grounded in class. The ramifications of the Union's debate and the eventual adoption of an official position against sterilisation may have had a significant impact on government policy. Yet while one might view these concerns with the welfare of mentally defective patients as indicative of a shift in Union policy towards the interests of the patients, an examination of the debate illustrates the equivocal nature of Gibson's opposition to sterilisation.

Medicalising treatment

Healthcare professionals' inability to develop biomedical treatments for patients diagnosed with mental deficiency marked the field as one lacking prestige, for many psychiatrists in the early to mid-twentieth century believed that situating mental healthcare within mainstream medical practice offered the best means of destigmatising mental illness and its treatment. The roots of these efforts stemmed back to the nineteenth century, when a number of psychiatrists sought to identify biological causes of mental illness, although this research tended to consolidate ideas regarding degeneration and incurability rather than inform new treatment approaches.[70] In the early twentieth century, the American psychiatrist Henry Cotton sought to revolutionise psychiatric treatment with his theory that chronic sepsis within the body caused mental illness, an idea which attractively linked psychiatry to the development of antiseptic surgery. Cotton focused on removing possible sites of infection from patients' bodies, ranging from the extraction of teeth and tonsils to the surgical removal of parts of the intestines, abdomen, cervix or colon.[71] Despite the high death rate of his surgical interventions, Cotton's theories exerted a strong appeal for psychiatrists in America and Britain who were keen to align their profession with general medicine.

The development of new physical treatments in the 1930s and 1940s, Joan Busfield argued, 'brought psychiatry closer to other areas of medicine and helped to increase its legitimacy as a field of medical practice'.[72] These treatment methods, which included insulin treatment, convulsion, malarial therapy, prefrontal leucotomy, sedatives and stimulants, were designed to alleviate psychological symptoms by inducing physiological change or by altering the structure of the brain. Proponents of physical therapies, such as William Sargant, claimed that mental illnesses had a somatic aetiology and wanted to bridge the gap between psychiatry and general medicine. In *An Introduction to Physical Methods of Treatment*, co-authored with fellow psychiatrist Eliot Slater, Sargant claimed that new treatment methods had transformed mental hospitals beyond recognition within a decade.[73] Physical treatments, asserted Sargant and Slater, 'produce their beneficial effects with greater speed and greater certainty than the older and more well-established psychotherapeutic methods'.[74] Psychiatrists could now interpret the emotional distress and social problems experienced by patients as a product of underlying biological malfunction rather than a cause of their disorder.

In the late 1940s and 1950s, two factors converged to create an atmosphere amenable to the dissemination of physical therapies within psychiatric practice. Although the Board of Control continued to regulate mental health services until the passing of the 1959 Mental Health Act, the nominal incorporation of psychiatric hospitals within the new NHS in 1948 presented an opportunity for psychiatrists to realign their professional activities with general medicine.[75] This was also an era of rising patient numbers, leading to overcrowding. As the resident population in mental hospitals peaked at 151,400 in 1954,[76] many psychiatrists may well have been inclined to agree with Slater and Sargant regarding 'the incapacity of highly individual and time-consuming methods to deal with a large-scale problem', viewing physical treatments as more efficacious in terms of 'speed, convenience and certainty'.[77] As will be examined in Chapter 6, Sargant served as the chief medical consultant for the BBC's first television series on mental illness in 1956, in which physical therapies played a pivotal role in trying to frame a positive representation of mental illness – and its treatment – to the public. Other major psychiatric textbooks such as *Clinical Psychiatry*, co-authored by William-Mayer-Gross, Eliot Slater and Martin Roth in 1954, also emphasised the organic aetiology of mental illness and the value of physical therapies, largely dismissing the influence of social and psychological factors in mental distress.[78]

Some mental healthcare practitioners viewed these treatments as a welcome means of reinvigorating the status of mental hospital personnel. As we saw in Chapter 1, some psychiatrists took this opportunity to write books for the public which attempted to demystify – and enhance the prestige – of their profession. The mental nurses' Union, meanwhile, hoped that the new therapies employed in mental hospitals would enhance the professional image of the mental nurse by allowing closer approximation to the role of the general nurse. Its journal carried reports on the experimental use of leucotomies and electroconvulsive therapy, and cited the government's Athlone Report on nursing, which insisted 'medical staff now require highly skilled mental nurses to assist . . . there is every justification for the recognition of mental nursing as a highly skilled branch of the profession and entitled to a worthy status'.[79]

Sargant's 1967 autobiography, *The Unquiet Mind: The Autobiography of a Physician in Psychological Medicine*, vividly recounts the attractions of the new physical therapies for the author.[80] Sargant consciously titled himself a physician rather than a psychiatrist to emphasise his view that mental illness was essentially the same as any other illness and should be treated according to the same principles that governed medical interventions in general hospitals. He presented himself as a risk-taker who bravely battled the oppressive medical establishment – military metaphors abound in the text – in a heroic bid to alleviate the sufferings of his patients. In such an adventure, casualties were unavoidable. 'Some doctors prefer to take few such risks at all', he acknowledged, 'but this means patients can remain hopelessly incarcerated for life in a mental hospital with sufferings that are too terrible to contemplate'.[81] Early in his account, Sargant recalled attending a party at which he had consumed a mix of gin and champagne, before returning to the hospital at dawn and undertaking a surgical procedure. 'I had learned my lesson', he recalled. 'Never on any account to get so drunk as to risk a patient's life'.[82] This anecdote, doubtless incorporated to amuse his readership, encapsulates how Sargant's reckless experimentalism tended to override concerns for patients' safety. He ridiculed psychological explanations for mental distress, extrapolating from a couple of examples to surmise that all psychological symptoms had a physical origin. Thus, he gleefully recounted how Dr Stoddart, his predecessor at St Thomas's Hospital, used to tell students that they feared Zeppelins and bombs because both weapons were phallic symbols which awakened homosexual impulses.[83]

In his autobiography, Sargant used the spectre of the gothic Victorian asylum, archaic medical practices and the deteriorated chronic psychotic to justify invasive medical interventions. Describing the time he had spent as a locum at Hanwell, Sargant implied that little had changed since the building had been opened. He described the 'hundred-year-old Hanwell Lunatic Asylum' as 'a gloomy building surrounded by a massive brick wall', 'a typical Victorian locked-up mental hospital',[84] 'a dead end, full of terrible suffering for which I could do nothing'.[85] Here, according to Sargant, nurses sought to lighten their load by heavily dosing difficult patients with bromides or paraldehyde. Lacking any effective means of treating mental disorder and theoretically responsible for around five hundred patients each, the doctors attended to minor physical ailments and recertified patients between leisurely meals and games of tennis, in which junior doctors were expected to cede victory to senior colleagues (a detail which demonstrated how hierarchy pervaded every aspect of mental hospital life). 'I suppose we had advanced somewhat since the eighteenth century when the habit of whipping prisoners, sometimes to drive the devil out of them, still continued', Sargant grudgingly conceded.[86] While at Hanwell, Sargant became convinced that insanity was 'a series of physically treatable disorders, offering a great number of treatment approaches'.[87] At St Thomas's Hospital, Sargant was disappointed to find that the only teaching medical students received in mental illness was the observation of patients in mental hospitals in 'advanced . . . stages of madness'; Sargant's use of the term 'madness', which he would have viewed as archaic, served to underscore his contrast between neurotic or depressed patients and 'these exhibits'.[88]

Following the inauguration of the NHS, Sargant described how he seized the opportunity to integrate the treatment of mental illness into general medical practice, a development facilitated by the new physical therapies. 'Mental illness and its treatment', he claimed 'had become at last a true part of general medical treatment'.[89] Promptly setting up a ward for in-patients and an out-patient unit, through which drugs, electric shock and modified insulin treatments were administered, Sargant insisted that patients should receive the same treatment as those on ordinary medical or surgical wards. Initially, he experienced difficulties with acute schizophrenic patients, whom female nurses with a general hospital training struggled to manage. Refusing to employ male nurses because this 'would have given our wards a different look from the rest', he sent such cases to mental hospitals. With the introduction of the tranquilliser chlorpromazine, Sargant explained how 'even the acutest schizophrenic' could be kept tranquillised 'while electric shock treatment and other methods speeded their recovery'.[90] Mental nurses, who had embraced the adoption of new physical treatments as a means of reinvigorating mental hospitals and cementing the prestige of their profession, viewed such practices with concern. In 1948, one member of the mental nurses' Union tabled a motion for the Trades Union Congress agenda which sought to establish the principle that only nurses qualified in mental nursing should staff wards in general hospitals allocated to patients with a mental illness.[91] Like his predecessors who had advocated treating incipient mental disorder outside of the asylum, Sargant stressed the importance of treating mental distress as early as possible if a cure was to be achieved. In the 'bad old days' before the introduction of physical treatments, he explained, repeated attacks of illness left patients 'scarred' and eventually in a chronic condition.[92]

This raises the question as to what Sargant envisaged should become of chronic patients. As the therapeutic measures advocated by Sargant have been credited with transforming psychiatric practice and facilitating the discharge of hitherto long-stay patients, one might expect to find Sargant championing the use of these measures in connection with long-stay patients. Yet his autobiography focuses almost exclusively on the applicability of these treatments to acute cases and how they might enable such patients to be treated outside the mental hospital. A rare example to the contrary surfaced when Sargant recollected a trip to Alabama, where he visited an institution for black veterans. On his visit to the back wards, where he found 'negroes strapped down in chairs, like poor King George III', Sargant alighted upon a plan: why not give some of these 'pitifully agitated patients . . . the benefit of modified leucotomy operations', a measure, Sargant noted, which was 'simpler and cheaper' than that which preceded it.[93] Sargant believed that his 'negro-rescue plan' also offered 'a wonderful chance . . . [to] do a controlled experiment' by comparing the results of fifty operative cases with fifty control cases, and he persuaded Walter Freeman to offer his services as surgeon for free.[94] Justifying his suggestion, Sargant argued that 'the negro's suffering could certainly not be any worse after the operation',[95] a rationale that failed to convince the Veterans' Hospital Association, which forbade the experiment. In some respects, the tale typifies the rhetorical devices present throughout Sargant's memoir; Sargant conjured an archaic vision of the brutal asylum where suffering patients were restrained 'like George III' to justify an invasive procedure. Yet the combination of the patients' ethnicity and chronicity amplified Sargant's latent experimental streak, producing a situation in which more interest appeared to be staked in the experiment than the well-being of the patients. By and large, Sargant believed that if mental illness had been left to run unchecked then the disease process would, in time, scar the patient. Physical therapies, he suggested, could have little impact when utilised at this late stage.

Ostensibly, Sargant supported mental hospitals, writing that 'the treatment given there may be very good'.[96] However, one barely has to read between the lines to arrive at a different conclusion. Sargant, for example, contrasted his strategy with the 'unfortunate misconception' that 'encouraging the admission of less seriously ill patients somehow increases the morale of chronic cases'. When this is attempted, Sargant argued, 'all that happens is that the newcomer's morale may rapidly descend nearer to the level of the chronic cases, simply because he now ranks as a similar mental hospital patient'. It was far preferable, Sargant insisted, to provide in-patient care in a general hospital if a patient was too unwell for out-patient treatment, so as to avoid 'mental-hospital stigma'.[97] What can one infer from this? Essentially that there is nothing to be done for the chronic patient and that it is futile to attempt to reform mental hospitals. Sargant's solution merely exacerbated the problems of those people he labelled as chronic mental hospital patients.

Reinforcing stigma: chronic psychotics

Enoch Powell's 1961 address to the annual conference of the NAMH embodied many of Sargant's aspirations. It can be viewed as the logical culmination of an incremental campaign to align psychiatric treatment with general medical treatment and, in breaking down the divide between mental illness and general illness, to obliterate the stigma of mental illness. After all, it is no coincidence that Powell delivered his speech, which heralded the demise of the asylum and unveiled the new policy of community care, to Britain's largest mental health charity.[98] Announcing cuts of 50 per cent or more in psychiatric hospital beds, Powell insisted that hospital spaces for mental illness should in future be sited in general hospitals.[99] He acknowledged that resources had been invested in psychiatric hospitals over recent years to make conditions 'less inadequate for the present generation of chronic mental patients'. Yet, he insisted, 'there comes a point where the very improvement of existing facilities militates powerfully against their supersession by something different and better'.[100]

If psychiatric hospitals and the medical personnel who staffed them had been rendered obsolete, as Powell asserted, one might wonder what was to become of the patients who inhabited these hospitals, whom Powell termed the 'present generation of chronic mental patients'. In a speech given, rather incongruously, at a symposium on 'The Future of the Mental Hospital',

Dr Geoffrey Tooth, medical officer of the Ministry of Health and one of the architects of Powell's closure plans, was disarmingly frank about the low priority assigned to the needs of long-stay patients. Admitting that he was 'almost entirely without inspiration' as to how such patients would be catered for in the future, Tooth nevertheless expressed the belief that 'the chronic and especially the brain-damaged psychotic who required no more than custodial care should not be mixed with those who were undergoing active treatment'.[101] If we turn to Ministry of Health documents, it becomes apparent that Tooth's statement was by no means a throwaway remark. One paper drawn up by the Ministry of Health for the Standing Mental Health Advisory Committee in 1960 observed that 'the rate of rehabilitation and discharge from the long-stay wards is likely to decline as the hard core of organically deteriorated patients is reached'.[102] Statements such as these give credence to Tom Butler's contention that postwar changes ushered in a new two-tier system of psychiatric care which privileged acute patients, although as we have seen these divisions stem back to the interwar years, if not before.[103]

Tooth's statement provoked the ire of James Bickford, Superintendent of De La Pole Hospital in Willerby from 1956 until 1981.[104] In a letter to the British Medical Journal, he accused Tooth of advocating 'third class treatment . . . for what he considers to be third-class patients'.[105] Around three-quarters of the patients in mental hospitals in England and Wales in the early 1960s had been resident for more than two years.[106] Thus, Bickford's concern that Tooth's comments pointed to the development of 'a very strange service for the mentally ill' – one in which the needs of the vast majority of patients had been overlooked – does not appear misplaced.[107] Nor was Bickford the only psychiatrist to express concerns regarding the fate of long-stay patients. Aubrey Lewis, Director of the Maudsley Hospital, wrote to the Ministry of Health's Chief Medical Officer George Godber to covey his misgivings.[108] He enclosed a paper from John Wing, Director of the Social Psychiatry Research Unit between 1965 and 1989, which suggested that only 15–20 per cent of long-stay patients could be discharged.[109] On these grounds, Wing argued that 'it would be a retrograde step to allow the conditions in mental hospitals to deteriorate still further in the belief that half of their beds will be empty in 15 years' time'.[110]

Wing did not publish this paper, described as a 'virulent attack' by Geoffrey Tooth. Wing, Tooth complained, had 'ignored the fact that the mortality rate in mental hospitals is higher than among corresponding groups in the general population'.[111] Indeed, waiting for long-stay patients to die appears to have constituted the Ministry's solution to the problem: commenting on the heightened death rate in mental hospitals, one Ministry paper observed that 'death alone . . . would eliminate these patients in about twenty-five years'.[112] However, in a paper for *The Lancet*, Kathleen Jones and Charles Gore challenged the Ministry's assumption that in sixteen years no long-stay patients would remain in mental hospitals. Surveying the in-patient population of Menston Hospital, Jones and Gore observed that many long-stay patients were relatively young and that most were diagnosed with schizophrenia, were unmarried and had few contacts with the outside world. Taken alongside the low staffing levels and limited occupational and therapeutic opportunities available within the Hospital, Jones and Gore did not envisage a rapid reduction of this patient population.[113] Tooth acknowledged that Menston might not meet his predicted trend, but insisted that the blame lay with the Hospital, which was too large, lacked staff and had not provided occupational activities. Gore and Jones, he stated, painted a 'depressing but typical picture of a mental hospital that has been steadily manufacturing "chronic" patients'.[114] He did not elaborate how the Hospital could surmount such problems, which doubtless stemmed from insufficient funds.

In his published work on this topic, Wing sought to devise rehabilitation methods which would enable patients to leave hospital and function in the community and the workplace, couching his concerns regarding government policy in a less overtly critical fashion. Wing believed that somatic factors were at work in the production of the symptoms of schizophrenia, but acknowledged that these factors were obscure and that patients' problems could not be resolved if they were understood as stemming solely from an illness. Instead, he argued, psychiatrists needed to explore the interactions between individuals and their social environments, to uncover people's aptitudes and capabilities as well as their impairments. 'Long-term hospital care may often have been due to severe clinical disabilities', he acknowledged. However, he asserted, 'it may, in itself, have produced social disabilities which prevented discharge, even though the clinical condition subsequently improved sufficiently to allow this'.[115]

Rehabilitation programmes inaugurated within psychiatric hospitals sought to reawaken patients' abilities to function independently. They were structured to meet the perceived needs of patients according to the severity of their impairments, their age range and preconceptions as to suitable gender roles. Nurses and occupational therapists working with elderly patients sought to engender a greater degree of self-care and awareness of their surroundings. At Glasgow's Gartnavel Hospital, gendered ideals shaped the nature of the social activity groups which patients were expected to join: in 1976, the available options were slimming, baking, beauty, flower arranging, lunch group, metal work or woodwork.[116] Married women patients were retrained in domestic skills such as cooking, laundry, shopping, budgeting and cleaning, often in household management units.[117] Many hospitals also established industrial rehabilitation units, in which patients undertook industrial sub-contract work, mostly of a repetitive and simple nature. Discussing the possibility that patients might find such work rather monotonous, the authors of a 1959 *Lancet* article concluded that 'a job does not seem to be so simple and repetitive to the deteriorated psychotic as to the normal person'.[118] Some hospitals sought to elicit a greater degree of self–care amongst the more refractory patients by reinforcing desirable behaviour, such as getting up, dressing and making the bed without assistance, via the distribution of tokens. Undesirable, noisy or violent conduct could result in the detraction of tokens.[119] These treatment approaches, which focused on managing and re-educating patients' behaviour, could not easily be conceptualised as medical interventions and were poles apart from the therapeutic innovations of the 1940s, 1950s and 1960s; indeed, they were not that dissimilar from methods of managing mental deficiency in the early decades of the twentieth century.[120]

By the time that Bickford dispatched his angry riposte to Geoffrey Tooth's disparaging remarks regarding the future of chronic patients, he had amassed a significant publication track record in medical journals regarding the needs of this patient cohort. This interest appears to have been sparked after Bickford joined De La Pole Hospital as Deputy Superintendent in 1953 and turned his attention to the conditions of the Hospital's long-stay patients. 'All psychiatrists agree that no effort must be spared to cure the patient when he first falls sick', Bickford noted in an article for *The Lancet* in 1954:

> So he is admitted to a modern, well-furnished, and comfortable ward; he is treated sympathetically and energetically, and conferences are held by the medical staff to ensure that he is treated by the most effective means available. If he fails to recover within some three to six months, his treatment changes . . . skill and energy are tacitly withdrawn. He becomes a chronic patient . . . He is moved from the admission ward to the main building where he is kept physically healthy . . . There will be no privacy, no curtains or carpets, no pictures on the wall . . . He is very lucky if he has any form of medical care directly from his doctor for more than half an hour in each year.

Psychiatrists, Bickford argued, appreciated 'the pleasant furniture and surroundings of the admission ward', and enjoyed interacting with patients 'who are well dressed and who can talk sensibly'. There was thus little incentive for the senior psychiatrists to 'surrender these pleasant things to work in the aesthetically unpleasing and culturally barren atmosphere of the chronic wards'.[121]

Yet, inverting the axiom that intervention should be targeting acute cases,

Bickford argued that long-stay patients were more in need of the psychiatrist's attention than acute cases, who would spontaneously remit or improve after receiving physical treatments, irrespective of the time devoted by psychiatrists. His objective was to discharge patients in a condition that would enable them to live and work within the community, and he scathingly attacked the 'facile distinction between "curable" and "incurable" patients' which many psychiatrists perpetuated.[122] At a time when his colleagues enthusiastically embraced monotonous industrial work as a therapy for long-stay patients,[123] Bickford implemented sports, physical training, and gardening programmes at De La Pole Hospital, seeking to ensure that every patient left their ward to venture outdoors each day. He described how this approach had been beneficially adopted to treat patients who had previously received 'every form of physical treatment which was thought likely to benefit them', to no avail.[124] 'Given help', he insisted, 'many so-called chronic patients prove themselves able to return to the community'.[125] These therapeutic changes were complemented by the establishment of exchange holidays with other mental hospitals,[126] hiring seaside camps to provide holidays to patients,[127] and camping trips for groups of patients in Europe.[128]

Similarly, at Claybury, Dennis Martin charted his efforts to help the resident long-stay patients.[129] As the average doctor was responsible for around three hundred patients, he explained, many chose to make their rounds of the chronic wards as quickly as possible so as to free up as much time as possible to spend with those patients who appeared to benefit most from assistance. Consequently, the quiescent chronic patient who caused no trouble helped facilitate this system of operation, enhancing the appeal of a disciplinary system in which patients submitted to the authority of nurses. Equally, subdued patients considerably eased the burden for nurses. Moreover, medical personnel had to contend with antiquated buildings which embodied the ideals of Victorian psychiatry and were frequently extended on an ad hoc basis to accommodate growing numbers of patients. Within this large institution, 'the individual is frequently lost sight of as a unique person to be cared for in a personal way'.[130]

Martin's assessment of the difficulties facing the doctor who wished to help his patients in a traditional, authoritarian hospital strikingly mirrors William's Sargant's synopsis of the barriers he encountered at Hanwell. Yet while Sargant abandoned Hanwell as 'a dead end . . . full of terrible suffering for which I could do nothing',[131] Martin turned his energies towards opening up communication, erasing hierarchies and dispensing with obsolete rules so as to unpick the authoritarian regime which institutionalised long-stay patients. While hoping to avoid the institutionalisation of new patients,

Martin also sought to reverse this process in long-stay patients so as to enable as many as possible to leave hospital. He claimed that even those who did not recover sufficiently to leave now enjoyed friendlier relationships with staff members and benefited from greater freedom to visit local shops and cinemas. For such patients, Martin believed, the ability to live in the hospital 'with the freedom and dignity of individual people, rather than as "chronic deteriorated patients"', was crucial. He objected to the way in which the term 'back wards' still connoted an 'implication of therapeutic neglect and hopelessness'.[132]

A 1962 television debate on the future of the mental health services captured psychiatrists' divergent attitudes towards government proposals to close down mental hospitals. The debate featured Sargant and two other speakers, who appear to be David Clarke, who instituted a therapeutic community approach within Fulbourn Hospital, and the psychoanalyst and Medical Director of the Cassel Hospital, Tom Main.[133] Discussion focused on the provision of psychiatric units in general hospitals and the introduction of community care. Predictably, Sargant extolled the merits of pharmacology, describing drugs as a 'new weapon' which enabled patients to be treated in general hospitals, and attributing relapse figures to patients' failure to take their medication. He also advocated leucotomies, which he insisted were now back in fashion. Tranquillisers, he insisted, often simply stifled 'the cries for help from the back ward'.

The other two participants were less sanguine about government plans. Responding to proposals that in future mental health services could comprise short-stay psychiatry units in general units for acute cases, medium-stay units for patients who did not recover quickly and 'long-stay units for the chronic population', one expressed surprise as he had been under the impression that a proportion of the beds in general hospitals would be utilised for chronic patients, enabling them to remain in the community rather than sending them to 'distant hospitals'.[134] 'One of the things we haven't discussed is the chronic patient', one speaker commented, observing that in his view Powell had committed a 'real bloomer' when he had predicted on rather slender evidence that the number of long-stay hospital patients would dwindle to nothing. These participants contested Sargant's assertion that discharge rates could be attributed to drugs, crediting the therapeutic community approach for regenerating many mental hospitals. Querying the extent to which the needs of all patients could be catered for solely via community care or treatment in general hospitals, one referred to the continuing need for the therapeutic community for people 'who have long-term crippledom'. On receipt of Ministry of Health circulars, he observed, 'one saw embarrassed medical officers of health running round saying "they tell me I've got to have bright ideas about psychiatric care.

Somebody tell me some bright ideas." And very few of them had got any forward-looking ideas as to how they were to help the psychologically crippled adults.'[135]

This use of the term 'crippledom' points to a convergence between the concepts of chronic mental illness and mental disability in the 1960s and 1970s, which originated from the work of psychiatrists preoccupied by the difficulties facing long-stay patients. Believing that social disabilities could pose more of a barrier to discharge than any residual clinical symptoms, John Wing used the term 'long-term mental disablement' to encompass 'those who are disabled by reason of mental retardation, dementia . . . and chronic mental illness'. 'To refer to those disabled by chronic schizophrenia as "mentally ill" induces an expectation that medical treatment is the chief factor determining the type of residential or day care needed', he explained, 'whereas it is generally agreed that social needs are often more important'.[136]

Discarded by some psychiatrists who sought to enhance their professional prestige by working with more promising patients, a number of long-stay patients with seemingly intractable problems were channelled elsewhere. An article from the *BJSPW* explained how the PSW employed in a mental hospital faced an 'overwhelming . . . amount of incurable illness' while her colleague working in the field of community care was 'likely to find that a high proportion of "hopeless" cases will come her way – semi-stabilised psychotics, chronics of all descriptions, psychopaths, epileptics, dullards – until the local authority office may even be regarded as a sort of benevolent dustbin'.[137] It was precisely these cases, whose difficulties had not been resolved by the application of biomedical therapies, which PSWs working in mental hospitals and for the local authorities tried to help through social interventions.[138]

As discussed in the previous chapter, PSWs, particularly those working in the less prestigious fields of hospital and community care, struggled to secure recognition of their professional status from other healthcare workers and the state. While many mental healthcare professionals sought to enhance their professional prestige by expanding their activities with more promising patients in community settings, PSWs found an opportunity to carve out a niche, albeit one which lacked prestige, by developing new approaches to assist individuals with enduring mental health problems. Conversely, their colleagues in child guidance clinics, who had enjoyed a more defined professional role from the outset, appeared to be moving in the opposite direction as clinics began to re-orientate their services towards less disturbed children.[139] An article in *Mother* claimed that child guidance clinics dealt with 'normal children', and sought to 'keep normal children normal'. Complaining that 'whenever they hear the word "psychiatrist" some people immediately think of mental disease', the article sought to reassure readers that normal emotional states and minor mental disturbances now fell within the remit of psychiatry.[140] The following year, *Good Housekeeping* advertised the work of clinics to its middle-class readership and sought to dispel prejudice. The types of problems discussed in the article such as thumb-sucking and bed-wetting were less disturbing than those described by PSWs in early articles, a change acknowledged in the article.[141] By focusing on normal and respectable families, PSWs may have de-prioritised those with more severe mental disorders. Indeed, while a number of PSWs sought to publicise their work with chronic patients in articles for their peers and other mental health professionals, the APSW displayed unease when the general press linked PSWs with this patient cohort. Thus, the Association criticised a report in the *Guardian* on music therapy in 1962 because it 'portrayed mental hospitals with only chronic and deteriorating patients'.[142]

Conclusion

The desire expressed by the APSW to promote representations of mental health services which transcended chronic patients in mental hospitals has recently been echoed by post-revisionist historians of psychiatry, who challenge the agency ascribed to psychiatrists by revisionists and the centrality of the asylum in mental healthcare. In this vein, Volker Hess and Benoît Majerus urge historians to turn their attention to extra-mural provisions and developments. In their view, work which focuses on institutional provision and seeks to explain psychiatric practice via the concepts of professionalisation and social control is outmoded and fails to account for many of the postwar developments.[143] Yet Hess and Majerus acknowledge that 'opening up institutions resulted in new problems, in particular with regard to caring for long-term hospitalized patients'. 'Old and chronically ill patients', they admit, 'especially in psychiatry, and despite all efforts for reform, continued to belong to a frequently neglected and in many respects marginalized group of patients'.[144]

Hess and Majerus are surely right to draw our attention to the significance of provisions and facilities sited outside the walls of psychiatric hospitals when tracing the history of mental healthcare in the twentieth century. However, their desire to sidestep the institution and, by extension, the long-term hospitalised and chronically ill patient, is both odd and troubling. It would be misleading, after all, to portray the asylum as a site bypassed by all medical reformers seeking to enhance the public image of their work; as we have seen, a number of mental healthcare reformers sought to remodel the asylum on the template of the general hospital, believing that the asylum could serve as a hub through which extra-mural services operated. It is also a troubling interpretation, as attempts to destigmatise incipient mental distress and increase the prestige of psychiatry were achieved in part by entrenching the stigma attached to asylums, chronic mental illness and mental deficiency. Thus, some practitioner-reformers used the image of the gothic Victorian asylum where patients were chained up and brutalised by unfeeling attendants as a rhetorical device to enhance the appeal of new 'medicalised' approaches. Analysis of extra-mural developments and the treatment of incipient mental disorder should co-exist alongside studies of the treatment of chronic mental illness, otherwise we risk compounding medical apathy with historical apathy. Given the demonstrable indifference displayed towards the plight of long-stay patients by Ministry of Health personnel as they crafted the policy of hospital closure, examination of major innovations from the perspective of the 'chronic psychotic' may well offer valuable insights into the objectives of policy change.[145]

Indeed, this analysis demonstrates that 'mental illness' served as a descriptive category which encompassed a heterogeneous group of people with very divergent experiences. Attempts to enhance the prestige of mental healthcare and encourage more people to seek treatment through the adoption of new therapeutic approaches could lead to the neglect of the needs of people with enduring mental health problems. When discussing appropriate methods of treating or managing particular patient cohorts, healthcare practitioners often distinguished between patients who were 'ill' and likely to respond to medical treatment; patients who were deviant and needed to be contained (a topic explored further in the next chapter); and chronic patients who had 'deteriorated' and would derive little benefit from further treatment. As a consequence, the boundaries between chronic mental illness and learning disability could at times be more porous than the boundaries between acute and chronic mental illness. These distinctions generated a hierarchy of mental disorder in which resources were directed towards 'promising' patients diagnosed with an acute neurotic disorder, at the expense of patients diagnosed with learning disabilities or chronic psychoses.

While a number of healthcare workers sought to enhance their professional prestige by focusing their work upon promising patients, other healthcare workers attempted to carve out areas of expertise by developing new therapeutic approaches to help patients with enduring mental health problems: patients whose symptoms had proved intractable in the face of the new physical therapies, and whose needs were sometimes neglected by those psychiatrists keen to emphasise the curability of mental illness.[146] To study such developments, we need to trace the connection or disconnection of intra- and extra-mural provisions, to analyse the 'medical' and the 'social' dimensions of care, and to turn our attention to the role of auxiliary and ancillary workers who delivered this care, such as nurses and social workers. Habit training, recreation, occupational therapy, social work and industrial therapy may not have attracted the same historical attention accorded to psychosurgery or pharmacology, but these practice, many of which originated as methods of treatment for mental deficiency in the first half of the century, were just as prevalent and demand analysis if we are to fully understand the history of postwar mental healthcare in Britain, particularly as it affected individuals who experienced severe or enduring mental health problems. Ruminating on the historiography of mental healthcare, Mathew Thomson complained of the 'bias towards the history of curing rather than caring'.[147] Thomson's observation points to the need to interrogate social approaches alongside biomedical approaches, to unpick the relationship between care and treatment; alleviation, recovery and cure. Biomedical approaches were arguably more likely to be conceptualised as potentially curative treatments which enhanced the prestige of psychiatry and facilitated psychiatry's integration within general medicine.[148]

Recent campaigns to destigmatise mental illness have sought to normalise mental distress by emphasising its prevalence and treatability. Arguably, however, stigma remains most entrenched around enduring mental health problems and perceptions that those suffering from mental health problems are liable to display violent behaviour. This raises the question as to whether healthcare professionals, in attempting to raise their own professional status by drawing attention to their success with acute or less severe cases of mental distress, exacerbated the stigma attached to enduring mental health problems, potentially reducing the resources and services available to such patients. The next chapter pursues this line of enquiry, exploring how gender shaped healthcare workers' representations of their patients.

Notes

1 W. A. F. Browne, *What Asylums Were, Are and Ought to Be* (Edinburgh, 1837), p. 229, reprinted in A. Scull (ed.), *The Asylum as Utopia: W. A. F. Browne and the Mid-Nineteenth Century Consolidation of Psychiatry* (London and New York, 1991).

2 For discussion of the role of the voluntary sector, see Chapter 5.

3 E. Powell, speech given to the NAMH (1961), text from http://studymore.org.uk/xpowell.htm.

4 A. Scull, C. MacKenzie and N. Hervey, *Masters of Bedlam: The Transformation of the Mad-Doctoring Trade* (Princeton, 1996), p. 3.

5 *Crichton Royal Asylum, 18th Annual Report*, 1857, p.40, quoted in Scull, MacKenzie and Hervey, *Masters of Bedlam*, p.118.

6 J. C. Bucknill, *The Care of the Insane and Their Legal Control* (London, 1880), p.x, quoted in Scull, MacKenzie and Hervey, *Masters of Bedlam*, p.210.

7 Scull, MacKenzie and Hervey, *Masters of Bedlam*, pp.214–23.

8 Ibid., pp.239–41.

9 On the concept of the field, see P. Bourdieu, *Distinction: A Social Critique of the Judgement of Taste* (1979; translation by Richard Nice 1984: Abingdon, 2005), pp.466–84.

10 See M. Thomson, *The Problem of Mental Deficiency: Eugenics, Democracy, and Social Policy in Britain, c. 1870–1959* (Oxford, 1998), p.284; M. Thomson, 'Status, manpower and mental fitness: mental deficiency in the First World War', in R. Cooter, M. Harrison and S. Sturdy (eds), *War, Medicine and Society* (Stroud, 1998), pp.149–66.

11 Thomson, *The Problem of Mental Deficiency*, p.2.

12 Such a clause was already incorporated within Scottish legislation.

13 'Incipient and unconfirmed insanity: deputation to the Lord Chancellor', *JMS*, 45 (1899), 415–17; 416.

14 J. Sibbald, 'The treatment of incipient mental disorder and its clinical teaching in the wards of general hospitals', *JMS*, 48 (1902), 215–26; 218, 217.

15 Ibid. On female nursing in male wards, see V. Long, '"Surely a nice occupation for a girl?" Stories of nursing, gender, violence and mental illness in British asylums, 1914–1930', in P. Dale and A. Borsay (eds), *Nursing the Mentally Disordered: Struggles that Shaped the Working Lives of Paid Carers in Institutional and Community Settings from 1800 to the 1980s* (forthcoming).

16 'The possibility of providing suitable means of treatment for incipient and transient mental disease in our great general hospitals', *JMS*, 48 (1902), 697–709; 699.

17 Ibid., 698.

18 Ibid., 708.

19 T. Clouston, *The Hygiene of the Mind* (London, 1906).

20 H. Pols, '"Beyond the clinical frontiers": the American mental hygiene movement, 1910–1940', in V. Roelcke, P. Weindling and L. Westwood (eds), *International Relations in Psychiatry: Britain, Germany and the United States to World War II* (Rochester, 2010), pp.111–33; p.126.

21 C. Beers, *A Mind that Found Itself: An Autobiography* (London, 1908).

22 See L. Westwood, 'Avoiding the Asylum: Pioneering Work in Mental Health Care, 1890–1939' (DPhil thesis, Sussex University, 1999); L. Westwood, 'A quiet revolution in Brighton: Dr Helen Boyle's pioneering approach to mental health care, 1899–1939', *Social History of Medicine*, 14 (2001), 439–57.

23 G. M. Robertson, 'The employment of female nurses in the male wards of mental hospitals in Scotland', *JMS*, 62 (1916), 351–62. Robertson's efforts to hospitalise the asylum are discussed in more detail in the next chapter.

24 G. M. Robertson, 'Discussion on the diagnosis and treatment of borderland cases', *British Medical Journal*, 2:3177 (1921), 827–31; 828.

25 S. Soanes, 'Rest and Restitution: Mental convalescence and the English Public Mental Hospital, 1919–1939' (PhD Thesis, University of Warwick, 2011).

26 S. Soanes, 'Reforming asylums, reforming public attitudes: J. R. Lord and Montagu Lomax's representations of mental hospitals and the community, 1921–1931', *Family and Community History*, 12 (2009), 117–29; 127.

27 *NAWU Magazine*, 17 (June–July, 1928), 1.

28 *NAWU Magazine*, 19 (November, 1930), 5.

29 *NAWU Magazine*, 19 (June–July, 1930), 8–9.

30 M. Jackson, *The Borderland of Imbecility: Medicine, Society and the Fabrication of the Feeble Mind in Late Victorian and Edwardian England* (Manchester, 2000), p. 150.

31 Thomson, *The Problem of Mental Deficiency*, p. 122.

32 Ibid., pp. 97–8.

33 *NAWU Magazine*, 19 (March, 1930), 6.

34 Thomson, *The Problem of Mental Deficiency*, p. 143.

35 See, for example, P. McCandless, '"Build! build!" the controversy over the care of the chronically insane in England, 1855–1870', *Bulletin for the History of Medicine*, 53 (1979), 553–74; C. Yanni, *The Architecture of Madness: Insane Asylums in the United States* (Minneapolis and London, 2007); L. Topp, J. Moran and J. Andrews (eds), *Madness, Architecture and the Built Environment: Psychiatric Spaces in Historical Context* (Abingdon, 2007).

36 Thomson, *The Problem of Mental Deficiency*, p. 71.

37 *MHIWU Journal*, 24 (July, 1935), 8.

38 Thomson, *The Problem of Mental Deficiency*, p. 107, 186.

39 Ministry of Health, *Report of the Departmental Committee on Sterilisation*, Cmnd. 4485 (London, 1934).

40 Jackson, *The Borderland of Imbecility*, p. 136.

41 These ideas helped construct feeblemindedness as a distinct eugenic concern in the early years of the twentieth century. see Jackson, *The Borderland of Imbecility*. For a discussion of these ideas in an American context, See J. W. Trent Jr, *Inventing the Feeble Mind: A History of Mental Retardation in the United States* (Berkely and Los Angeles, 1994), pp. 131–83.

42 Thomson, *The Problem of Mental Deficiency*, pp. 127–8.

43 Ibid., p. 138.

44 *Report of the Interdepartmental Committee on Mental Deficiency, 1925–1929* (London, 1929).

45 *Report of the Departmental Committee on Sterilisation*.

46 *NAWU Magazine*, 18 (August, 1929), 3.

47 Thomson, *The Problem of Mental Deficiency*, p. 226.

48 For an overview of McCardie, see A. Lentin, 'McCardie, Sir Henry Alfred (1869–1933)', *Oxford Dictionary of National Biography*, Oxford University

Press, 2004: www.oxforddnb.com/view/article/34677, accessed 10 October 2011.

49 *NAWU Magazine,* 19 (August, 1930), 1.

50 Thomson, *The Problem of Mental Deficiency,* p. 97.

51 *NAWU Magazine,* 18 (October, 1929), 2.

52 L. Westwood, 'Avoiding the Asylum', 138ff.

53 Montgomery wrote the revised and enlarged edition of *Notes for the Mental Nurse in Training,* published by the NAWU in 1927 and reissued in 1933.

54 *NAWU Magazine,* 18 (September, 1929), 16.

55 *NAWU Magazine,* 18 (October, 1929), 12.

56 Morgan, who opposed a 1931 Bill that sought to legalise voluntary sterilisation, was subsequently appointed medical adviser to the Trades Union Congress in 1932. On Morgan's role in the Parliamentary debate on the 1931 Bill, see Thomson, *The Problem of Mental Deficiency,* pp. 60, 66–7. On Morgan's subsequent work for the Trades Union Congress, see V. Long, *The Rise and Fall of the Healthy Factory: The Politics of Industrial Health in Britain, 1914–60* (Basingstoke, 2011), pp. 98–101.

57 *NAWU Magazine,* 18 (November, 1929), 11. The class-based concerns of the early eugenics movement in Britain have been examined by G. R. Searle, *Eugenics and Politics in Britain 1900–1914* (London, 1976).

58 *NAWU Magazine,* 18 (December, 1929), 12.

59 MRC, COHSE Archive, MSS.229/CO/1/3, National Executive Committee minutes, 6–8 December 1955. Flanaghan gave evidence to the Royal Commission on the Law Relating to Mental Illness and Mental Deficiency in 1955. At the end of his career, he was working as an assistant chief male nurse at Winwick Hospital and had served for thirty years as a registered male nurse. See COHSE Archive, MSS.229/6/C/CO/3/12, 'Law relating to mental illness and mental deficiency: minutes of 18th day' (1955).

60 *NAWU Magazine,* 19 (December, 1930), 10.

61 *MHIWU Journal,* 20 (January, 1931), 10.

62 *MHIWU Journal,* 20 (January, 1931), 10.

63 *MHIWU Journal,* 20 (March, 1931), 10.

64 *MHIWU Journal,* 20 (November, 1931), 3.

65 Berry worked for a number of years in Australia, where he combined research in mental deficiency with studies of Australian Aboriginals, reflecting the desire of many doctors to view mental deficiency as a reversion to a more primitive race. See K. F. Russell, 'Berry, Richard James Arthur (1867–1962)', *Australian Dictionary of Biography* (1979): http://adb.anu.edu.au/biography/berry-richard-james-arthur-5220/text8703, accessed 8 February 2013.

66 *MHIWU Journal,* 23 (August, 1934), p. 11. Similar 'humanitarian' arguments were mobilised in Germany to justify killing psychiatric patients: see M. Burleigh, *Death and Deliverance: 'Euthanasia' in Germany 1900–1945* (Cambridge, 1994)

67 *MHIWU Journal,* 21 (July, 1932), 6.

68 Thomson, *The Problem of Mental Deficiency*, pp. 193–4.
69 See D. Mitchell, 'Parallel stigma? Nurses and people with learning disabilities', *British Journal of Learning Disabilities*, 28 (2000), 78–81.
70 For an overview, see E. Shorter, *A History of Psychiatry: From the Era of the Asylum to the Age of Prozac* (New York, 1997), pp. 69–112.
71 See H. Cotton, 'The relation of chronic sepsis to the so-called functional mental disorders', *JMS*, 69 (1923), 434–65. For an assessment of Cotton's work, his influence in Britain and the broader context in which he practised, see A. Scull, *Madhouse: A Tragic Tale of Megalomania and Modern Medicine* (New Haven and London, 2005).
72 J. Busfield, 'Restructuring mental health services in twentieth-century Britain', in M. Gijswijt-Hofstra and R. Porter (eds), *Cultures of Psychiatry and Mental Health Care in Postwar Britain and the Netherlands* (Amsterdam, 1998), pp. 9–28; p. 16.
73 The emergence of these treatments are outlined in Shorter, *A History of Psychiatry*, pp. 190–224, and more critically in P. Fennell, *Treatment without Consent: Law, Psychiatry and the Treatment of Mentally Disordered People since 1845* (London, 1996), pp. 129–50.
74 W. Sargant and E. Slater, *An Introduction to Physical Methods of Treatment in Psychiatry* (Edinburgh, 1948), p. 1.
75 Mental hospitals were nominally included within the regional hospital boards and came under the formal control of the Ministry of Health, but in practice psychiatric services appear to have been poorly integrated. See J. V. Pickstone, 'Psychiatry in general hospitals: history, contingency and local innovation in the early years of the National Health Service', in J. V. Pickstone (ed.), *Medical innovations in Historical Perspective* (Houndmills, 1992), pp. 185–99.
76 K. Jones, *Asylums and After. A Revised History of the Mental Health Services: From the Early 18th Century to the 1990s* (London, 1993), p. 161.
77 Sargant and Slater, *An Introduction to Physical Methods*, pp. 189, 188.
78 See Shulamit Ramon's analysis of the 1956 edition of Henderson and Gillespie's *A Textbook of Psychiatry* and the first (1954) edition of Mayer-Gross, Slater and Roth's *Clinical Psychiatry*: S. Ramon, *Psychiatry in Britain: Meaning and Policy* (London, 1985), pp. 163–78.
79 *Health Services Journal* (February, 1946), 4.
80 W. Sargant, *The Unquiet Mind: The Autobiography of a Physician in Psychological Medicine* (London, 1967).
81 Ibid., p. 159.
82 Ibid., p. 28.
83 Ibid., p. 51.
84 Ibid., pp. 1, 2.
85 Ibid., p. 13.
86 Ibid., p. 4.
87 Ibid., p. 12.
88 Ibid., p. 144.

89   Ibid., p. 147

90   Ibid., p. 148.

91   COHSE Archive, MSS.229/CO/1/1/2, National Executive Committee minutes, 15–27 August 1948.

92   Sargant, *The Unquiet Mind*, p. 154.

93   Ibid., p. 129.

94   Ibid., p. 130.

95   Ibid., p. 129.

96   Ibid., p. 146.

97   Ibid., p. 148.

98   For discussion of the role of the voluntary sector, see Chapter 5.

99   Powell, speech given to the NAMH.

100 Ibid.

101 'Future of the mental hospital', *British Medical Journal*, 5259 (1961), 1078–9.

102 The National Archives (TNA), MH 133/424, 'Trends in the mental hospital population and their effect on future planning', 2 December 1960.

103 T. Butler, *Changing Mental Health Services: The Politics and Policy* (London, 1993), p. 37.

104 For an overview of Bickford's career, see P. Fisher, 'James Bickford', *Guardian* (3 April 2009), www.guardian.co.uk/theguardian/2009/apr/03/obituary-james-bickford.

105 J. A. R. Bickford, 'Chronic sick of psychiatry', *British Medical Journal*, 5263 (1961), 1358–9.

106 J. K. Wing, D. H. Bennett and J. Denham, *The Industrial Rehabilitation of Long-Stay Schizophrenic Patients: A Study of 45 Patients at an Industrial Rehabilitation Unit: MRC Memorandum No. 42* (London, 1964), p. 1.

107 Bickford, 'Chronic sick of psychiatry', 1359.

108 TNA, MH 133/424, letter from A. Lewis to G. Godber, 7 March 1961.

109 TNA, MH 133/424, J. K. Wing, 'Future planning of hospital services for the mentally ill', March 1961.

110 Ibid.

111 TNA, MH 133/424, memo from G. Tooth to G. Goodman, 29 December 1961.

112 TNA, MH 133/424, 'Trends in the mental hospital population and their effect on future planning', 2 December 1960.

113 C. P. Gore and K. Jones, 'Survey of a long-stay mental hospital population', *The Lancet*, 2:7201 (1961), 544–6.

114 Memo from G. Tooth to G. Goodman, 29 December 1961.

115 G. W. Brown, M. Bone, B. Dalison and J. K. Wing, *Schizophrenia and Social Care: A Comparative Follow-Up Study of 339 Schizophrenic Patients* (London, 1966), p. 3.

116 The Mitchell Library, Glasgow, NHS Greater Glasgow and Clyde Archives, Gartnavel Royal Hospital Archives, HB 13/11/81, notes of meeting of Rehabilitation Committee to discuss occupational/industrial therapy, 22 April 1976.

117   See D. Gittins, *Madness in Its Place: Narratives of Severalls Hospital, 1913–1997* (London, 1998), pp. 107–9.

118   S. D. Collins, S. J. Fynn, F. Manners and R. Morgan, 'Factory in a ward', *The Lancet*, 274:7103 (1959), 609–11. For an analysis of industrial therapy, see V. Long, 'Rethinking post-war mental healthcare: industrial therapy and the chronic mental patient in Britain', *Social History of Medicine*, advance access, published online 10 March 2013.

119   See R. C. Winkler, 'Management of chronic psychiatric patients by a token reinforcement system', *Journal of Applied Behavior Analysis*, 3 (1970), 47–55.

120   See, for example, Jackson, *The Borderland of Imbecility*, pp. 165–202, and Thomson, *The Problem of Mental Deficiency*, pp. 139–47.

121   J. A. R. Bickford, 'Treatment of the chronic mental patient', *British Medical Journal*, 263:6818 (1954), 924–7; 924.

122   Ibid., 924.

123   See Long, 'Rethinking post-war mental healthcare'.

124   J. A. R. Bickford, 'The forgotten patient', *The Lancet*, 266:6897 (1955), 969–71; 969.

125   Ibid., 971.

126   J. A. R. Bickford and H. J. Miller, 'Exchange of patients by mental hospitals: a therapeutic holiday', *The Lancet*, 274:7093 (1957), 96–7.

127   J. A. R. Bickford, 'Shadow and substance: some changes in the mental hospital', *The Lancet*, 271:7017 (1958), 423–4.

128   E. Beadle, A. G. Chisholm and J. M. Todd, 'Travelling abroad with long-stay psychiatric patients', *The Lancet*, 283:7328 (1964), 322–3.

129   D. V. Martin, *Adventure in Psychiatry: Social Change in a Mental Hospital* (Oxford, 1962).

130   Ibid., p. 24.

131   Sargant, *The Unquiet Mind*, p. 13.

132   Martin, *Adventure in Psychiatry*, p. 133.

133   Wellcome Library, William Sargant Collection, PP/WWS/J.1/3, BBC, 'The future of the mental health services', 1962. Sargant's role in the debate is evident; the other two participants have been deduced through the names by which they are referred to – 'Tom' and 'David' – and the description of the participants' positions and perspectives in the synopsis of the programme.

134   Ibid. It is unclear whether this speaker is Main or Clarke.

135   Ibid. Again, the speaker cannot be identified.

136   J. K. Wing, 'Trends in the care of the chronically mentally disabled' in J. Wing and R. Olsen (eds), *Community Care for the Mentally Disabled* (Oxford, 1979), pp. 1–13; pp. 3–4.

137   K. I. Jones and P. M. Hammond, 'The boundaries of training', *British Journal of Psychiatric Social Work*, 1:2 (1948), 172–7; 173–4.

138   This is discussed in more detail in V. Long, ' "Often there is a good deal to be done, but socially rather than medically": the psychiatric social worker as social thera-

pist, 1945–70', *Medical History*, 55 (2011), 223–39; V. Long, '"A satisfactory job is the best psychotherapist": employment and mental health, 1939–60', in P. Dale and J. Melling (eds), *Mental Illness and Learning Disability since 1850: Finding a Place for Mental Disorder in the United Kingdom* (Abingdon, 2006), pp. 179–99.

139 See D. Thom, 'Wishes, anxieties, play and gestures: child guidance in inter-war England', in R. Cooter (ed.), *In the Name of the Child: Health and Welfare, 1880–1940* (London, 1992), pp. 200–19.

140 MRC, APSW Archive, MSS.378/APSW/14/4/58, 'When parents can't cope', *Mother* (February, 1961).

141 E. Elias, 'Please, can you help me?', *Good Housekeeping* (March, 1962), 89.

142 APSW Archive, MSS.378/APSW/14/1/38, APSW Public Relations Working Party minutes October 1962, p. 2. The PRSC became the Public Relations Working Party in 1962 when Miss Barnes was appointed Public Relations Officer.

143 V. Hess and B. Majerus, 'Writing the history of psychiatry in the twentieth century', *History of Psychiatry*, 22 (2011), 139–45.

144 Ibid., 140.

145 This argument is made at greater length in Long, 'Rethinking post-war mental healthcare'.

146 See Long, '"Often there is a good deal to be done"'.

147 Thomson, *The Problem of Mental Deficiency*, p. 2.

148 For a discussion of the concepts of care, recovery and treatment in mental health-care, see Long, '"Often there is a good deal to be done"', 237–9.

4

MAD, BAD AND DANGEROUS TO KNOW? MEN, WOMEN AND MENTAL ILLNESS

A 'female malady'?

In the previous chapter, we saw how some healthcare professionals generated stigmatising images of chronic patients while seeking to improve services for, and reduce the stigma attached to, acute mental disorder. Focusing on the mental nurses' Union studied in Chapter 2, this chapter builds upon these ideas, exploring how some nurses exploited the image of the dangerous madman to further their own interests. It commences by tracing the historiographical debate on gender and mental illness, before considering the argument that the image of the violent madman was a product of the community care era. The chapter then analyses how members of the Union represented patients in early issues of their journal, examining how the Union mobilised the image of the violent and depraved madman in an attempt to prevent women from nursing male patients. It explores how psychiatric nurses reignited these discourses and fuelled stigma by arguing for the retention of and investment in institutional provision following the inclusion of psychopathy into the remit of nursing under the 1959 Mental Health Act, and the government's decision to abolish mental hospitals and establish services in the community.

Examination of the ways in which the image of the madman has mobilised debate over the course of the twentieth century offers a counterbalance to existing literature, which has traced connections between madness and femininity. This body of work evolved out of Phyllis Chesler's 1972 monograph, *Women and Madness*. Radicalised by the upsurge in feminist activity in the late 1960s, and motivated by the misogyny she experienced as a practitioner within the psychology profession, Chesler interwove historical examples and contemporary accounts to argue that a patriarchal psychiatric profession diagnosed women who deviated from gender roles as mad. Men's disturbed behaviour, she claimed, was less likely to be interpreted as symptomatic of madness, unless they were perceived to act in a feminine way.[1] These ideas were developed and applied to historical accounts by Elaine Showalter in her influential 1987 monograph, *The Female Malady*.[2] In the eighteenth century, Showalter asserted, the insane were viewed as 'unfeeling brutes, ferocious animals that needed to be kept in check with chains, whips, strait-waistcoats, barred windows, and locked cells'. By the early years of the nineteenth century, she claimed, the 'symbolic gender of the insane person shifted from male to female'.[3] Reconfiguring madness as a form of sickness characterised by loss of reason, reformers drew upon the more appealing image of the vulnerable madwoman, cementing associations between female irrationality and male rationality.

Showalter's account contributed towards the revisionist historiography of psychiatry of the 1970s and 1980s, which sought to demolish the whiggish interpretation of the rise of the asylum as a triumph of humanitarian interests and medical progress. Yet Showalter also identified a significant limitation in the revisionist literature. Michel Foucault, she observed, had 'brilliantly exposed the repressive ideologies that lay behind the reform of the asylum', yet failed to explore the gendered dimensions of this repression. 'Even the most radical critics of psychiatry', Showalter noted, 'are concerned with class rather than gender as a determinant of the individual's psychiatric career and of the society's psychiatric institutions'. Her objective was to 'supply the gender analysis and feminist critique missing from the history of madness'.[4]

Further works by Jane Ussher and Lisa Appignanesi did much to cement the idea that women were more liable to be labelled as mad. Displaying the unmistakable influence of Showalter's and Chesler's work, Ussher encapsulated the central thesis of her 1991 monograph in its title: *Women's Madness: Misogyny or Mental Illness?* Drawing upon historical examples, Ussher asked, 'Why is it *women* who are mad? Why is it that it has *always* been women? Is this madness actually the result of misogyny, as many feminists would claim, and are the symptoms not madness at all, but anger or outrage?'[5] A footnote to this section admitted that 'men are diagnosed as mad, and receive psychiatric treatment', but asserted 'it is women who have dominated in the psychiatric statistics for centuries, and women who are regulated through the discourse of madness'.[6]

Ussher viewed 'the oppression of "mad" women . . . as just another form of misogynistic torture . . . misogyny makes women mad either through naming us as the "Other", through reinforcing the phallocentric discourse, or through depriving women of power, privilege and independence. Or misogyny causes us to be named as mad. Labelling us mad silences our voices.'[7] On page 10 of this 352-page book, Ussher offered her last statement on men and mental illness. Men, she accepted, 'may be mad – but are likely to be positioned as bad. They are likely to manifest their discontent or deviancy as criminals. Whilst women are positioned within the psychiatric discourse, men are positioned within the criminal discourse . . . I will leave the case of men here.'[8]

The trope of the 'female malady' was resurrected once more in 2008 by Lisa Appignanesi, who explained:

> I decided to focus on women as a way into this history of symptoms, diagnoses and mind-doctoring for various reasons. Perhaps the first is simply that there are so many riveting cases of women, and through them a large part of what we recognize as the psy professions was constructed . . .
>   There is more. Contemporary statistics always emphasize women's greater propensity to suffer from the 'sadness' end of madness.[9]

Doubtless successful in bringing the ideas of other scholars to a wider, non-academic audience, Appignanensi's work is perhaps best viewed as a work of synthesis which may well leave historians disappointed. Reviewing the work for *History of Psychiatry*, Lesley Hall pertinently observed: 'without some better understanding than we currently have about the definition of men as mad, lunatic, insane, and how the observation of mad, bad, sad men contributed to the development of psychiatry and associated disciplines, can we really say anything particularly useful about psychiatry and women?'[10]

Showalter's frequently reprinted account has exerted a tenacious hold on the undergraduate psyche, finding expression in the seemingly endless stream of earnest assignments which explain how the asylum functioned as a tool of patriarchal oppression through which perfectly sane women were locked up for failing to conform to norms of feminine behaviour. Amongst historians, however, this interpretation has been under attack for some time. Critics observe that the authors of many of these works are not historians by training and are prone to extrapolate from a narrow range of art and fiction to make ill-grounded and poorly evidenced historical assertions about women and madness which cannot be substantiated when archival records are examined. In 2004, an edited volume by Jonathan Andrews and Anne Digby drew together many of these reinterpretations. In their introduction, the editors explained that:

> Gender perspectives on the history of British and Irish psychiatry and asylums were once dominated by a somewhat exclusive focus on women; on distorted, if not misogynistic, psychiatric constructions of femininity, and of specific, female-directed forms of treatment; on the creation of mental illness as a predominantly feminine disorder, and on male-orchestrated abuse of women and chauvinism within psychiatry and psychiatric institutions.[11]

The volume adopted a 'post-revisionist critique', attacking what it described as 'the overly ideologised and unconvincingly theorised approaches to issues of class and gender in asylum and psychiatric history'.[12] Chapters within the volume were based primarily on empirical archival research and queried Showalter's assertion that women outnumbered men within asylums.

When I commenced work on my doctoral thesis, it had not occurred to me that gender would figure prominently in my analysis. But as my research progressed, I struggled to reconcile Showalter's thesis with my own research findings which suggested that representations of mental illness in twentieth-century Britain have been shaped by the image of the violent male patient. As the feminist historiography of the 1970s and 1980s had suggested, discarding gender as a category of analysis would impoverish our understanding of the history of madness. But, following Joan Busfield, I would argue that it is 'the interrelationship of *gender* and madness, not just of women and madness in isolation', which demands historians' attention.[13] Disaggregating data on gender and mental illness from the 1970s and 1980s, Busfield points out that the 'feminine' nature of madness is dependent upon how one defines what constitutes mental illness. 'It is less "madness" that is identified as the female malady than the broader territory of more "minor" psychiatric conditions', Busfield concluded.[14]

The violent madman: a product of the community care era?

Conventionally, mental health campaigners identify the mid-1980s as the era in which the stereotype of the dangerous madman emerged, framed by a growing disillusionment with community care. In 1985, the journalist Marjorie Wallace published a series of stories on schizophrenia in *The Times* under the title 'The forgotten illness'. Wallace painted a bleak picture in which families struggled to cope with highly disturbed relatives who had been dumped in the community. Four of the twenty-three patients described in Wallace's articles were women and were presented as pitiable figures. Discussing the case of his daughter who had suffered from episodes of schizophrenia for thirty years, John Blake appeared most distressed by the change in his daughter's physical appearance, explaining 'she could have been a beautiful woman, she had such a pretty face. Now she looks drab and disorderly.'[15] Representations of violent male patients predominated however. Michael, Wallace explained, 'became a schizophrenic at 23, throwing up his career as an artist': an absurd choice of wording which implies that Michael wilfully chose to abandon his pursuit of art to embrace a 'career' as a schizophrenic. Wallace described how Michael subsequently spent 'several turbulent years in and out of hospital and terrorizing his family'. '"He used to line up the knives and point them in my direction wherever I moved", his mother recalls. "He even threatened us with an axe."'[16]

In the following year, Wallace founded SANE. Frequently reviled by service users and more libertarian voluntary sector groups, SANE sought to enlist public support for its calls to reverse the policy of community care by issuing a series of provocative posters in 1988 which conjured the image of a submerged army of violent, delusional individuals poised to lash out at any moment. The most discussed depicted a bearded man and carried the text 'he thinks he's Jesus, you think he's a killer. They think he's fine – stop the madness'.[17]

In 1994, another body, the Zito Trust, was established with very similar objectives to SANE – to campaign for greater powers to control and manage patients suffering from severe mental illness. This organisation was founded following the murder of Jonathan Zito by Christopher Clunis, a man suffering from schizophrenia. This murder has conventionally been portrayed as a turning point in public attitudes to community care, transforming scandals about the abuse suffered by the mentally ill at the hands of practitioners and the public into scandals about the violence unleashed by former asylum patients on unsuspecting members of the public. Writing in the early and mid-1990s, the Glasgow media group argued that inaccurate media depictions linking violence and mental illness had led to hostile public attitudes towards those with psychiatric disorders that in turn threatened the social integration of health service users. An analysis of media content carried out by the group in 1993 revealed that the bulk of media content 'situates mental illness in the context of violence or harm and represents the public as "potential victims of random mania"'. 'Such representations', the group concluded, 'alter perceptions of the "dangerous" nature of mental illness as well as affecting beliefs about the risks of random attacks by the "maniacs" who are presented as populating the world'.[18]

The impact of this coverage is heightened by the fact that positive representations of mental distress are generally situated in low-impact media. Thus diagnostic categories such as schizophrenia and psychopathy, owing to their media associations with violence, receive more coverage than other types of mental distress. Mental health campaigners express concerns that media representations of dangerous, violent patients cut adrift by healthcare professionals to run amok in the community lead the public to believe that sufferers of mental illness pose a risk, in turn reshaping mental healthcare policy. In the twenty to thirty-four age bracket more men were admitted for in-patient treatment than women, a statistic which suggests that the perception of dangerous young male patients has informed treatment procedures.[19] In 1998, the Health Secretary Frank Dobson claimed that

> Care in the community has failed. Discharging people from institutions has brought benefits to some. But it has left many vulnerable patients to try and cope on their own. Others have been left to become a danger to themselves and a nuisance to others. A small but significant minority have become a danger to the public as well as themselves.[20]

Arguing that the rights of patients had to be balanced with public safety, the government introduced draft mental health bills in 2002 and 2004 which contained new compulsory treatment and detention powers. Most contentiously, the bills proposed removing the treatability test: this would have enabled people to be confined against their will, even if their condition would not have benefited from treatment.[21] This latter proposal was watered down following pressure from mental health charities. However, the 2007 Mental Health Act introduced supervised community treatment orders (designed to prevent the 'revolving door' and minimise risk), and more than 1,200 people in England were made subject to compulsory treatment outside hospital five months after the powers were introduced under the Act.[22]

From this one might reasonably deduce that irresponsible press reporting in the 1980s and 1990s gave disproportionate coverage to a handful of tragic but statistically insignificant cases and, in so doing, generated the stereotype of the dangerous madman. This fuelled public fears about mental illness, led to a disproportionately high rate of in-patient care for young men and induced the government to enact new legislation driven by risk management rather than patients' interests. It is a compelling narrative, but not one which can be convincingly substantiated, as representations of the violent male patient can be traced back to the early years of the twentieth century. Take, for example, a press cutting from 1902 ostensibly written to praise the work of the MACA, a charity which offered convalescent care and work placements to discharged asylum patients (this work is discussed in the next chapter). The writer's main contention was that premature discharge led to 'many of the daily tragedies which startle the newspaper reader. A certain number of homicidal maniacs are let loose upon society every week . . . frequently this outburst – or rather, this recurrence – of mania means a murder, sometimes a massacre. The homicidal maniac who *Shocked the World as Jack the Ripper* had been . . . in a lunatic asylum.'[23] One can well imagine that the individual who added this clipping to the charity's press-cuttings did so with a heavy heart, given that the article's main intention was to generate panic among its readers that discharged patients were dangerous, violent and by no means cured.

Brutish, brutal and brutalising: asylums, patients, nursing and masculinity[24]

Cutting nails, chronic males,
    Courtyard evolution:
You bet you can get 'bumped off' at
    A mental institution.[25]

In Chapter 2, we saw how asylum attendants founded a trade union in 1910 to campaign for higher wages, shorter working hours and a reduction in the rules and restrictions which regulated their work. The above verse, penned by a member of the Union and published in the Union's journal in 1934, illustrates how representations of asylum patients could be mobilised by Union members seeking to secure their goals. Early representations of asylum patients within the journal were usually deployed by the Union to advance conditions of attendants rather than those in their care. Not that an outwardly hostile attitude to the patients was taken: an article ironically entitled 'A Patient's Paradise' reflected awareness of the shared fortunes of patients and attendants, describing the hard physical labour expected from patients and the poor food they received in return. This theme recurred in an article which described the poor food given to patients because medical superintendents preferred to spend money on the outward appearance of asylums, inciting the editor Herbert Shaw to interpolate a sardonic aside: '[Why do the patients need good food? They aren't Superintendents.]'[26] The very first editorial of the journal commented: 'we seriously maintain that if the Lord Chancellor and the Lunacy Commissioners are sincerely anxious for the welfare of the patients, the very first thing to which they should turn their attention is to see to it that the conditions of asylum service are such as to attract and retain the best types possible of men and women ... they allow the public money to be wasted ... in giving medical superintendents huge salaries'.[27] Dingwall, Rafferty and Webster note that, early in the twentieth century, asylum attendants in the pauper asylums 'shared the conditions of the patients. Both were equally subject to the same complex web of rules and to the expectation of automatic and unquestioning obedience.'[28] These early critiques on behalf of the patients may indicate how the poor working conditions of attendants led them to sympathise with the patients.

A more usual strategy adopted by the Union at this time to obtain improved conditions and pay, however, was to focus on the unpleasantness of the patients. Complaining of the visiting committees of asylums in 1912, one writer argued, 'asylum staffs have quite enough to do to attend to the antics of deluded and degraded "mental-deficients" and moral perverts under them'.[29]

Frequently, contributors to the journal described how attendants had to 'manage' or pacify difficult patients through an astonishing array of personal qualities. 'The staffs at asylums', argued one correspondent in 1913, 'have to exercise . . . the caution of a lion tamer, the cunning of Sherlock Holmes; they have to cajole, wheedle, threaten, persuade, fascinate, charm, captivate, pacify, soothe, calm, appease, relieve, discipline, coax and humour the patients'.[30] This article represented patients as alien, foreign, devious and different from normal people, in need of management. The use of the metaphor of a lion tamer adds an air of animality to the implied description of the patient. This idea of how to handle patients could have been drawn from the main text for training attendants, where the terms 'nursing' and 'management' or 'control' of patients appear to be interchangeable.[31] Nor had things radically changed by 1929 in a description of the job of the mental nurse, when the author claimed that 'her patients may be unpleasant, abusive, filthy in habits and language, or ungrateful, suspicious, unwilling and resistive . . . her sympathy, kindliness and tact must be abundant to overflowing for a mental patient . . . is amenable to nothing else'.[32]

Contributors to the journal often advanced the argument that attendants' calls for better wages and conditions were justified by the violent and anti-social behaviour of the patients. An attendant's response to an earlier 'joke' article about the slothful life of the asylum attendant bitterly attacked his work, and the patients at the heart of his job:

> We have such fun, washing and dressing the patients, often belching in one's face and worse . . . in some asylums . . . they have an endless amount of fun provided by patients wandering round the table, falling in fits, and occasionally throwing a spittoon onto the table . . . then . . . the bedding of the patients. Oh! The fun we have; it makes our sides split – undressing, bathing, pulling, struggling; it really is delightful. Then sometimes we get a black eye, a kick on the shin, or a tooth or two knocked out.[33]

This author depicted patients as violent and anti-social, not ill. Other articles explicitly responded to allegations published in the medical and general press that asylum attendants assaulted patients. Thus in 1928, the journal carried a report of an incident in which an attendant had been attacked by a patient:

> The nurse was knocked unconscious and the patient lifted the chair to strike another, and perhaps, a fatal blow, when the patient playing cards sprang to the rescue . . . The nurse had to have six stitches in his head . . . These are the everyday 'emoluments' of the mental nurse which are not advertised by those critics of the service whose principal concern is to expose the alleged 'brutality' of the mental nurses.[34]

In this article, the author placed two conjectures in the account; that the next blow from the patient would perhaps have been fatal, and that such events were 'everyday'. These phrases shifted the meaning of the story to fit the desired conclusion – that any individual undertaking such work deserved better conditions and pay, not because they were skilled professionals but because they managed dangerous, violent inmates.

As these examples illustrate, the theme of violence and risk permeated discussions of attendant-patient interactions within the Union journal. In 1920, patients' violent, anti-social behaviour was emphasised and given a gendered aspect by the NAWU in a battle reflecting the composition and power structure within the organisation. Although by the end of 1920 women's membership had increased to almost 46 per cent of the total membership,[35] Union delegates to the annual conference and branch executives were almost entirely male. It also appears that the authorship of the journal was dominated by men. During the First World War, a number of mental hospitals employed women on the male wards of mental hospitals to combat manpower shortages. Some medical superintendents maintained the system after the cessation of hostilities, nominally on medical grounds, although the lower wages paid to women may also have prompted this decision. These developments brought simmering tensions between male and female attendants and nurses to a boil, as the Union contested female nursing of male patients. Both psychiatrists and the trade unionists argued that the presence of female nurses would have a profound effect upon the male patients they cared for, although the two groups drew very different conclusions about the effects of female nursing.

While the practice of female nursing was something of a new phenomenon in English asylums, born out of the exigencies of the war, Scottish asylums had been experimenting with the system since the end of the nineteenth century. Indeed, by 1916 Dr George M. Robertson, the most prominent advocate of female nursing on male wards, felt justified in describing the practice as a 'firmly established feature of the Scottish system of care for the insane', adopted in the vast majority of Scottish asylums.[36] Robertson argued that women showed 'superior aptitude and skill' for the duties of nursing, because of their mothering instinct. He acknowledged that some male attendants were 'kind and devoted nurses',[37] yet as another participant in the debate put it, 'it is a misuse and a waste of male attributes to see a stalwart young man training as an attendant doing his year in the sick wards, feeding an advanced general paralytic, say, with sop, and carrying out other nursing duties, which, without any shadow of a doubt, are women's work'.[38] Robertson believed that men lacked the natural qualities which made women such good nurses, reinforcing his views by referring to men who worked in asylums as 'attendants', and women as 'nurses'.

Robertson suggested that male patients would respond more favourably to a woman's influence. Female nurses, according to Robertson and his supporters, awakened the chivalrous instinct in male patients. The presence of women on the ward thus encouraged male patients to control themselves better and to use less foul language. Moreover, Robertson argued, female nurses preferred to work with male patients, who were less inclined to disregard their instructions than female patients (at no stage was the logic reversed to suggest that male nurses should attend to female patients). Speaking in support of Robertson's paper at a quarterly meeting of the Medico-Psychological Association, Dr Legge described how he had begun to introduce female nurses on male wards at Mickelover Asylum. The system, he argued, 'got rid of some things one was ashamed to have'. He explained how he no longer had to be concerned with complaints from patients, because 'it would be obviously ridiculous for a male patient to aver that a woman had struck him'.[39] Regarding the proprieties of women nursing men, Robertson noted that female nurses in general hospitals nursed male patients and, provided the same decencies were observed, he could see no difficulties emerging. He also maintained that male patients with sexual proclivities should remain under the care of male nurses.

For Robertson, female nursing was part of a grander scheme to hospitalise the asylum, refashioning its purpose, structure and operations upon the template of the general hospital. His proposals can thus be situated within the interwar mental health reform movement which sought to raise the status of psychiatry, discussed in the previous chapter. Robertson averred that insane people were sick and required nursing. Invoking a historical narrative which would justify his proposals, Robertson argued that male attendants were an anachronism left over from the time when 'madhouses . . . were prisons for the safe custody of a dangerous class. Little wonder, then, that the methods adopted in them were those of a prison, that "keepers" alone were employed on the male side.'[40] Robertson's arguments were not unanimously accepted by his fellow psychiatrists. At a quarterly meeting of the Medico-Psychological Association, Dr Soutar objected that Robertson had failed to differentiate between the purposes of asylums and hospitals. While the inmates of hospitals were 'sick physically; and . . . amenable to direct dietetic and medicinal treatment', asylum patients were 'abnormal but not sick', 'misfits'.[41] If women's influence was so invaluable to asylum treatment, Soutar joked, then all asylum superintendents (Robertson included) should 'at once tender their resignations, and ask that women doctors might be appointed in their stead'.[42] However, the majority of psychiatrists swung behind Robertson's ideas (at least in theory); as Dr Drapes asserted, 'members should not give up the idea that every insane person was a sick person'.[43] An editorial comment in the

JMS, which reviewed the debate, decided that most doctors who approached the subject would 'come to the conclusion that Doctor Robertson has proved his point', and predicted that sooner or later, the system would 'be generally if not universally adopted throughout the asylum service'.[44]

Asylum superintendents such as George Robertson justified their decision to replace male attendants with female staff by drawing on medicalised concepts of mental disturbance as an illness which required skilled nursing, a supposedly natural female skill, in a hospital setting. Male attendants contributing to the Union journal, however, did not portray the insane as sick patients who would respond to the maternal instincts of skilled female nurses by exercising restraint and self-control. Instead they depicted male patients as violent, anti-social misfits, likely to attack female nurses or subject them to indecency. Moreover, the journal represented female nurses who engaged in such work not as professional and skilled hospital nurses but instead as morally degraded by the dirty work they had undertaken. The Union journal first discussed the issue of female nurses working on male wards in January 1920 and continued to attack the practice in virtually every monthly issue throughout 1920. Arguments focused on the 'depraved' behaviour of male patients and the supposed vulnerability of female nurses to violent attacks from male patients.

In his January article, the Union's General Secretary George Gibson incorporated a report he had sent to the annual conference of the Labour Party. Female nurses, Gibson claimed, could not manage the violent behaviour exhibited by male patients. Painting a lurid picture of the sexually depraved behaviour of male patients, he launched an attack on the reputation of female staff who undertook this work. Gibson substantiated his argument by drawing upon passages from the *Handbook for Attendants Upon the Insane* relating to 'self indulgence', 'indecent conduct', 'filthy and dirty habits' and dangerousness posed by (male) patients to (female) staff to condemn the 'revolting' and 'degrading' system of female nursing of male patients. Quoting from the *Handbook*, Gibson cautioned his readers that 'many seemingly quiet patients are, at times, liable to become dangerous to themselves and others'.[45] Admittedly, the overall tone of the *Handbook*, authored by doctors and published in conjunction with the Medico-Psychological Association, provided some ammunition to Gibson and his colleagues; as noted earlier, it was this book which conflated the terms 'management', 'nursing' and 'control'.[46] By abstracting passages from the *Handbook* and changing the emphasis of the text through type fonts and the interpolation of sarcastic observations, Gibson created a stigmatising image of the male patient and the female nurse who would choose such a job. For example, Gibson quoted from page 344 of the *Handbook*:

'p.344 – . . . Bad sexual practices are, unfortunately, *common among the insane*, and ought to be prevented as far as possible. The possibility of *any* patient indulging in bad habits should be borne in mind, *and a constant watch for signs should be kept up*.'*47

Starring this passage, Gibson inserted his own observation: '*Surely a nice occupation for a girl?*'48 Within the context of the *Handbook*, this passage was gender-neutral and would read as applying to both male and female patients. However, by placing the quotation in an article on male patients, Gibson encouraged readers to infer that the quote referred to male patients. Moreover, by choosing to emphasise the words 'common among the insane', Gibson tainted all male patients, while the aside comment, by implication, attacked the reputation of women who chose to undertake the work. The Union also linked poor recovery rates and a patient suicide to the practice of female nursing on male wards, effectively attacking the nursing standards of their woman members. Instead of allowing women or 'girls' to voice their opinions on what he described as 'the degrading system' and the 'revolting duties' they undertook, Gibson used paternalistic language to speak for them. 'There is no medical superintendent, nor any male member of the Board of Control, who would *permit* wife or daughter to undertake such work', he asserted, 'and having equal *veneration* for all women, I protest emphatically against the employment of female labour in the male lunatic wards'.49

The Union failed to find any female nurses to censure the system, although several wrote in attacking the Union for criticising the character of female nurses, accusing the men of 'selfishness and jealousy', and of branding the profession a degradation.50 One female critic perceptively commented on the harmful stigmatisation of male patients that the Union was undertaking, asserting that 'it is an insult to a great number of patients to infer that all mental cases are depraved'.51 The *Nursing Times*, which represented the interests of the general nursing profession, was quick to see a different side to the argument: 'we confess to a feeling of great distrust when we hear of complaints by male attendants in asylums of the "demoralising" influence of women nurses in male wards. Why this solicitude for the women? . . . Not a single complaint of any kind has been made by the female nurses.'52 This position was doubtless influenced by the rather strained relations between asylum attendants and general nursing, discussed in Chapter 2.

Seeking to muster support for its campaign, the Union encouraged its members to send copies of the articles to the local press, and suggested that branches contact local associations of discharged soldiers and sailors to 'acquaint them with the fact that the continuance of this system of female nursing in asylum wards is depriving many ex-servicemen of the opportunity of securing employment in a public service'.[53] This strategy initially met with some success. In Wakefield, the Union organised a joint protest with the local ex-servicemen's branch. Union coverage also reached the national press: *John Bull* picked up on the story, attacking the practice of female nursing in male wards after reading the Union's journal, 'in whose columns the revolting nature of the duties involved are emphasised with lurid force'.[54] While nominally the Union stated that its intention was to protect women, the prime objective appears to have been protecting men's jobs and pay levels: equally, psychiatrists advocating female nurses were doubtless motivated in part by the attractions of a cheaper labour force, although a desire to improve the low status of psychiatry within the medical profession at large by refashioning asylums on the template of general hospitals was doubtless also a factor.

The Union had sought to mobilise the support of ex-servicemen for their campaign. Ex-service personnel would, however, play a more multifaceted role as the story unfolded in the national press. Parallel to the debate over the issue of women nursing on male wards, the Union discussed the allegations of cruelty by attendants made in the journal *Truth* by a former patient who had been invalided from service after a nervous breakdown. This article belonged to the genre of tales of wrongful confinement and violent staff that had figured prominently in the *Pall Mall Gazette* in the 1870s.[55] However, the story attracted more attention because it had been written by a former soldier. As Peter Barham has argued in *Forgotten Lunatics of the Great War*, public concern for the well-being of working-class soldiers who experienced mental health problems as a consequence of their wartime service helped dismantle the barriers which segregated asylum inmates from the community at large.[56] The article in *Truth* depicted the mental hospital as a place of incarceration where 'inmates' were 'detained' by 'brutal and ignorant warders' or 'gaolers'.[57] The writer of this article based his argument on the contention that insanity was a form of sickness that would respond to medicalised treatment in hospital settings: an objective shared by many psychiatrists and general nurses, but opposed by the male-dominated Union. In the article, the writer depicted shell-shocked cases as patients suffering from an incipient stage of mental disease who needed to be restored to health. Violence was abundant again in this narrative, yet here the violence was ascribed to male attendants, not patients. The author referred to the 'variety of forms of physical violence' used by attendants to control patients. Those described in the article included throttling, half-drowning, hitting the back of the patient's head against the floor, and what the author referred to as 'obscene methods of torture the nature of which

I can only leave to the imagination of the reader'.[58] The author restricted these allegations of cruelty to male nurses, argued that most patients would be better off with female nurses.[59]

In February 1920, the Union rejected these allegation in an article entitled 'Truth and Exaggeration', pointing out that nurses faced severe penalties for assaulting a patient, and arguing that patient testimony was unreliable. Despite denying the charges, the author felt it necessary to provide some excuses for poor nurse behaviour, citing 'the confinement of nurses within asylum walls in the atmosphere of insanity for 80 to 100 hours per week' and 'the provocation which may be received' that 'maybe only those who have been engaged in attendance upon the insane can fully appreciate'.[60] This response, and a Union publicity stunt in which George Gibson invited a journalist from the *Sunday Chronicle* to look round another military mental hospital and report favourably on it, failed to stem the tide of people writing to *Truth* with their own allegations of neglect and abuse suffered at the hands of asylum nurses. Indeed, the publicity stunt may have been counterproductive, as *Truth* subsequently related the story of Mrs X., who alleged that her ex-soldier husband had been subjected to brutal treatment in this same institution.[61] The focus of reports in *Truth* remained upon the discharged servicemen, contrasting 'admirable hospitals' in Kensington where 'the nursing was in the hands of skilled women nurses' with the 'dark cells and padded room of the lunatic asylum, with brutal warders cowing the unfortunate occupants by physical force, to which the NCOs and men were condemned after their nervous systems had been wrecked by exposure to an unheard-of strain'.[62]

The media flurry generated by George Gibson's condemnation of women nursing male patients illustrates how mental health workers, motivated by occupational concerns, could trigger a debate on the nature of mental illness within the general media. Treatment of the issue within the Union's journal was followed by further press coverage. However it proved difficult to control the direction and impact this might have. Diane Gittins, in her work on Severalls Hospital, has discussed fears of the polluting powers of the mad and madness, suggesting that those who worked with the mentally ill were perceived to be contaminated by association.[63] Nor were healthcare workers necessarily immune from such fears. In his 1985 memoir, the psychiatrist R. D. Laing recalled the day when one of his colleagues brought some buns baked by patients on a refractory ward to the doctors' sitting room, and offered them round. Of the seven or eight doctors present, 'only two or three were brave, or reckless, enough to eat a bun baked by a chronic schizophrenic . . . the psychiatrists were afraid of catching schizophrenia'.[64]

Male nurses writing in the magazine emphasised how the polluted identity of male patients could contaminate female nurses, enforcing the stigma
of asylum patients and their carers in the public mind. They used male
patients, and, to a lesser extent, female nurses, as voiceless targets, victims of
harmful representations, to further their occupational aims. Sociologist Jenny
Kitzinger has argued that the way in which a topic is covered may frame the
way that similar events are discussed and represented in the media in the
future, an observation that appears to characterise the events discussed in
this chapter.[65] In the debate surrounding the alleged mistreatment of shell-
shocked patients, some of the themes that emerged in the first debate relating
to insanity, nursing, and violence were deployed. Factors arising from the First
World War played a part in creating and shaping these debates. The shortage of available male staff promoted discussion amongst psychiatrists of the
system of female nursing on male wards while the plight of shell-shocked soldiers mobilised public interest. In *Truth*, it was the figure of the ex-serviceman
and not the pauper lunatic who attracted sympathy and respect.[66] Meanwhile,
the Union argument against female nursing was based partly on an appeal that
women were depriving ex-servicemen of jobs.

A contested view of the nature of insanity underpinned these stories.
Insanity was viewed by some psychiatrists and the journal *Truth* as a form of
illness, requiring skilled, hospital-trained female nurses, imbued with maternal
instincts, to treat the sick patients. The use of female nurses, it was believed,
would negate the risk of violence towards male patients. However, for other
psychiatrists and the male leaders of the Union, insanity was portrayed as a
form of social deviance and loss of control. The introduction of female nurses
to male wards would produce exhibitions of sexual deviance and violence that
women could not control. While claiming to represent the interests of their
female members, the male executive of the Union derogatorily portrayed
women who nursed male asylum patients as morally degraded by the dirty
work they had undertaken, in order to gain benefit for themselves. Throughout
the year, male writers in the journal launched an unremitting campaign to
remove women from male wards by attacking the character of such female
nurses and labelling male patients as violent and sexually depraved. In so doing
they exacerbated the stigma of mental illness and smeared it by association to
the nursing staff.

The representations of male patients disseminated by the Union's journal
and by leaders of the Union failed to represent the interests of patients and
undermined the interests of many Union members, reflecting the imbalance
of power between men and women in the Union in an era in which women
were underrepresented in the trade union movement throughout Britain.[67]

Prejudice persisted towards woman within the Union, especially women in positions of authority, and attacks on the character of matrons were in particular prolonged and bitter. In 1913, a male correspondent to the Union's journal criticised a matron who had ordered a male attendant on duty. In his view, the matron should have been 'kept in her place by the medical officer, and not allowed to use her opinion'.[68] A motion on the Union's 1930 conference agenda attacked the authority of matrons over male staff in mental hospitals.[69] In 1942, the journal published a thinly veiled attack on female nature in an article which ostensibly focused upon matrons. Disingenuously claiming to defend victimised female nurses, the author blamed the poor working conditions in many mental hospitals upon matrons, arguing that 'the inability of most women to take positions of responsibility and behave with human tolerance to subordinates of their own sex was no small part of the problem'. Another backhanded insult was aimed at women when the writer claimed 'it is gratifying to see our female colleagues at last realising the need of organisational action', suggesting women were too slow to see the advantages beforehand. Perhaps it was unsurprising that more women at that particular branch had chosen not to join the Union.[70] An impression of female nurses' attitudes towards the Union can be gleaned from a letter written in 1936 from a nurse who had been assisted in a legal case by the Union. Although she thanked the Union for its help, the nurse added 'frankly, I had begun to begrudge paying my monthly subscription as I nursed a suspicion that female nurses were inadequately catered for'.[71]

One of the main functions of the Medico-Psychological Association was to defend the interests of its members. Psychiatrists were however unsympathetic to the new attendants' Union, attacking the Union's indifference to patient welfare and staff training. Although Dr Soutar had objected to Robertson's plans to hospitalise the asylum in 1916 on the grounds that asylum patients were abnormal, not sick, he nevertheless rejected the Union's approach. In 1919 he attacked the Union's industrial viewpoint, remarking that fortunately there were still some attendants 'who have in them the true spirit of nursing, who recognise that they are not, like factory hands, merely industrial workers. That spirit – the nursing spirit of sacrifice and readiness to serve the sick – is active in many of our asylum nurses and attendants.'[72] Soutar's critique illustrates a belief often expressed by doctors and general nursing organisations about the incompatibility of professional ideals and efforts to improve the material conditions of workers. As we saw in Chapter 2, the Union's tactics to advance the conditions of their members stood in sharp contrast to organisations that represented female nurses in general practice, such as the College of Nursing.

Professional crisis and a new stigmatisation of the (male) psychiatric patient

Chapter 2 examined how the Union shifted its strategy in the 1930s, advancing the claims of psychiatric nurses for improved status and conditions on the basis that psychiatric nursing was a skilled medical profession. The introduction of new therapies such as electroconvulsive therapy, insulin coma therapy and psychosurgery facilitated these developments, enabling the Union to equate psychiatric nursing with general nursing. Depictions of male patients as violent and sexually perverted disappeared from view, which confused the long-serving mental nurse C. H. Bond, who wrote in to the Union's journal in 1948 to express his shock that the Union had discarded its opposition to female nursing of male patients. 'Surely some of our old London District Council members remember ... the degradation being imposed upon females nursing male mental patients?' he asked.[73] The issue appeared to die away in 1959, when a motion to bar women from nursing in male wards was overturned at the annual conference. Proposer Mr Higgins claimed that 'a female nurse working on male wards would be a witness to degrading scenes by chronic patients'. This image of the patient was seen as embarrassingly dated and a threat to the professional image the Union was then trying to create to most of those present; the resolution was dismissed by one delegate as 'restrictionist and . . . as obsolete and outmoded as the padded cell or straitjacket'.[74]

However, psychiatric nursing began to face serious problems, and the Union's response to these difficulties undermined its claims to champion a patient-centred view, suggesting that psychiatric nurses' primary concern remained their working conditions. Psychiatric nurses viewed the inclusion of psychopathic disorder within the Mental Health Act with grave concern, and at the Union's 1959 conference, members debated a resolution which suggested that 'sex perverts, psychopaths, criminal patients and some other dangerous mental patients who can easily abscond from ordinary mental hospitals' should be detained in a special secure hospital in each region. The proposer argued that if a dangerous patient absconded from a normal mental hospital and 'murdered a child or some innocent person ... then public opinion would soon put the clock back and the many would suffer for the few'. This resolution followed in the wake of a string of newspaper reports concerning the escapes of Rampton patients.[75] In the interests of preserving open door policies for the majority of mental patients by appeasing public opinion, this delegate suggested a new form of custodialism for certain categories of patients by raising the spectre of the (sexually) violent patient. Two further resolutions at this conference dealt with concerns for the safety of staff if prisoners were admitted to ordinary mental hospitals.[76]

The other bone of contention for Union members was Health Minister Enoch Powell's 1961 announcement that 75,000 hospital beds would close over a period of fifteen years. The Union bitterly opposed this, arguing that the shortage of mental nurses would worsen as individuals sought to leave a profession with no future, and that mental hospitals would be downgraded as they faced closure, a view which Ministry of Health officials gave credence to.[77] Dingwall, Rafferty and Webster note that the effect of Powell's policies was liable to make mental nurses' work more onerous as the younger and least 'damaged' patients were discharged, leaving hospitals to care for the most severely disordered and elderly.[78]

As morale worsened, writers in the Union's journal suggested that nurses in psychiatric units should be paid 'danger money', returning to arguments advanced by the Union soon after it had first formed.[79] In 1961, the Union's General Secretary Jack Jepson raised alarms about attacks on mental hospital staff, which Jepson claimed had resulted from Powell's policy of placing psychiatric patients into Broadmoor, Rampton and Moss Side only as a last resort. 'It may be a counsel of perfection for the report to say it is wasteful to provide security precautions for patients who do not need them', Jepson commented, 'but nurses who have been attacked by informal patients who seemed harmless will need to be convinced'.[80] An article in 1963 told a 'classical case' of a man sent to a mental hospital from the law courts, and admitted as an informal patient: 'he left the hospital, went home and assaulted his wife. He decided to return to the Hospital, but got drunk before he arrived. He attacked the staff nurse in charge and left, only to be returned to the same ward by a probationer officer.'[81] Anger at Powell's policies prompted one Union writer to depict psychiatric patients as incurable, violent criminals in an article of September–October 1961, which dubbed Powell 'the executioner' and argued that the policy of discharging patients from hospitals on prescriptions was creating a nation of drug addicts:

> In 1954, 54,000 patients were admitted to our mental institutions. Today the figure is 90,000, of which 80,000 are discharged and returned to the community. Do not delude ourselves with the idea that this great mass of patients goes home cured or even half cured. The truth is that a large number leave behind them a trail of violence, robbery, assault, rape and murder.[82]

The Union conveyed similar messages at its 1965 conference in Aberdeen, where a motion calling for the establishment of maximum security hospitals captured the tabloid imagination. 'Wards where dangers lurk', reported the

Daily Record, informing readers that staff and patients in mental hospitals were being '"severely mauled" by patients with aggressive and criminal tendencies'.[83] Reporting the story under the title 'Nurses "knocked about"', the *Birmingham Post* informed its readers that 'many mental nurses were suffering from injuries received from patients'.[84] A motion passed at the same conference which opposed the integration of male and female wards attracted even more media interest. 'Conference told of sex and the insane', the *Glasgow Times* reported, while the *Scotsman* printed the story under the title 'Sex "encouraged" in mental hospitals', and the *Daily Mail* informed readers, 'Vice girl at work in hospital'.[85] These stories did not go wholly unchallenged. In his address to the conference, the Scottish Secretary William Ross chided his audience. 'I have been looking at the headlines you have been getting', he informed his listeners, 'and I wondered if it was Peyton Place you were talking about'.[86]

Nor did the situation improve by the end of the 1960s. Indeed, the furore created by Barbara Robb's exposé of the ill-treatment of elderly patients in mental hospitals in her book *Sans Everything: A Case to Answer* led to investigations of nursing practices at many mental hospitals.[87] Robb acknowledged that 'there are many wonderful nurses' and that 'grim, inadequate buildings, bad organisation, over-crowding, shortage of money and shortage of staff' in part accounted for the neglect of elderly patients. Nevertheless, Robb insisted, 'psychiatric hospitals tend to attract a higher proportion of apathetic, ignorant or, frankly, mentally ill doctors and nurses than others'.[88] She drew upon testimony from six nurses to substantiate her assertions. One respondent recalled overhearing a charge nurse 'snarl at an old man lying in bed: "Die, you bastard, die." The old man replied: "It takes time, charge."'[89] In a contribution to Robb's volume, the journalist C. H. Rolph described one nurse's account of the treatment meted out to elderly patients in her hospital as 'a catalogue of cruelty, callousness, filth and depersonalization such as I have not seen since I was reviewing the reports of the Nuremberg trials'.[90]

Although a subsequent White Paper dismissed most allegations,[91] the Union complained of a 'witch hunt atmosphere' and derided Robb's book as 'knock everything'.[92] Even the Royal College of Nursing, which tended to focus less on the working conditions of nurses than the Union did, chose the occasion of its 1970 conference to attack psychiatric nurses' conditions of work. Although the Chairman of the Psychiatric Committee claimed that nurses were demoralised 'by not being able to provide the service they wished for their patients', he subsequently shifted his attack to suggest that the patients posed the main limitations to nurses' work. Nurses, he claimed:

Serve when they are spat at, kicked scratched and bitten, they serve as they separate patients locked in fights as they ward off physical assaults on themselves.
They tolerate verbal abuse and serve as they retrieve towels, socks and other
clothing from lavatory pans. And they serve as they climb on slippery roofs to
bring patients back to safety.

Another resolution at the conference re-established the division between
mentally and physically ill patients, as delegates voted to ensure as a matter
of policy that the two groups of patients were not placed in the same ward.[93]

Conclusion

Members of the psychiatric nursing Union often proclaimed their interests
in the welfare of their patients and decried what they viewed as the public
prejudice attached to mental illness and its treatment. However, these assertions can appear somewhat disingenuous because the Union itself periodically
played an active role in stigmatising asylum patients as violent and brutish, and
the asylum as a hazardous and hellish environment. If we turn to examine these
stigmatising representations, we find few examples of the 'cultural image of
women as mental patients' which Showalter discussed.[94] Instead, the image of
the violent, chronically ill male mental patient predominated throughout the
twentieth century, and has played a pivotal role in debates on healthcare policy
and perceptions of risk and mental illness. This raises the question as to what
extent psychiatric nurses and other healthcare workers have fuelled the stereotypes which anti-stigma campaigns now seek to dismantle. It also unseats the
hypothesis that the expansion of community care in the 1980s precipitated an
inversion of earlier scandals in which patients had been portrayed as the helpless victims of abusive staff in brutal mental hospitals.[95]

Why did the Union adopt this approach? We could point to gender inequalities and castigate the Union's strategy when contrasted to the professionalisation route adopted by general nurses. Arguably, however, we might arrive
at a richer historical analysis if we eschew the desire to seek an easy moral conclusion and turn our attention to the broader field of mental health in which
mental nurses' occupational strategies were forged. The Union's strategies
were enmeshed within this field, shaped by the aspirations and relative power
of other healthcare workers. Psychiatrists sought to advance a medicalised
model in which the asylum was reconfigured into a hospital and the attendant into a skilled (female) nurse, although this ethos was rather undercut
in the *Handbook for Attendants upon the Insane*, authored by doctors, which
emphasised control rather than care. In response to the hospitalisation model
promoted by psychiatrists, asylum attendants, positioned near the bottom

of the professional hierarchy within the field of mental health, pragmatically sought to defend their interests and improve their wages by emphasising the occupational hazards of their work, focusing on the figure of the violent madman. In so doing, they represented themselves as keepers of dangerous lunatics. However, these competing visions of the nature of mental illness and what constituted an appropriate method for caring for such individuals were not contested on an equal footing; attendants lacked the professional authority of doctors and could not exert the same influence on government policy or medical practice.

Between the 1930s and 1950s, the status of the occupation rose as new legislation and therapeutics enhanced the image of the mental patient and the mental hospital. The Union now fought for the humanisation of the patient, promoting the image of the professional, medically trained psychiatric nurse who cared for the sick. However, these trends went into reverse in the early 1960s following proposals to close hospitals and transfer care into the community. Frustrated with a career that appeared to offer no future, and stuck working in decaying buildings earmarked for closure with a higher proportion of challenging patients as more promising cases were discharged, the Union reverted to its earlier strategy. These developments illustrate that we cannot account for change within the ethos of mental healthcare occupations through recourse to any comfortable whiggish narrative of progress and increasing humanitarian interest in patients' welfare.

Within the interconnected field of mental health, stigma was impossible to contain; it ricocheted and rebounded from the figure of the asylum patient to tar the image of the asylum and the asylum attendant. This reflects Duncan Mitchell's observation that mental nurses to some extent shared the stigma of their patients,[96] although I would argue that nurses were instrumental in generating this stigma, describing their patients as violent deviants and constructing a dichotomy which separated mental patients from other people. The Union's failure to recognise just how interconnected asylum nurses and patients were in the public mind thus appears to have been a significant tactical error. Thus, the Union may have succeeded in protecting the jobs of male attendants when it campaigned to stop the practice of women nursing male patients in 1920. However, examination of press coverage illuminates the interconnections between risk, mental illness and masculinity in newspaper stories, illustrating how patients were able to draw on and invert this discourse to accuse male attendants of brutality. Moreover, the Union's decision to represent patients as violent deviants requiring control, rather than sick patients requiring medical care, made it difficult for mental nurses to establish themselves as a professional group with specialised expertise and an ethical concern for those they cared for. Indeed, these scandals created the impression that asylums were brutish places, perhaps perpetuating stigma in the public mind and the media about mental illness and asylum treatment.

Notes

1 P. Chesler, *Women and Madness* (1972: New York, 1973), pp. 75–6.
2 E. Showalter, *The Female Malady: Women, Madness and English Culture, 1830–1980* (1987; London, 2001).
3 Ibid., p. 8.
4 Ibid., p. 6.
5 J. Ussher, *Women's Madness: Misogyny or Mental Illness?* (London, 1991), p. 6.
6 Ibid., p. 14.
7 Ibid., p. 7.
8 Ibid., p. 10.
9 L. Appignanesi, *Mad, Bad and Sad: A History of Women and the Mind Doctors since 1800* (London, 2008), pp. 6–7.
10 L. A. Hall, 'Essay review: does madness have a gender?', *History of Psychiatry*, 20 (2009), 497–501; 498.
11 J. Andrews and A. Digby, 'Introduction: gender and class in the historiography of British and Irish psychiatry', in J. Andrews and A. Digby (eds), *Sex and Seclusion, Class and Custody: Perspectives on Gender and Class in the History of British and Irish Psychiatry* (Amsterdam and New York, 2004), pp. 7–44; p. 8.
12 Ibid., p. 13.
13 J. Busfield, 'The female malady? Men, women and madness in nineteenth century Britain', *Sociology*, 28 (1994), 259–77; 259.
14 J. Busfield, *Men, Women and Madness: Understanding Gender and Mental Disorder* (Houndmills, 1996), p. 19.
15 M. Wallace, 'The tragedy of schizophrenia: keeping patients in the community can tear their families apart', *The Times* (16 December 1985), p. 10
16 M. Wallace, 'The tragedy of schizophrenia: where the progressive vision of community care falls down', *The Times* (17 December 1985), p. 8.
17 Text reproduced in N. Crossley, *Contesting Psychiatry: Social Movements in Mental Health* (Abingdon, 2006), p. 195.
18 G. Philo, G. McLaughlin and L. Henderson, 'Media content', in G. Philo (ed.), *Media and Mental Distress* (London, 1996), pp. 45–81; p. 80. The quotation cites a headline from the *Herald*, 13 April 1993.
19 S. Payne, 'Outside the walls of the asylum? Psychiatric treatment in the 1980s and 1990s', in P. Bartlett and D. Wright (eds), *Outside the Walls of the Asylum: The History of Care in the Community, 1750–2000* (London, 1999), pp. 244–65; p. 248.
20 'Health: Dobson outlines Mental Health Plans', 29 July 1998, http://news.bbc.co.uk/1/hi/health/141651.stm.
21 Mind, 'Updated mental health bill must promote civil rights, not damage them,

says alliance', 23 March 2006: www.mind.org.uk/news/1866_updated_mental_health_act_must_promote_civil_rights_not_damage_them_says_alliance.

22 P. Lombard, 'Mental Health Act: demand for community orders swamps services', *Community Care*, 30 March 2009: www.communitycare.co.uk/articles/30/03/2009/111151/mental-health-act-demand-for-community-orders-swamps-services.htm.

23 Wellcome Library, MACA, SA/MAC/H.2/2, article from unknown paper, unknown author, 1902. Emphasis in original text. Casebook (Jack the Ripper) attributed this article to George R. Sims and situates it as one within a series of articles written by Sims on the Ripper: see www.casebook.org/press_reports/dagonet.html, consulted on 22 November 2010.

24 The material in the section is also given consideration in V. Long, '"Surely a nice job for a girl?" Stories of nursing, gender, violence and mental illness in British asylums, 1914–1930', in P. Dale and A. Borsay (eds), *Nursing the Mentally Disordered: Struggles that Shaped the Working Lives of Paid Carers in Institutional and Community Settings from 1800 to the 1980s* (forthcoming).

25 From 'The Song of the Charge' by a correspondent from Fishponds, *Mental Hospital and Institutional Workers' Union Journal* (hereafter *MHIWU Journal*), 23 (August, 1934), 6.

26 *NAWU Magazine*, 2 (May, 1913), 65–7.

27 *NAWU Magazine*, 1 (October, 1912), 3.

28 R. Dingwall, M. Rafferty and C. Webster, *An Introduction to the Social History of Nursing* (London, 1988), p. 127.

29 *NAWU Magazine*, 1 (October, 1912), 9. The reference to moral perverts was perhaps an allusion to the category of 'moral imbeciles', described in the mental nurses' handbook as 'persons who from an early age display some mental defect coupled with strong, vicious, or criminal propensities on which punishment has little or no detrimental effect': Medico-Psychological Association, *Handbook for Attendants on the Insane* (London, 1908), p. 216. By substituting 'pervert' for 'imbecile', the writer conveyed an impression of sexual depravity, reflecting how some nurses viewed this category of patient.

30 *NAWU Magazine*, 2 (May, 1913), 3.

31 *Handbook for Attendants on the Insane*, pp. 335–6.

32 *NAWU Magazine*, 18 (March, 1929), 2.

33 *NAWU Magazine*, 2 (May, 1913), 2.

34 *NAWU Magazine*, 17 (March, 1928), 9. This article was satirically entitled 'More "Emoluments"', a reference to the earlier tradition of paying part of the attendant's wages in goods or services.

35 M. Carpenter, *Working for Health: The History of the Confederation of Health Service Employees* (London, 1988), p. 75.

36 G. M. Robertson, 'The employment of female nurses in the male wards of mental hospitals in Scotland', *JMS*, 62 (1916), 351–62; 351.

37 Ibid., 360.

38   'The Medico-Psychological Association of Great Britain', *JMS*, 62 (1916), 445–55; 455.

39   Ibid., 449.

40   Robertson, 'The employment of female nurses', 352.

41   'The Medico-Psychological Association', 447–8.

42   Ibid., 448.

43   Ibid., 453.

44   'Female nursing of male insane', *JMS*, 62 (1916), 416–21; 421.

45   *NAWU Magazine*, 9 (January, 1920), 8.

46   For a brief overview of the history of the *Handbook*, see H. R. Rollin, 'The Red Handbook: an historic centenary', *Psychiatric Bulletin*, 10 (1986), 279.

47   *NAWU Magazine*, 9 (January, 1920), 8. Gibson took this quotation from an unspecified edition of the *Handbook for Attendants upon the Insane*, although he italicised parts of this quotation. His italicisations have been reproduced here.

48   Ibid., 8. Italic type in original text. Starred comment by George Gibson.

49   Ibid., 9. Italic type in article.

50   *NAWU Magazine*, 9 (February, 1920), 11.

51   *NAWU Magazine*, 9 (September, 1920), 14.

52   *NAWU Magazine*, 9 (February, 1920), 2. Reprinted from the *Nursing Times*, issue and page number not given.

53   *NAWU Magazine*, 9 (September, 1920), 8.

54   *NAWU Magazine*, 9 (February, 1920), 9. Reprinted from *John Bull*, issue and page numbers not given.

55   For examples of wrongful confinement articles, see 'Legal difficulties in cases of alleged lunacy', *Pall Mall Gazette* (8 June 1870), p. 10; 'Certificates of lunacy', *Pall Mall Gazette* (31 May 1870), p. 10. For examples of tales of staff cruelty, see 'The treatment of lunatics: its known and permitted horrors', *Pall Mall Gazette* (15 January 1870), p. 6; 'In a lunatic asylum', *Pall Mall Gazette* (9 May 1870), p. 6.

56   P. Barham, *Forgotten Lunatics of the Great War* (New Haven and London, 2004).

57   Anonymous, 'Army mental hospitals: a little light on a national scandal', *Truth*, 87 (January, 1920), 95–7; 96, 97. The author described the mistreatment of shellshock patients, but argued that the same conditions applied to pauper lunatics who were cared for in the same institutions by the same staff.

58   Ibid., 97.

59   Ibid., 96.

60   '"Truth" and exaggeration: mental hospital treatment', *NAWU Magazine*, 9 (February, 1920), 6.

61   'The Lord Derby War Hospital', *Truth*, 87 (February, 1920), 235–6.

62   'The Mental Hospital Scandal', *Truth*, 87 (February, 1920), 183–5; 183.

63   D. Gittins, *Madness in Its Place: Narratives of Severalls Hospital 1913–1997* (London, 1998), pp. 21–4 and pp. 48–9.

64   R. D. Laing, *Wisdom, Madness and Folly: The Making of a Psychiatrist 1927–1957* (1985: London, 1986), p 116.

65 J. Kitzinger, 'A sociology of media power: key issues in audience reception research', in G. Philo (ed.), *Message Received: Glasgow Media Group Research 1993–1998* (Harlow, 1999), pp. 3–20.

66 On distinctions between pauper lunatics and ex-servicemen who suffered from mental disorder, see F. Reid, 'Distinguishing between shell-shocked veterans and pauper lunatics: the Ex-Services' Welfare Society and mentally wounded veterans after the Great War', *War in History*, 14 (2007), 347–71.

67 For a detailed account of the relationship between women workers and the trade union movement, see S. Boston, *Women Workers and the Trade Unions* (London, 1980), especially pp. 96–184.

68 *NAWU Magazine*, 2 (May, 1913), 9.

69 *NAWU Magazine*, 19 (September, 1930), 5.

70 *Mental Health Services Journal*, 31 (November–December, 1942), 23.

71 *MHIWU Journal*, 26 (November, 1936), 11.

72 'The Medico-Psychological Association', 127.

73 *Health Services Journal*, 1 (January, 1948), 10.

74 *Health Services Journal*, 12 (July–August, 1959), 23.

75 These articles mainly concerned escapes and attempted escapes from the institution, such as 'Four Rampton patients caught: window bar cut to aid escape', *The Times* (22 December 1958), p. 4. In one incident, the two escaped men were found guilty of assault and robbery; see 'Rampton men accused: "intent to murder"', *The Times* (23 January 1957), p. 5, and 'Prison sentences on Rampton men: judge's concern with protecting the public', *The Times* (5 March 1957), p. 5. In 1958, it was reported that a nurse had been assaulted; see 'Ministry statement on Rampton incident: "no question of mass break-out attempt"', *The Times* (21 May 1958), p. 7. In 1963, however, a student nurse was alleged to have assisted a patient to escape; see 'Rampton escape aided by nurse', *The Times* (10 August 1963), p. 4.

76 *Health Services Journal*, 12 (July–August, 1959), 46.

77 Discussed in the previous chapter.

78 Dingwall, Rafferty and Webster, *The Social History of Nursing*, p. 139.

79 Correspondence from E. Buck and W. D. Chanbelen, *Health Services Journal*, 14 (March–April, 1961), 21–2.

80 *Health Services Journal*, 14 (July–August, 1961), 2.

81 *Health Services Journal*, 16 (July–August, 1963), 2.

82 *Health Services Journal*, 14 (September–October, 1961), 8.

83 'Wards where dangers lurk', *Daily Record* (23 June 1965), p. 9.

84 MRC COHSE Archive, MSS.292/6/C/CO/10/1, 'Nurses "knocked about"', *Birmingham Post* (27 June 1965).

85 COHSE Archive, MSS.292/6/C/CO/10/1.

86 COHSE Archive, MSS.292/6/C/CO/10/1, 'Much ado about sex says Ross', *Aberdeen Press and Journal* (26 June 1965). Peyton Place was a reference to the 1956 novel, 1957 film adaptation and 1960s television series with sexual themes.

87 See G. Smith, 'Tyranny over the unloved old', *The Times* (3 July 1967), p. 8; 'Mental nurse to go after inquiry', *The Times* (4 November 1967), p. 3.

88 B. Robb, *Sans Everything: A Case to Answer* (London, 1967), p. xiv.

89 M. Osbaldeston, 'Nobody wants to know', in ibid., pp. 13–18; p. 13.

90 C. H. Rolph, 'Cruelty in the old people's ward', in ibid., pp. 3–7; p. 5.

91 'Hospitals cleared of cruelty', *The Times* (10 July 1968), p. 1.

92 'Mental hospitals staff defended: "witch hunt atmosphere"', *The Times* (20 June 1968), p. 3.

93 'Mental nurses demoralized by conditions', *The Times*, (19 October 1970), p. 4.

94 Showalter, *The Female Malady*, p. 249.

95 See, for example, M. Muijen, 'Scare in the community: Britain in moral panic', in T. Heller, J. Reynolds, R. Gomm, R. Muston and S. Pattison (eds), *Mental Health Matters: A Reader* (Houndmills, 1996), pp. 143–55.

96 See D. Mitchell, 'Parallel stigma? Nurses and people with learning disabilities', *British Journal of Learning Disabilities*, 28 (2000), 78–81.

5

'THE PERSONAL TOUCH': VOLUNTARISM, THE PUBLIC AND MENTAL ILLNESS

Moving from professional narratives and asylum care towards the community, this chapter explores the interactions of voluntary, professional and state action in the field of mental health throughout the period 1870 to 1970. While a range of voluntary organisations were active in the field of mental health by the second half of the twentieth century, this chapter focuses on the MACA: the only association in this sector whose history spans the entire period under study.[1] This long, unbroken chronology offers an unrivalled opportunity to explore how it affected, and was in turn affected by, other agents in the field of mental health, illuminating the interconnections between state provision, healthcare professionals, patients, the public and voluntarism. Engaging with a broader literature on the role of voluntary organisations in the twentieth century, this chapter demonstrates how professional groups worked through the Association to advance their objectives. Moreover, the strategies adopted by the MACA in different eras can be contextualising by drawing a comparison to the path taken by the NAMH, utilising the literature generated on the history of this organisation.[2]

Dependent upon public support to continue its activities, the MACA retained a role within the network of service provision by adapting to shifts in state policy, generating images of mental illness for public consumption at odds with the dominant paradigm. In the late nineteenth and early twentieth centuries, the Association pioneered convalescent care and acted as an employment bureau, helping former patients bridge the gap between the asylum and the community. While many psychiatrists in this era viewed mental illness as an incurable hereditary condition, the Association elicited support from the public for this work by depicting its clients as suffering from a curable condition brought about by social strain. In the 1950s when biomedical psychiatric promoted the view that mental illness was curable, the Association

reconfigured its service to provide long-term support for people who experienced enduring mental health problems. However, despite the Association's emphasis on the personal touch, MACA personnel portrayed their clients as objects of philanthropy rather than equals.

Voluntarism, the state and mental illness

While professional groups in the field of mental healthcare frequently stated that the public should be enlightened about mental illness and its treatment, their attempts to secure this state of affairs were pursued alongside their efforts to secure their professional objectives. However, voluntary groups established to provide services to those who suffered from mental health problems, or to combat public prejudice against such people, appear initially to be unencumbered by such considerations. Established solely to meet their objectives and operating independently of the state, charitable groups exemplify the principles of the public sphere, seeking to achieve what they believed to be in the public interest – or so one might assume.

However, closer examination of the composition of voluntary groups and their interactions with public bodies and the state belie many of these suppositions. Indeed, recent literature has stressed the interaction of voluntary and statutory bodies in the provision of welfare services, undercutting the idea of a disinterested voluntary sector which acted outside the aegis of the state. Thus, Jane Lewis dismissed a narrative which views the emergence of the welfare state as the culmination of a shift from individualism to collectivism, insisting that Britain has 'always had a mixed economy of welfare, in which the state, the voluntary sector, the family and the market have played different parts at different points in time'.[3] Such a perspective is now widely accepted, and in a recent review of the literature Bernard Harris took the relationship between the state and the voluntary sector as axiomatic, focusing his analysis on the ways in which this relationship has changed over time.[4] Thus, in the nineteenth century, poverty and its relief was a major preoccupation for both the state and charities, and local authorities often provided funds to support charitable institutions. However, Harris argued, the activities of the two sectors assumed a distinctive character; voluntary groups were more likely to focus their efforts on the relief of poverty emanating from exceptional circumstances.[5]

Similarly, one cannot presume that charitable activities dwindled as state involvement in welfare provisions expanded in the early years of the twentieth century. As the frontiers of state activities moved, Geoffrey Finlayson argued, 'the frontiers of voluntarism also moved'. Yet, he insisted, the balance between the voluntary sector and the state shifted in favour of the state, prompting many voluntary groups to shift their agendas 'towards the state . . . seeing the state as a source of funds, or as providing a basic service, leaving them to develop a more specialized role'.[6] While public bodies distributed funding to voluntary agencies to provide services on their behalf, some individuals active in the voluntary sector expressed their belief that the function of the voluntary sector was to pioneer new services until such time as the state accepted responsibility for these services.[7] Following the inauguration of the NHS, the relationship between the state and the voluntary sector underwent further permutations. Seeking to implement comprehensive, nationwide provision, the government claimed both the responsibilities and the costs for delivering the new services. In these circumstances, a number of voluntary groups continued to specialise in providing services which fell outside the remit of state provisions. However, in its report of the future of voluntary organisations in 1978, the Wolfenden Committee identified new trends within the sector, including the emergence of mutual-help groups and the development of pressure groups.[8]

This framework helps us to analyse and contextualise the work undertaken by the MACA. Established in 1879 as 'The After-care Association for Poor and Friendless Female Convalescents on Leaving Asylums for the Insane', the MACA was the first association established to assist those affected by mental disorder and embodied many of the preoccupations which shaped charitable aid in this era.[9] It emerged during a period of extensive philanthropic activity, in part a response to the depression of the late nineteenth century that generated high unemployment, low wages and social unrest. That many of these problems were met through philanthropic aid and localised provision rather than centralised state services was not accidental. It reflected the value placed by Victorian society on a citizenship of contribution, a concept which provided an outlet for the expression of religious faith through philanthropy. This concept of citizenship sought to promote social harmony in an unequal society by emphasising people's social interdependence and offered middle-class women opportunities to participate in the public sphere.[10] Viewing poverty as a failing of the individual to support himself or herself, those distributing aid nevertheless distinguished between the deserving poor, whose misfortunes stemmed from factors outside of their control, and the undeserving poor. Philanthropic bodies such as the Charity Organisation Society set about their work with the aim of enabling clients to support themselves.[11] Yet, while the Charity Organisation Society ostensibly subscribed to the principle that assistance should be offered only to the deserving poor, it found such distinctions to be difficult to police in practice.[12]

A brief examination of early leading figures within the MACA reveals that many had acquired considerable expertise of different aspects of mental illness and its treatment before joining the Association. The Reverend Henry Hawkins, founder of MACA, had begun work as an asylum chaplain in 1859 and when he formed the MACA was serving as chaplain of Colney Hatch Asylum, a post he held until his retirement in 1900.[13] The parliamentary reformer Lord Shaftesbury, who served as President from 1880 until his death in 1885, secured the passing of the 1845 Lunatics Act and served as a Lunacy Commissioner.[14] In 1886, the Association appointed Dr Daniel Hack Tuke, a respected figure within the profession, as chair of its newly constituted council. Hack Tuke was a great-grandson of the founder of the York Retreat, an institution associated with pioneering moral therapy. Although he never worked as an asylum superintendent, he was elected President of the Medico-Psychological Association in 1881, served as a co-editor of the *JMS* from 1880 and, with John Charles Bucknill, co-authored the *Manual of Psychological Medicine*, which was first published in 1858.[15] Following Shaftesbury's death, the Association persuaded the philanthropist Lord Brabazon, Earl of Meath, to act as President and, in the same year, the Association employed its first paid Secretary, Mr H. Thornhill Roxby, to recruit local lady visitors to inspect clients.[16]

The MACA provided convalescent homes for women discharged as recovered from asylums who might otherwise have nowhere else to go, and assisted former asylum patients in finding employment so as to save them from the workhouse and prevent a possible recurrence of their disorder. It expanded its work to include men in 1894, and in 1904 it established branches outside the London area. In these early years, the MACA successfully attracted the interest and participation of asylum medical superintendents and Poor Law guardians in its work. It also numbered many clergymen and lady philanthropists amongst its membership.

In 1914, the MACA extended its work to incorporate patients 'on trial' from asylums who had not officially recovered. In the following year, Miss Ethel Vickers replaced H. Thornhill Roxby as Secretary of the Association, retaining this position until her resignation in 1940. Vickers's appointment appears to have had a significant impact on the extent of the MACA's work. From forty-one individuals assisted in 1887, the annual number of applications rose to 373 in 1914, a figure that had remained stable since 1907. After Vickers replaced Thornhill Roxby, the number of individuals helped rose rapidly. Thus, the Association considered 508 individual cases in 1916, 944 in 1922, 1,936 in 1927 and 4,269 in 1938. Following Vickers's retirement, annual caseloads fell to 2,509 within two years.[17] Examination of surviving case files reveal that Vickers played an active role in these, and in 1931 the Council paid tribute to Vickers's contribution: 'She *is* the Association: the two are synonymous terms . . . Could all those she has helped and established present themselves, the square outside would not hold them.'[18] The expansion of the MACA's activities can also in part be attributed to the largesse of the industrialist Sir Charles Wakefield, Lord Mayor of London between 1915 and 1916, President of the Bethlem Royal Hospital and MACA's President from 1920 to 1940, who donated significant sums of his own money to the Association.[19] London County Council's interest in the services provided by the Association and its willingness to fund the MACA to provide care for some of its patients also contributed to the expanding caseload work.[20]

While the MACA had been the first voluntary body established in the field of mental health, other groups were founded in the early twentieth century: the Central Association for Mental Welfare (founded 1913), the National Council for Mental Hygiene (established 1922) and the Child Guidance Council (formed 1927). As the agendas of these groups expanded, the services each offered began to overlap. In 1937, the Feversham Committee on the voluntary mental health services, whose membership was drawn from government bodies, local authorities, voluntary bodies and medical professionals, sought to bring together the work of these four charities and remove inefficient duplications. It urged local authorities to co-ordinate voluntary and statutory mental health services within their area so as to ensure that voluntary bodies could undertake extra-mural work not covered by state services, and to consider paying voluntary bodies to provide such services.[21] Priscilla Norman, who spent much of her life working voluntarily for mental health issues, recollected in her autobiography that negotiations were fraught with antagonism, fuelled by 'dear Evelyn Fox's explosive temperament'. Fox, the Secretary of the Central Association for Mental Welfare, observed Norman, 'saw things clearly from her point of view, but the three other organisations saw this move as a swallowing up of their identities by this dynamic personality'.[22] However, Fox was by no means the only impediment to a unified voluntary mental health sector; the MACA had little inclination to relinquish its independence or personalised service, and dissented from the recommendations of the 1939 Feversham Report, while the remaining three charities formally amalgamated in 1946 to form the NAMH, with Lord Feversham, chair of the Committee which had recommended the merger, serving as the first Chairman.[23] That year, the MACA annual report unambiguously stated the Association's independence.[24]

The approach adopted by the newly formed NAMH, meanwhile, continued to reflect the mental hygiene ethos which had characterised its founding organisations. As we saw in Chapters 2 and 3, the mental hygiene movement relied upon emerging professional groups such as psychiatric social workers to help achieve its objective of preventive mental healthcare. While the MACA focused on providing personalised services to individuals who had experienced mental illness, the NAMH sought to educate the public about mental health. In so doing, its objectives were twofold: to alleviate the stigma attached to mental illness, and to help promote mental health and prevent mental illness.[25] To meet its educational objectives, the NAMH organised courses for health and education professionals, arranged mental health exhibitions, published books, pamphlets and a journal, held an annual conference and monitored coverage of mental health in films. The NAMH also continued to operate a number of services established by its founding bodies, including agricultural hostels for men diagnosed as mentally handicapped; holiday homes for individuals diagnosed as mentally defective and for mental hospital inmates; convalescent homes; a home for 'pre-delinquent' children and a home for old people.[26]

The death of Sir Charles Wakefield and the retirement of Ethel Vickers in 1940 ushered in a new group of long-serving officers, helping to maintain continuity in the MACA. Princess Arthur of Connaught served as President until 1949, succeeded in 1958 by the Duchess of Kent who also served as Patron for the NAMH. The Duchess continued to work for the MACA until her death in 1965. Miss Russell, a PSW who had been appointed Assistant Secretary in 1936, took over from Vickers in 1940 and stayed in office until her retirement in 1960, when her position was filled by Mrs E. Clifton. Russell was awarded the MBE in 1953. Dr Henry Yellowlees was also an influential figure in the Association, serving as Chairman of the Council from 1938 to 1956. Yellowlees authored a book for the general public on psychiatry, which is discussed in Chapter 1, and his involvement in the MACA doubtless stemmed from his desire to educate the public about mental health matters.[27]

In 1948, the MACA chose not to change its direction in response to the inauguration of the NHS, arguing that 'the new Acts have barely survived their birth, and it is therefore impossible to state with any accuracy how widespread the changes will ultimately become'.[28] However, in 1954 Yellowlees acknowledged that better state provisions for former hospital patients and the unemployed rendered many of the charities' activities obsolete and suggested more work should be undertaken with elderly, chronic patients.[29] In the 1960s, the Association began to call vocally for many more hospital patients to be cared for in the community. By the end of the 1960s, the MACA struggled to keep their homes open as maintenance grants from local authorities for patients in the Association's care failed to increase in proportion to running costs. The scope of this chapter is not sufficient to cover the change in direction made by the Association in the 1980s.[30]

Creating and publicising a 'suitable case' for aid

Publicity was an integral dimension of the MACA's work as it required funds to support its activities. An examination of the publicity produced by the MACA thus offers some insight into the MACA's perceptions of the public and the representations of mental illness it felt would elicit support, while allowing us to examine whether the MACA's representations of the deserving charitable case drew upon a common philanthropic language. From its inception in 1879 though to the 1920s, the MACA courted public support through case studies published in its annual reports. Each report described between ten and twenty individuals helped by the MACA, detailing the individual's gender, age, family background, institutional history, help given by the Association and the outcome of the case. One subscriber commented in 1887, 'the list of cases read to us from the report is in itself the most efficient plea that the charity can put forward for the sympathy and support of the public with this movement'.[31] These vignettes drew together a series of interconnected ideas: the vulnerability of friendless but respectable women; the desirability of restoring people to their rightful place in society as wage earners and the financial savings which could be reaped by supporting the MACA's work. A counter-discourse characterised a small proportion of cases, which depicted individuals with flawed personalities who required the charity's guidance and control.

Outlining the Association's work and aims, Thornhill Roxby described the women helped by the MACA as 'governesses, highly educated ladies, quite destitute, for whom the workhouse surroundings are very unsuitable'.[32] The plight of governesses often featured in the Association's annual reports, as for example, in 1893 when the Association described the case of 'a governess, daughter of an officer who is now dead; high qualifications. Was in a London Asylum. Grant of money made through the Charity Organisation Society who knew the case to be thoroughly deserving.'[33] The emphasis placed by the MACA on the plight of the governess may appear disproportionate if we consider Joseph Melling's findings that only twelve amongst more than two thousand women admitted to the Devon County Asylum between 1845 and 1914 were governesses.[34] However, the MACA's focus on vulnerable respectable women, in particular the figure of the respectable governess fallen on hard times, may have helped the Association to attract contributions and indicates why the majority of the subscribers were women, for, as F. K. Prochaska has argued, women preferred to contribute to causes that helped with 'pregnancies, children, servants and the problem of ageing and distressed females'.[35] The figure of the Victorian governess generated concern because of her marginal position on the edge of respectable society. She was a decent woman reduced to paid work, often an unmarried young woman in a sexually vulnerable position away from the protection of her family.[36] Governesses relied upon social connections to secure positions and, as Joseph Melling has observed, their relatives thus viewed admittance to an asylum as a last resort which would significantly inhibit future employment prospects.[37]

At a time when poverty was increasingly attributed to degeneration, the MACA took care to differentiate its clients from the perceived social residuum.[38] It thus represented its cases as respectable and deserving individuals, attributing their breakdowns to social pressures as opposed to hereditary flaws. In so doing, the MACA differentiated its clientele from individuals labelled as feeble-minded, constituted in this period as an ominous eugenic threat.[39] A case printed in the first report, for example, attributed mental breakdown to a social cause and concluded in suitable employment: 'A most respectable girl. Became ill through worry and deprivation in helping her father – a small tradesman who lost his capital. Is now in service in a house of a member of the committee.'[40] Another case in the same report described a 'very highly educated lady, quite destitute. Assisted by a gift of clothing. Has obtained situation as a governess.'[41] These cases typified the MACA's rhetoric, depicting respectable but destitute women whom the Association enabled to support themselves. Thornhill Roxby emphasised this aim, arguing 'it is so important to enable these saddest of sad cases to once more take their places among the workers of the world'.[42] More than 80 per cent of the 481 case studies printed in the annual reports between 1897 and 1914 concluded with the helped individual obtaining work.[43]

Council members involved in the MACA in the late nineteenth century were anxious to demarcate the individuals they helped from chronic asylum patients. In the annual report of 1888, the MACA claimed that some applicants had been declined as 'they would never be fit for the struggle of life again'.[44] The psychiatrist G. H. Savage reinforced this point at the annual meeting when he raised the spectre of the chronic patient, asking 'how often one ought to help a patient who had broken down more than once'. Those who suffered from 'recurrent insanity', Savage suggested, should be bypassed 'in favour of sufferers who were of a more hopeful character'.[45] Savage resigned his post as physician superintendent at Bethlem Royal Hospital in this year to focus on private practice, and professional considerations doubtless sparked his desire to distinguish between the hereditarily insane and potential clients whose disturbance could be ascribed to environmental or social cases.[46] Other doctors present at the meeting contested Savage's views. Calling for asylums to be renamed 'Brain Hospitals', Dr E. White claimed that many of the cases helped by the MACA had broken down through no fault of their own and insisted that mental illness should be viewed in the same way as any other illness.[47]

These discussions paralleled the debate amongst psychiatrists discussed in Chapter 3 as to whether a change in the law enabling incipient cases of mental disorder to be treated outside the asylum was desirable, or whether this would reinforce the stigma of the asylum, illustrating how the voluntary sector could serve as a forum for airing professional concerns. Nevertheless, Savage's sentiments were also expressed by lay personnel within the MACA; Thornhill Roxby, for example, insisted at an early meeting that the Association 'took no cases where recovery was not certain'.[48] Notwithstanding such assurances, descriptions of respectable cases assisted back into employment co-existed in the Association's publicity materials alongside cases in which the Association had attempted to reform the personality of the individual through 'befriending', suggesting that the MACA considered some of its clients to be impaired. This ideology bears comparison to that of the Charity Organisation Society, which urged its visitors to befriend those they visited and to use these personal relationships to build character, in the belief that recipients would squander any alms received if they lacked will and character.[49] In this vein, a 1901 newspaper report of the MACA's work claimed that the former asylum inmate 'cannot be trusted all at once to take up his former interests and anxieties without their effect upon his intellect being watched less any sign of irregularity should betray itself';[50] while, in the following year, Thornhill Roxby described many former patients as 'poor and friendless, and with peculiarities in appearance and habits, weak in judgement and needing help in life'.[51] One case from the MACA's 1887 report described 'a young woman from one of the metropolitan asylums. Very badly brought up; was placed in service by the Association, after having been in a cottage home. But did not give satisfaction. Was placed in a training home by the Association where it is hoped she may in time become useful.'[52] Similarly, a case from 1917 related 'another striking example of personal influence', describing a young woman who, prior to committal to an asylum, 'had been four times in prison with a very bad record. This girl, after weeks of patient endeavour, responded to the better influence brought to bear . . . she has voluntarily undertaken the support of her child . . . her situation is down in the south, away from her unsuitable friends.'[53]

It is difficult to ascertain from the brief vignettes published within the annual reports how MACA personnel interacted with their clients. However, we can gain some insight into this matter by examining the MACA's case files, in which the accounts of convalescent home owners, relatives, employers and clients compete to define events and negotiate the course of action to be taken.[54] Alice T.'s file stretches over nine years, commencing with Alice's reception into a convalescent home in 1915 where the homeowner, Mrs Balls, conveyed Alice's views to MACA Secretary Miss Vickers, who oversaw the case.[55] Alice, like many other MACA clients, was placed in domestic service, a field of work which remained a major employer of women in the interwar years but which was perceived to lack the appeal of other sectors of the female labour market.[56] She doubtless benefited from the wartime labour market, which opened up more opportunities in the domestic service field as other women took work in the industrial sector.[57] Her first placement was unsuccessful, but Miss Vickers conceded to another potential employer that this might not have been Alice's fault. The MACA then secured work for Alice in a boarding house, a position she chose to leave, as she did not enjoy the post. Her employer, however, had a favourable opinion, stating 'I only wish I could have kept her, she seems a very good maid and thorough'. Miss Vickers then placed Alice in February 1917 with Mrs B., but the situation had deteriorated by March, when Mrs B. informed Miss Vickers that Alice was 'off her head'. In April, Mrs B. readmitted Alice – who had seemed depressed and threatened to jump out of a window – to Colney Hatch Asylum. Aggrieved at the inconvenience Alice's problems had caused her ('it has been a very unpleasant experience for me'), Mrs B. appeared indifferent to the fate of her former servant, grumbling to Miss Vickers that 'it has been too much expense for my poor pocket'.

While in the asylum, Alice received a letter from Miss Vickers which conveyed sympathy for Alice's plight and best wishes for her recovery. In response, Alice expressed her wish to 'get out and earn my own living again which I am so longing to do . . . I am sure there is plenty of work for women now.' This mentality appealed to the MACA, which received Alice on her discharge in October 1918 before placing her with Mrs Q. In just over a month, this placement broke down; Mrs Q. complained that Alice was 'defiant and rude', and demanded her removal. She insisted that Alice's lack of skills in domestic service was to blame, but Alice believed that the problem stemmed from Mrs Q.'s inability to accept that she had recovered. Mrs Q., she protested, 'treats me as if I am silly and a lunatic . . . I have told her I am supposed to be free now.' A neighbour of Mrs Q. suggested that Mrs Q.'s refusal to pay Alice prompted the dispute. This latter piece of evidence indicates that Mrs Q. may have hoped to profit from Alice's status as a former asylum patient to gain cut-price labour, suggesting that at least some individuals who employed MACA clients were inspired by a desire to fill gaps in their household as cheaply as possible, rather than by any philanthropic impulse. Certainly, neither Mrs B. nor Mrs Q. appears to have accepted the MACA's rhetoric that it assisted cases who had recovered, treating Alice with suspicion. Alice's case ended on a positive note when she was employed by Mrs Marriott, who gave money to the Association and had 'no objection taking a girl who had mental troubles'.

The case notes focused on the employment of Alice, and Miss Vickers's efforts to encourage Alice to stay in her positions. While Alice was involved in decisions about her case, MACA personnel at times adopted a condescending attitude. In 1919, MACA worker Miss Wheatley described thirty-one-year-old Alice as 'quite a nice girl' although 'just lately has proved herself rather tiresome' to one potential employer. While this rather infantilising description doubtless in part reflected the class distinctions between the Association's staff and volunteers and those it assisted, it also contrasts with the image of the respectable and recovered client depicted in the Association's printed reports, evoking instead the belief that discharged patients needed to be watched and guided. Admittedly, Alice T.'s case file is one of only a handful to have survived from this era and it is thus impossible to vouch for its representativeness; nevertheless, the surviving cases do suggest that the neat closure achieved in the printed case studies of the Association's annual reports was rather deceptive.

In its efforts to resettle patients into social and economic life, the MACA's work could be viewed as a natural extension of the functions of the asylum, which also sought to enable its patients to take their place in society. Indeed, Stephen Soanes has observed how the MACA's founder Henry Hawkins sought to enlist the support of asylum superintendents by implying that the MACA's convalescent facilities helped the recovering patient safely bridge the gap between the therapeutic asylum and full participation in social and economic life, without sinking into the social residuum.[58] This attempt to form a collaborative relationship between the asylum and the MACA parallels the more pessimistic 'productive alliance' Peter Bartlett has identified which operated between the asylum and the Poor Law. Bartlett argues that the asylum was viewed primarily as a Poor Law institution, containing members of the 'social residuum' whose insanity was instigated by alcoholism or immorality. In this view, mental disorder was caused by a collusion of social factors and personality weakness and the asylum's function was to reform the personality of the patient.[59] The emphasis placed by the MACA in its publicity upon restoring its clients to employment suggests that one factor which motivated the Association may have been a desire to instil discipline into an unproductive workforce.

The MACA may not have been able to demonstrate that all its clients were highly respectable workers who had broken down through no fault of their own. However, it did publicise its ability to place unproductive people into employment, thus saving the local authorities money. From the outset, the Council of the MACA included Poor Law guardians and in 1890 the MACA sought to persuade more guardians to join on the grounds that 'much mutual good may be arrived at by co-operation between public and private bodies whose work is to benefit the poor'.[60] Taking practical steps to foster such collaboration, the MACA wrote to boards of guardians in England and Wales in 1898, asking for information on cases discharged from asylums to workhouses which might benefit from the MACA's services. By 1916, twenty-four boards of guardians provided an annual subscription to the MACA. A 1930s pamphlet urged donations from 'those who understand that patients helped and tided over this critical period of their life are a real economy to the community'.[61] This example illustrates how the MACA interacted with state bodies such as Poor Law agencies, a trend that accelerated through the Association's life.[62]

While the MACA had been established to assist recovered mental patients, it targeted its publicity to attract funding and support from different audiences. Consequently, it did not always portray itself as primarily representing the interests of ex-patients and those suffering from mental illness. The variety of concerns represented by the Association, such as the costs of maintaining paupers, the desire to raise the status of the psychiatric profession, notions of religious duty and the opportunity for women to exercise power, illustrate that even charitable organisations ostensibly concerned with public interest might fulfil a range of private interests too.[63]

State intervention and its impact on voluntary organisations

Reflecting on changes wrought in the field of welfare by the expansion of state provision at the 1954 annual general meeting of the MACA, the Chairman Henry Yellowlees remarked that 'it is now quite unthinkable that a patient should be turned out from a public mental hospital nominally recovered but weak in body and confused in mind, without friends, without money, without employment, without adequate equipment and clothing, and with only this charity to befriend him'.[64] Government agencies, Yellowlees remarked, now undertook many of the functions formerly the preserve of the MACA. Thus, labour exchanges and disablement resettlement officers now – in theory – found work for former patients,[65] while PSWs and almoners visited patients in hospital and once they had returned home.

The foundation of the NAMH in 1946 had been prompted in part by the formation of the welfare state which had fundamentally altered the context in which charities operated, prompting voluntary groups to rethink their functions. Yellowlees now proposed that the MACA should likewise alter the direction of its work and change its clientele in order to maintain its relevance. He argued that the Association's work with convalescent patients met with little need. Pointing to the 'great increase in the number of harmless and quiet chronic patients, owing to the success of modern treatments in at least removing violent, noisy and aggressive symptoms in cases where full recovery is impossible', Yellowlees reasoned that the Association could retain its original objectives by changing course, suggesting that 'if by caring for a chronic patient we are setting free accommodation for a recoverable one, we are surely acting in accordance with the spirit of our original constitution'.[66] By providing extra-mural care for long-stay hospital patients, the MACA's work in many respects anticipated the later shift towards community care in the 1960s and 1970s.

At first glance, Yellowlees's proposal appears to mark a dramatic rupture with the MACA's earlier work. However, the Association had started to diversify its work some years earlier. In 1924, the MACA began to provide convalescence for 'early' care clients: individuals who were ill but had not yet been certified. As discussed in Chapter 3, the treatment of this cohort had long been a subject of debate amongst psychiatrists, many believing that such patients were best treated outside the asylum. In 1933, MACA visitors started to act as social workers in hospitals, though this area of work began to decline in the late 1930s as the numbers of qualified PSWs started to increase. In the same year, the Association began to board out London County Council patients defined as 'chronic cases' who needed supervision to cope with life outside of hospital. These patients made up 101 cases in 1936 and 446 by 1940, a figure that remained stable up until 1970. From 1935, the MACA started to provide holidays for patients not well enough to leave hospital. In 1938 1,174 such individuals were helped, but the numbers quickly fell as the MACA decided to give preference to providing places for those patients leaving hospital who required permanent care. As Stephen Soanes notes, these developments in the 1930s stemmed in part from new legislation which changed the MACA's income streams. Boards of guardians, who had hitherto subscribed to the MACA, were disbanded as the Poor Law fell into obsolescence following the 1929 Local Government Act, while the 1930 Mental Treatment Act, which empowered local authorities to fund the MACA for the provision of convalescence, prompted London County Council to subscribe to the MACA in return for the delivery of new services.[67]

Similarly, the new direction announced in 1954 alerts us to the intersections of the state and the voluntary sphere, illustrating once more how the MACA's provisions were sensitive to, and entwined with, shifts in state policy and financial support. Moreover, the MACA was not the only voluntary group in the field of mental health to diversify its provisions. In the interwar years, the Central Association for Mental Welfare, for example, expanded its activities to provide holiday homes for mental hospital patients, while the Guardianship Society established an after-care committee.[68] Notwithstanding the MACA's claims to provide a distinctive function – a claim which it used to justify its decision not to merge into the NAMH – these developments point to overlaps within the voluntary sector for mental health.

Reorienting its services towards chronic patients gave the MACA a renewed and distinctive purpose. However, it necessitated a rethink of the publicity strategy, as the MACA could no longer sell its work on the strength of the number of people returned to economically productive employment. While the MACA had not hitherto flinched from discussing some of its more challenging cases in its publicity material, these had been interspersed with examples of model respectable cases. As Chapter 3 illustrated, the optimism of postwar psychiatry had been achieved largely by highlighting promising acute cases which responded to treatment, and concealing the plight of chronic patients. The MACA's new direction thus raised potential pitfalls, for, as Yellowlees acknowledged, 'nobody pretends that work for chronic patients is anything like so interesting or spectacular as work with convalescent or recoverable cases'.[69] Case studies printed in the annual report, such as that of A. G., emphasise this shift in focus. A. G. had been admitted to a mental hospital in 1950 and first began to take holidays with the MACA in 1960. In 1964, the MACA arranged to take over his long-term care from the hospital. 'He is . . . unlikely ever to be independent', the MACA reported, 'but gradually widening his interests'.[70]

How did the MACA's perceptions of its cases change in the postwar era, as it began to reorient its services towards chronic patients? We can begin to address this question by turning to the records of a long-stay home for elderly and chronic female patients which the MACA operated between 1948 and 1962. Within this file, the MACA social worker Miss C. (who was responsible for visiting four MACA homes) offered her perspective on the residents and the homeowners Mrs M. and Miss H., both qualified mental nurses.[71] The file confirms that the MACA had indeed begun to cater for a different client group. Of the twenty-six women resident on 5 November 1953, only six were under sixty years of age and eleven were over seventy years old. The descriptions given of these women do not refer to their medical condition with the exception of four women (all under sixty) who were referred to as MD (mentally deficient). Instead, Miss C. discussed the work carried out in the house by the women and sketched out her view of their personalities. She described Celia, for example, as a 'champion grumbler, arthritis etc. does nothing', and characterised Gwen as 'self-satisfied. Does some polishing'. Seventy-six-year-old Alice was simply described as 'old and miserable beyond description'. Although no register exists for this home in the archive, a register for a comparable home for chronic male patients indicates the diagnostic categories of residents catered for by the MACA at this time: chronic melancholia, paraphrenia, schizophrenia, anxiety neurosis and inadequate personality.[72] The deciding factor for selecting individuals to send to this home may have rested less on their medical diagnosis and more upon how 'well behaved' patients were. As the first social worker to the home explained in November 1948, 'both Mrs M. and Miss H. are inclined to be a bit difficult about the type of patient they have and do not seem to have much patience with difficult ones'.

The atmosphere in this particular home did not appear to be a particularly happy one. On 1 September 1954, Miss C. visited to find the patients 'sitting in separate and faintly hostile groups. The garden looked lovely and several patients said what a nice place it was but the people in it were not nice, although the matrons were and so on.' Both matrons, Miss C. observed, 'seem to have very quick tempers; they seem to get furious about quite small things'. 'I do think they both think they are running the home very well and that their methods are the right ones', Miss C noted:

> They make no secret of shouting at patients when naughty and even say it would be better if social workers gave them a good scolding too instead of appearing so sympathetic. Certainly about half the patients do seem contented: these of course are the 'good' ones who help a bit in the house or are genuinely incapable, or are just silly and thick skinned.

This account suggests that some MACA staff continued to view their clients as naughty children. One might speculate that the matrons had acquired this attitude while working in mental hospitals, where high patient numbers and a shortage of doctors fostered a disciplinary and hierarchical environment.[73] If so, it once again illustrates how professional practices permeated the practices of the voluntary sector. In July 1953, Miss C. reported that the matrons used 'shouting when angry and threatening return to hospital – they say it is the only thing to do'. Similarly, in August 1959 the matrons remarked to Miss C. that 'Mrs W. was much better since they had told her she would have to make her own arrangements if she did not improve'. The matrons' attitude towards the residents appears to have coloured the attitudes of the residents to one another. In January 1953, Miss C. saw ten of the patients privately and 'all thought all the other patients were too mental for them and each was evidently the only sensible one there in her own estimation'. Here we might observe how each resident's insistence on her own sanity, a form of self-presentation which she achieved by emphasising the craziness of her fellow residents, correlated with the narrative strategies adopted by former patients in their published memoirs, discussed in Chapter 1. The matrons' attitude also seems to have affected Miss C.'s judgement. In October 1955 she noted that the patients 'all think they should not be in this place "with this lot", and I have now taken to telling them almost as bluntly as Miss H., that they are all here for the same reason'.

Perhaps the matrons found working with chronic and elderly patients unrewarding, as the residents rarely seem to have displayed their appreciation or demonstrated an improvement in their medical condition. This challenge would face psychiatric nurses a decade later, as younger patients were discharged from hospital following the shift towards community care.[74] In March 1953, Miss C. wrote, 'they have a great many defectives and senile patients . . . a lot of the patients have to be helped in the bath, few of them seem to have any "life" in them and they do not seem to appreciate what is done for them'. In the instances where some improvement was evident, the matrons seem to have been very pleased. In August 1959, Miss C. reported how one resident returned from a weekend with a friend saying, '"it's so nice to be home again". Matrons were compensated for all sorts of disappointments by this compliment.'

Despite the radically altered clientele of the Association and the expectation that residents of the home would never be self-supporting, many older criteria for assessment, such as character, work and usefulness remained in currency. These assessments also drew on typical representations of femininity, focusing upon the attention individual women paid to their appearance and their willingness to undertake domestic chores. Correspondingly, researchers assessing the clinical conditions of long-stay female patients in mental hospitals in this era studiously noted the minutiae of patients' make-up, hairstyle, weight and dress.[75] When considering the closure of the homes, Miss C. described Isabel as 'very clean, tidy and presentable, indeed quite pleasant in appearance . . . Works quite hard and willingly cleaning stairs and passages etc . . . definitely useful.' Alice, meanwhile, was regarded as a success for a chronic patient:

> Has taken about two years to pull round since admission from depression, diffidence, lack of initiative, inability to make up mind, but is now a nice, friendly, quietly helpful, reliable person . . . She is clean, tidy, and dresses nicely, helps a bit in things like wiping the dishes, and also is reliable in taking messages, keeping an eye on a patient in bed or other socially useful things.

As a result of the MACA's decision to care for the chronically impaired, the Association increasingly chose to represent itself as providing a sanctuary or haven for those who would never recover sufficiently to be self-supporting.

This theme was teased out in an interview conducted for publicity purposes in the late 1970s with Annie, a MACA resident since 1951:

Interviewer – Do you feel that this place represents something very valuable?
A. – Oh I'm sure it does . . .
Interviewer – Not only to you but to others.
A. – I'm sure it does, it's a haven really, really is.
Interviewer – Could you say again, it's a haven really, yes this is a valuable place.
A. – It really is, it's quite a haven really
Interviewer – Could you make that into a statement without me talking?
A. – Well, I think it's valuable for people to be in a place like this, because it's quite a haven, it has been to me.[76]

By representing MACA homes as a haven, the Association sought to differentiate itself from the service provided by the state. A 1968 appeal on ATV claimed 'there are many remaining in mental hospitals only because there are not enough homes and hostels where, with sympathy and skilled support, they can be helped to regain their self-respect and confidence in their own ability to live happy normal lives'.[77] The MACA managed to preserve a thread of continuity in its ideology by retaining a focus on the importance of the personal touch, or 'befriending', which it argued differentiated its services from those provided by the NHS. Henry Yellowlees made this point forcefully in 1954 when he announced the change in the Association's clientele, insisting that the MACA remained unique because its work demanded 'personal contact with individual patients'.[78] Dr T. P. Rees, Superintendent of Warlingham Park Hospital and an advocate of liberalising the regime of psychiatric hospitals, made the same point in 1961. Rees stressed the unique role that could be played by a charity outside of the state, speaking of 'the great advantage of the human touch which characterises the voluntary association'.[79] Equally, the MACA could lay claim to innovating new approaches to mental illness, a point made by neurologist Sir Russell Brain when he addressed the MACA's annual meeting in 1955:

You were pioneers when you first came into existence and you have the opportunity of maintaining the pioneer spirit still. A voluntary Association has a power of initiative and flexibility which the state most inevitably lacks. You can think of new ideas and try them out and then, if they are successful, persuade the state to adopt them, as, indeed, you have done in the past.[80]

In 1962, NAMH chairman Lord Feversham credited the NAMH and the MACA for bringing about the government policy of community care. It was after all at a NAMH annual meeting in 1961 that Health Minister Enoch Powell first unveiled government proposals to close down the mental hospitals – the 'water towers' speech discussed in Chapter 3. The two charities, Lord Feversham argued, 'had preached that the only people who should be in mental hospitals should be those requiring hospital treatment', and in his view the state was now 'promoting the idea, which the MACA was the first to conceive, that all who could should leave the hospitals and live and work in the community'.[81] Certainly this is one interpretation, although it could be argued that MACA homes provided what Powell sought to abolish – long-term care for people who struggled to live independently. Indeed, Powell may have favoured the MACA's work because their homes provided a convenient repository for long-stay patients who needed to be discharged from psychiatric hospitals if hospital closures were to be achieved. He was certainly happy to acknowledge the MACA's role as pioneers in community care. At the official opening of a MACA home at Croydon in 1961, Powell stated that he 'regarded the hostel as something symbolic and as an early example of coming developments in the health service'. Voluntary organisations, he insisted, 'were not being used by officials to save trouble and expense, but to give "that something extra" . . . This is part of the benefit of the intermingling of the official and unofficial. It is no criticism of the official to say that sometimes the others can do something as well, if not a little better, as the official.'[82] In turn, the MACA Chairman Mr W. King described Powell as 'a man who had seen a vision and was now seeking to make it a reality. He had removed many of the old fashioned and forbidding hospitals.'[83] There were, however, limitations to this co-operation between the MACA and the state. By the end of the 1960s, the MACA found it increasingly difficult to maintain its homes as maintenance grants from local authorities for patients failed to increase in proportion to running costs.

If we turn to the NAMH, the other organisation accredited for inspiring the policy of community care, similar financial problems are evident in this era. In its report for 1964–1965, the NAMH stated that its expenditure had outstripped income for the second year running, by £3,162: in the previous year the deficit had been £10,417. This deficit, it explained, had arisen in part because the Ministry of Health had reduced the grant it gave to the NAMH.[84] Connecting its financial difficulties to state policy, the NAMH arranged its conference that year on the theme 'The Price of Mental Health'. The report drew upon statistics to emphasise the economic and human costs of mental illness, and the disjuncture between the extent of the problem posed to the country by mental ill-health and the resources allocated by the government to resolve such problems. Thus, the report noted that, in terms of human costs, over 5,000 people in England and Wales committed suicide every year and 40,000 attempted it, while, on the economic front, nearly 28 million working days were lost each year through mental disorder. Yet, while nearly half the hospital beds in the country were occupied by mental patients, the Medical Research Council spent only 8 per cent of its budget on research into mental disorder. These inequalities filtered down to the care that patients received in hospital. While the net in-patient cost per week in an acute (non-teaching) hospital was £33 6s 4d, the sum expended per patient per week in a mental hospital and a subnormality hospital was £10 9s 5d and £9 1s 8d respectively.[85] Thus, while Powell was happy to credit the voluntary sector for pioneering new approaches, and ostensibly claimed to value the services these charities provided, this may have been a tactic to exploit charitable provision, saving trouble and expenditure.

Lord Feversham's support for the government policy of community care might appear to indicate a new desire in the NAMH to engage with state policy. Yet a close link with the state had been forged from the very inception of the NAMH. The Association had, after all, come into existence at the prompting of a government committee, whose Chair – Lord Feversham – subsequently became the first Chair of the NAMH. In this vein, Nick Crossley argued that the NAMH was 'a political creation whose status as a voluntary rather than a statutory organisation was blurred to say the least', pointing to the NAMH's reliance on central government funding, the shared message of public education which the NAMH and the state collaborated to undertake, and the role played by NAMH's Chairman Lord Feversham in parliamentary debates on mental health legislation, most notably the 1959 Mental Health Act.[86] Crossley observed how public education, which underpinned the mental hygienist discourse that informed the NAMH, gained a new significance for MPs as they considered how the proposed shift to community provisions envisaged by the 1959 Act could be accomplished without greater public tolerance.[87] However, by the end of the 1960s the NAMH began to express a more critical view of government policy. In 1971, NAMH's Chair Christopher Mayhew launched the new 'MIND' campaign; the NAMH's new first objective was to 'create concern for mental health and to challenge apathy and neglect'.[88] Mayhew, a serving Labour MP who defected to the Liberal Party in 1974, had presented part of the BBC's first television series of mental health issues a decade earlier; this is discussed in the next chapter.[89] The campaign critiqued not only an apathetic public but an apathetic government too. It sought to 'place the whole question of mental health in the forefront of national politics; to stimulate citizen participation in the mental health services at a local level . . . We shall question the quality of community care, that beautiful, empty phrase . . . Public opinion must be rallied to the cause.'[90] In 1972, NAMH rebranded itself as MIND and shortly thereafter opened a legal and welfare department which sought reforms to the very piece of legislation it had campaigned to enact just over a decade previously – the 1959 Mental Health Act.[91]

The new direction adopted by MIND can be viewed within the broader context outlined at the beginning of this chapter: the growth of pressure groups in the postwar era. Within the field of mental health, MIND's reconfiguration was influenced by the anti-psychiatry movement.[92] NAMH had displayed an interest in some of the ideas expressed by those identified as leading figures within the anti-psychiatry movement, reviewing key works within its journal *Mental Health* and inviting R. D. Laing to address its 1966 annual conference. However, throughout the 1960s the NAMH remained largely in alliance with the psychiatric profession. Indeed, as Nick Crossley has noted, anti-psychiatry had a more indirect impact upon the NAMH. The upsurge of anti-psychiatry was embraced by Scientologists, who could now situate their pre-existing critique of psychiatry within a broader cultural vein. Believing the NAMH to be in cahoots with psychiatrists, Scientologists launched a series of legal challenges against the NAMH. In 1969, Scientologists adopted a different tack, seeking to infiltrate and take over NAMH by joining the Association en masse, a strategy which the NAMH managed to curb by forcing those Scientologists who had joined to resign their membership.

Crossley argues that the new course adopted by MIND in the 1970s reflected its desire to refresh its image in the wake of the scientology debacle and elicit donations from a public audience which viewed its work as old-fashioned. In this sense, a more direct connection can be hypothesised between MIND's agenda and the anti-psychiatry movement. As Colin Jones has identified, proponents of anti-psychiatry made few novel observations regarding mental illness and its treatment; it was not the message which was significant but the way it was delivered and the audience it was directed at. In short, anti-psychiatry resonated with more widely articulated cultural concerns, and can thus be viewed as both emanating from, and in turn informing, the culture of the 1960s.[93] So the financial problems experienced by the NAMH could be attributed to a new cultural climate in which the NAMH's objectives seemed old-fashioned, although the decline in state funding, as opposed to declining contributions from the public, appears to have lain at the heart of NAMH's financial problems. Jonathan Toms advances a different interpretation, attributing MIND's adoption of a patients' rights strategy not to financial considerations but to a concept of mental health which crystallized in the 1960s, characterized by emotional well-being. Stemming from the development of the therapeutic community, this approach stressed the importance of healthy interpersonal relationships as a means of securing mental health, leading to a rejection of authoritarian efforts to mould behaviour which had informed the mental hygiene movement.[94]

Intriguingly, despite MIND's ostensible shift towards a patients' rights agenda, the charity's Chairman Christopher Mayhew recalled his profound discomfort in the company of patients, who, in his view, had 'much to ask and little to give'. Mayhew had visited prisoners, who he had found 'outgoing, communicative and sometimes very funny'. He also enjoyed the company of psychiatrists and nurses, admiring 'their patience and cheerfulness, and their cool familiarity with the uglier sides of insanity – hostility, incontinence, sometimes violence'. Mental patients, however, left him 'feeling drained' and emptied his 'reserves of compassion'.[95] Mayhew's observations rather call into question the extent to which MIND officials embraced their new agenda. MIND displayed a similar ambivalence when faced with the incipient service user movement. When staff and patients at the Paddington Day Hospital went on strike in 1971 to protest against proposals to introduce conventional therapeutic approaches in places of the therapeutic community approach then operating,[96] MIND organised a press conference to support the cause. MIND did not, however invite patients involved in the protest to the press conference and, although it agreed to the request to admit the patients, it did not give the patients an opportunity to participate.[97]

A 'social' approach

At the MACA's AGM in 1948, the Secretary Miss Russell, a qualified PSW, 'stated that the MACA is the oldest organised body concerned with psychiatric social work'.[98] Russell, alongside Kathleen Laurie, a trained PSW hired as the Association's employment officer between 1939 and 1940, appears to have introduced the Association to theories current among the psychiatric social work profession, many of which focused on the social factors believed to affect mental disorder. While seeking to identify antecedents to their profession in the history of the MACA, both women also sought to integrate approaches from their professional training within the MACA's practices. Thus, Laurie echoed themes which had long characterised MACA objectives, noting in a report of her work that it would 'show a saving of Government money' and would help in 're-establishing people in normal life'.[99] Yet her approach was also informed by her belief that work itself could both cause mental distress and facilitate recovery. Laurie believed that an individual placed in the wrong job could experience dissatisfaction and frustration. Skilled workers placed in an undemanding position would lose interest and be less effective than an unskilled worker, who in turn would struggle if placed into a job which they lacked the capacity to fulfil. Either scenario, Laurie argued, could lead to a loss of confidence, emotional or intellectual dissatisfaction and maladjustment. These ideas had been formulated in the fields of industrial welfare and industrial psychology by practitioners concerned that the deskilling of labour entailed by new production methods and mechanisation led employees to view employment as simply a necessary means to obtain money for satisfactions outside of work.[100]

Earlier MACA workers had stressed the advantages of finding 'suitable work' for its clients. Laurie developed this idea further, suggesting that an 'employment history' be taken to establish the 'psychological motive' behind the individual's breakdown and to uncover where difficulties in employment arose in the past.[101] Arguing that *recovery and yet a certain impairment are not incompatible*', Laurie addressed a longstanding contradiction within the MACA as to whether its clients were fully recovered or required surveillance. Claiming that a person could be taught to deal with their delusions, she outlined a scenario in which an individual might have 'quite a dangerous or stupid attitude to one person (possibly his wife) and towards no one else. One such man is a good works foreman and is a reliable worker, but at all costs he must be kept away from his wife. His judgement on everything else in life is utterly sane and sound. To his wife he is still really dangerous.'[102]

Laurie then created a social treatment plan which took account of any remaining symptoms and sought to remove any aggravating conditions, for example by placing people whose home environment was hostile into a residential post. However, notwithstanding Laurie's preoccupation with the impact different types of work could have on mental health, certain continuities can be detected. For example, Laurie perpetuated the MACA tradition of equating recovery from mental illness with gainful employment. Moreover, she placed 220 of the 285 women she helped into domestic work. This may, in part, have pragmatically reflected difficulties encountered in securing work for women in other sectors during the interwar depression, but it does bring the novelty of Laurie's approach into question.

Laurie's activities in the field of employment typified the type of interventions which the MACA specialised in, summarised by the Association in 1953 when it commented that its work 'begins and ends outside the hospital precincts . . . efforts are concentrated on getting the patient back to normal living conditions after medical treatment or on preventing the necessity for treatment'.[103] However, the MACA's insistence that it confined its work to social care rather than medical treatment was a little disingenuous given its belief that the mental hospital was not the most appropriate locus of care for many patients. In its 1950 annual report, the MACA presaged the direction it subsequently adopted:

An Association professing to care for patients outside hospital, naturally asks itself how many of these patients could it suitably provide with other accommodation? Of a total number of 132,000 mental hospital patients, it has been estimated that 16 per cent could be adequately cared for in homes other than mental hospitals. This means that 21,000 beds are being taken up in hospital unnecessarily.[104]

Matrons and wardens had long played an influential role in the Association, providing care for convalescent cases boarded out by the Association. In the wake of the MACA's decision to provide care to chronic patients within the community, these individuals continued to play a significant role in delivering the Association's work, acting as the main point of contact between the MACA and its clientele and thus embodying the 'personal touch' which the MACA claimed distinguished its work. In 1959, the Chairman commented that the matrons and wardens 'have the immediate care and guidance of the patients for whose welfare the Association exists. It was not too much to say that the fate of the patients is largely in their hands.'[105] Social workers employed by the MACA served as intermediaries between the Association, its matrons and wardens and its clientele. Their role could prove rather fraught when dealing with matrons who owned their homes, and might not always take kindly to intervention. Miss H. and Mrs M., whose residential home was discussed earlier in the chapter, viewed their home as their private property and resented suggestions as to how they should manage their patients. In March 1953, the matrons threatened not to take any more MACA patients and in October 1954 they wrote to Miss C. complaining that she had strayed into their private quarters on a visit to their house. Miss C. had no success in trying to moderate the matrons' rather disciplinarian attitude towards the patients.[106]

By 1967, the MACA owned ten homes of its own and employed registered mental nurses to act as matrons and wardens. These homes provided places for 247 patients, outnumbering the MACA's provision for patients in privately owned homes. The MACA cited the retirement of previous matrons, new regulations affecting the running of registered homes for the mentally disturbed and the unsuitable location of many previous homes that had been far from centres of employment and out-patient clinics as reasons for this change in policy.[107] However, perhaps it also hoped to gain more control over the running of the homes by employing the matrons and wardens. The MACA sought to encourage interaction between the community and the residents in its new homes, claiming in its 1966 report that 'there have been many acts of kindness on the part of local residents'.[108] Quite how successful this integration with the community was is not clear. Local opposition surfaced in Thanet in 1976 when the Council enforced the closure of a number of homes. In some instances, the Council claimed that the homes failed to meet fire safety stand-ards. However, the Council insisted that other homes should close because they were in the 'holiday zone', complaining of 'the problems created by the influx of ex-mental patients into Thanet'. The matron of one of the homes blamed local opposition for the closures.[109]

While the MACA developed community provisions to meet the needs of long-stay patients, arguably it continued to view and treat its clientele as suf-fering from a medical disorder and did not fully engage with the ideas of social psychiatry, let alone anti-psychiatry, in the 1960s – although any attempt to do so would doubtless have been circumvented to some degree by the mindsets of the matrons and wardens who managed the MACA's homes. Addressing the MACA's annual general meeting in 1969, Dr Ross Mitchell, who had been appointed as a consultant psychiatrist at Fulbourn Hospital in Cambridge in 1966, urged the MACA to abandon the illness model of mental disorder and expand the field of its work into social therapy. Under the leadership of Dr David Clark, Fulbourn Hospital adopted social therapies and the therapeutic community approach in the 1950s and 1960s. Mitchell helped enact these changes, implementing a rehabilitation programme in the Hospital's long-stay wards.[110] Mental aftercare, he observed, was 'based on the "illness model" of mental disorder'. However, the social model of mental illness hypothesised that mental disorders arose out of the interaction between individuals. 'When we move out of the "mental illness model" to the "social model"', he explained to his audience, 'organisations like your own are faced with the challenge of par-ticipating away from tertiary care and into the exciting field of primary care'.[111]

Not 'educating the public'

As a voluntary organisation, the MACA relied upon public support to con-tinue and expand its work. It was thus obliged to depict its work in a favour-able manner and as a consequence promote certain messages about mental disorder to the public. However, while believing that the public should be educated to hold a more enlightened view of mental disorder, the MACA did not see itself as the right organisation to do this, observing in its 1946 annual report that its activities were 'purely of a practical nature'.[112] This stood in marked contrast to the objectives of the NAMH, which believed that public ignorance of available treatments created stigma and unnecessarily delayed therapy, leading to more incurable illness. It focused on promoting mental health through public education and saw itself as 'standing midway between the statutory services and the lay public', acting as a bridge between the state and the public.[113] Nick Crossley argues that the Association in its early years sought to impose its beliefs upon others using social power rather than discussion, framing their ideas as incontestable fact.[114]

As discussed earlier, the MACA relied heavily on its annual reports as its main form of publicity during the late nineteenth century and the first two decades of the twentieth century. The records of its propaganda committee, established in 1921 and operative until 1929,[115] provide further insights into the MACA's publicity strategy and its perceptions of the public. These records reveal how the Association targeted specific groups, fostering the flattering idea that its supporters were more enlightened than the general public regarding the problems posed by mental illness and the value of the MACA's work. Thus, appeals directed at churchgoers inferred that helping the mentally afflicted was a religious duty, while campaigns directed at people who subscribed to other charities emphasised that the MACA was a unique charity catering for people unable to defend themselves. The MACA targeted those with direct connections to asylum patients: healthcare workers and those with a friend or family member receiving treatment in an asylum. Eliciting support from boards of guardians, the MACA emphasised its value for money. It also approached large business such as Lloyds and the Stock Exchange for support, sending letters to the press and rotary clubs.[116] This was a rational option for the MACA prior to the introduction of the NHS, as the Association could argue that their work helped maintain a stable workforce and thus saved businesses and industry money.[117] The MACA reiterated these themes in other publicity materials, which throughout the 1930s combined humanitarian arguments with an emphasis on the cost-effective nature of its work. Thus, the cover of one pamphlet proclaimed in large, bold type, 'ADMINISTRATIVE EXPENSES ONLY 8.08%'.[118]

Above all, MACA publicity in the early to mid-twentieth century was dominated by the message that having a mental illness was so stigmatising that it had to be concealed. Consequently, those who had recovered were unable to talk about their experiences, thus necessitating intervention from a third party. Extracts from speeches made at the AGM in 1919, for example, claimed that the MACA:

> Does work for those who cannot ask for themselves, and their disabilities are of a kind which we cannot advertise. These people have to seek the help of an asylum, and you can quite understand that, when they are recovered and fit to go out again, they rather shrink from anybody knowing they ever had an illness which necessitated their being sent off.[119]

How did reforms in mental healthcare in the interwar years, discussed in Chapter 3, impact upon the MACA? A letter sent by the MACA Treasurer to

The Times in 1938 illustrates that the MACA was not removed from the tensions and ambiguities of mental healthcare reform which in practice tended to distinguish between promising acute cases and chronic cases. Initially, the letter embraced the main tenets of mental health reform, suggesting that new physical therapies and the provision for voluntary admissions to mental hospitals under the 1930 Mental Treatment Act would destigmatise mental disorder. Contradictions began to surface when attitudes towards certification came under consideration. At the beginning of the letter, the Treasurer argued that certification should no longer be viewed as a shameful process, attacking 'the fear of the mentally afflicted which, except for those very few persons who are members of mental hospital visiting committees, and medical officers, undoubtedly is present in ordinary people; only gradually is certification ceasing to be a stigma upon the family history'. However, the next statement, which sought to promote early treatment for incipient mental illness, suggested ambiguously that certification was still viewed as stigmatising: 'How many are there who are aware that the Mental Treatment Act provides for admission to mental hospitals without certification, thus avoiding stigma, if stigma there be?' A similar tension emerged when the Treasurer emphasised the favourable treatment given to new and promising patients in separate accommodation, 'divorced as far as possible from the main institution'. The letters serves as a reminder that, while the MACA focused on the provision of care outside the walls of the asylum, its work was profoundly influenced by what took place within those walls.[120]

From 1944, the MACA began to use radio broadcasts to publicise its cause to the charitable public. In the first broadcast, MACA's Chairman Henry Yellowlees related the story of MACA home residents in Luton who had been taught to carry out some of the processes for a war factory. Reiterating a well-worn theme, Yellowlees insisted that the MACA's clients, who had 'struggled out of the dark shadows of mental disease', were capable of productivity and usefulness if provided with the opportunity. 'Once they realise . . . that they can still be of use', he argued, 'their self-respect returns in a flash and they hold up their heads once more'.[121] This traditional MACA theme of helping former patients back into a socially useful and economically productive place in the community resonated during wartime, particularly as the plight of soliders disabled in combat heightened awareness of the need for rehabilitation and sheltered work.[122] The appeal raised £1,363 4s 9d.

A 1955 appeal emphasised the continuities between the Association's current work and the aims of the original founder of the MACA.[123] In this broadcast, Yellowlees explained how the Reverend Henry Hawkins 'said that something *must* be done to befriend and re-equip ex-patients, to give them convalescent care, and thus ease and hasten their return to completely renewed usefulness and regained happiness'. 'Today', Yellowlees claimed, 'we take convalescent patients from mental hospitals and bridge the gap between discharge from hospital and full normal activity in the outside world'. The broadcast also reiterated the emphasis placed on befriending: 'we rehabilitate – or to use our founder's simpler word, we befriend – sufferers from the saddest of all human ills', and Yellowlees summarised the MACA's work though the Bible phrase 'Beauty for ashes, the oil of joy for mourning, the garment of praise for the spirit of heaviness'. The appeal focused on individuals who had recovered from mental disorder, but also described the MACA's work with people suffering from chronic mental disorder. A 1961 appeal broadcast revisited familiar ground, describing people affected by mental illness as 'victims of the saddest ill which afflicts mankind – the malady of the mind'.[124]

A 1968 ATV television appeal marked a radical break with earlier radio broadcasts.[125] The appeal did not use biblical texts or pleas to help the 'mentally afflicted', although the broadcast was produced by the religious programmes department. Instead, the appeal used statistics to create a series of mental illness 'facts' and 'risks' that affected everyone, an approach which characterises contemporary anti-stigma campaigns such as Time to Change. The title of the appeal, 'One in Five', referred to the number of families thought to be affected by mental illness at some stage. A flyer for the programme listed this figure alongside the number of women and men who would at some stage be committed to a mental hospital (one in nine and one in fourteen respectively) and the statistic that psychiatric patients took up 47 per cent of all hospital beds. Everyone, the Association suggested to its audience, was at risk from mental illness. Deviating from earlier appeals which had implied that sufferers of mental illness were too stigmatised to speak for themselves, a MACA client was enlisted to take part in a discussion to help the appeal. Yet continuity with earlier themes persisted: the final programme featured images of four MACA cases at work – a clerk, a typist, a waitress and an assembler at an engineering works. In so doing, it harked back to the emphasis upon employment which characterised the case studies printed in the Association's annual reports from the nineteenth century.[126] The appeal claimed that 'these people have in common the fact that they have received treatment, have recovered and are now working again with the supportive and understanding care that our hostels provide'. A new element within the appeal was the suggestion that chronic patients should receive care in community homes to help them 'regain their self-respect and confidence in their own ability to lead happy normal lives'.

Conclusion

While organisations like the Medico-Psychological Association, the mental nurses' Union and the APSW were established primarily to advance the interests of mental healthcare professions, the MACA was formed to advance the interests of the discharged mental patient. It is thus tempting to view charities such as the MACA as ideal public spheres; formed from private individuals voluntarily trying to do what is in the common good. Yet it is difficult to substantiate this idea when the operation of voluntary organisations are examined for, as Steve Sturdy has argued, charities frequently 'conformed only poorly to . . . ideals of inclusiveness, transparency and formal equality', and were often 'appropriated and privatised by particular interest groups intent on self-advancement and the pursuit of social influence'.[127] Moreover, as historians of voluntarism have demonstrated, an examination of the operation of charities over the course of the twentieth century reveals how charitable operations and state operations became enmeshed, and the MACA was by no means exempt from this trajectory.

One could conclude, therefore, that this analysis demonstrates how the interpenetration of voluntarism and the state debased the public sphere and allowed private interest to insidiously gain a stranglehold, inhibiting democratic participation and bearing out Jürgen Habermas's influential critique.[128] Yet, examining the co-operation of voluntary bodies with the state in the twentieth century, Geoffrey Finlayson offered a different perspective, arguing that voluntary organisations released energies that might otherwise have remained dormant. Such organisations, he argued, offered people the opportunity to participate in the public sphere and public policy free from the constraints of compulsion, at a time when they had little access to formal political structures. This enabled participants to become actively involved citizens instead of merely being entitled to services whose organisation they were excluded from. Pointing to the vibrancy of voluntary bodies in the interwar years and their capacity to adapt to changing circumstances, Helen McCarthy and Pat Thane argue that voluntary groups' capacity to engender social and political change should not be underestimated.[129] We might, perhaps, then argue that the interaction of the state and the public sphere, represented here by the MACA, facilitated democratic debate and the participation of private individuals for the common good, engendering new ideas about mental illness and its treatment.[130] In annual meetings, MACA members debated the issues surrounding mental illness. These debates were replicated on smaller, localised scales in the interactions between MACA staff, MACA clients, employers, homeowners, subscribers, local residents and social workers.

However for most of the period under study, the very people whose interests were most affected by these debates continued to be represented as child-like patients: entitled to receive, but not to participate or contribute their own opinion, except when manipulated for publicity purposes. In part, this reflected MACA's view that mental illness was so stigmatising and so discrediting that it had to be concealed at all costs, necessitating advocacy from a third party.

The MACA viewed the problems it sought to resolve as private and personal, not public and national, and this remit shaped its engagement with the public. Its appeals for help frequently castigated public ignorance and prejudice towards mental disorder, but did not seek to tackle this stigma, as the MACA did not share the NAMH's interest in educating the public. The MACA, however, relied on donations from the public to support its work. Thus, while the plight of those it helped may well have motivated MACA members, they often alluded to other interests and concerns which could be served by donating to the MACA. Pamphlets in the 1930s, for example, balanced the social benefit gained by the individuals helped with the utilitarian benefits of supporting a cost-effective Association that kept its clients away from public support. From the Association's inception though to the 1968 ATV 'One in Five' campaign, the MACA equated recovery with gainful employment, suggesting that their work could transform unproductive people into industrious citizens who would not burden state resources.

As a charitable organisation operating in an era of increasing government intervention in social affairs, the MACA had not only to interact with state provisions but to differentiate its services from those provided by the government so as to justify its continued operation. In order to survive, the MACA chose to adapt, and, in so doing, it inaugurated provisions which the government later hailed as a precursor to its own policies; these findings resonate with McCarthy and Thane's argument regarding the role of voluntary bodies in driving social and political change.[131] The representations put forward by the Association about the nature of mental illness were designed to promote the services that the Association offered at any point in time, and this led the MACA to invert dominant representations of mental illness. In the late nineteenth century, when mental disorder was frequently depicted by medical practitioners as hereditary, chronic and incurable, the MACA portrayed its clients as suffering from a curable condition brought about by social strain. In attempting to decrease the stigma of the voluntary or early case patient, the MACA may have worsened the stigma attached to chronic mental illness. Yet in the mid-twentieth century, when psychiatrists increasingly represented mental disorder as a curable illness from which individuals could recover and resume their place within the community, the MACA began to publicise the image of the chronically ill individual who would need permanent care, albeit outside of the hospital.

For most of the period under study, the MACA sought to generate a sense of continuity in its provisions by grafting new directions on to its traditional ideologies of befriending and the 'personal touch', linking appeals for help to notions of religious duty towards the mentally afflicted sufferer. In 1968, when the government had embraced the policy of community care but had slashed the funding it provided to voluntary groups providing community services, the MACA changed tack, creating a campaign for ATV that was based not on the figure of the friendless isolated and voiceless victim of mental disorder but on statistics. This suggested that mental health and ill health posed a risk and responsibility to everyone, a message which continued to underpin current anti-stigma campaigns. Moreover, the MACA no longer sought to speak on behalf of the mentally ill and represent their interests to the public, but enabled some MACA clients to share their perspectives and experiences, and represent their own interests.

Notes

1 Now operating under the name 'Together'.
2 The archives of NAMH (later known as MIND) were inaccessible to researchers at the time of writing.
3 J. Lewis, *The Voluntary Sector, the State and Social Work in Britain: The Charity Organisation Society Family Welfare Association Since 1869* (Aldershot, 1995), p. 3.
4 B. Harris, 'Voluntary action and the state in historical perspective', *Voluntary Sector Review*, 1 (2010), 25–40.
5 Ibid., 27–8.
6 G. Finlayson, 'A moving frontier: voluntarism and the state in British social welfare 1911–1949', *Twentieth Century British History*, 1 (1990), 183–206; 204.
7 Harris, 'Voluntary action', 33.
8 Ibid., 35.
9 For a brief overview of the Association, see J. Smith, 'Forging the "missing link": the significance of the Mental After Care Association archive', *History of Psychiatry*, 8 (1997), 407–20; for a longer history commissioned by the Association, see S. Strong, *Community Care in the Making: A History of MACA 1879–2000* (London, 2000). See also V. Long, 'The Mental After Care Association: Public Representations of Mental Illness, 1879–1925' (MA thesis, University of Warwick, 2000).
10 See G. Finlayson, *Citizen, State, and Social Welfare in Britain, 1830–1990* (Oxford, 1994); B. Harris, *The Origins of the Welfare State: Social Welfare in England and Wales, 1800–1945* (Basingstoke, 2004), pp. 59–75.

11   See A. W. Vincent, 'The Poor Law reports of 1909 and the social theory of the Charity Organisation Society', *Victorian Studies*, 27 (1984), 343–63.

12   See Lewis, *The Voluntary Sector*, p. 11.

13   Together, 'Henry Hawkins: Founder of Together', www.together-uk.org/uploads/pdf/history/henryhawkins.pdf, accessed 08 November 2011.

14   See K. Jones, *Asylums and After. A Revised History of the Mental Health Services: From the Early 18th Century to the 1990s* (London, 1993), pp. 78–92.

15   A. Digby, 'Tuke, Daniel Hack (1827–1895)', *Oxford Dictionary of National Biography*, Oxford University Press, 2004: www.oxforddnb.com/view/article/27804, accessed 15 November 2011.

16   Brabazon was a prominent philanthropist who also served as Honorary Secretary of the Hospital Saturday fund. See J. Springhall, 'Brabazon, Reginald, twelfth earl of Meath (1841–1929)', *Oxford Dictionary of National Biography*, Oxford University Press, 2004; online edition, January 2011: www.oxforddnb.com/view/article/32019.

17   Other factors such as the outbreak of the Second World War and the formation of the NAMH also had an impact.

18   Wellcome Library, MACA Archive, SA/MAC/B.1/43, 'The MACA Annual Report 1931', p. 7. Emphasis in original text. The titles of the report varied as the name of the organisation underwent small changes, but I have standardised references to 'The MACA Annual Report'.

19   T. A. B. Corley, 'Wakefield, Charles Cheers, first Viscount Wakefield (1859–1941)', *Oxford Dictionary of National Biography*, Oxford University Press, 2004; online edition, January 2011: www.oxforddnb.com/view/article/36679.

20   Jones, *Asylums and After*, pp. 127–8.

21   'Voluntary mental health services: the Feversham Committee's Report', *British Medical Journal*, 2:4099 (1939), 239–41.

22   P. Norman, *In the Way of Understanding – Part of a Life: Lantern Slides in a Rough Time Sequence* (Godalming, 1982), pp. 63–4. Evelyn Fox was Secretary of the Central Association for Mental Welfare.

23   See S. Soanes, 'Rest and Restitution: Mental Convalescence and the English Public Mental Hospital, 1919–1939' (PhD Thesis, University of Warwick, 2011), pp. 261–4.

24   MACA Archive, SA/MAC/B.1/58, 'The MACA Annual Report 1946', p. 3.

25   See N. Crossley, *Contesting Psychiatry: Social Movements in Mental Health* (Abingdon, 2006), pp. 69–90.

26   Ibid., pp. 79–84.

27   H. Yellowlees, *To Define True Madness: Commonsense Psychiatry for Lay People* (1953; Harmondsworth, 1955).

28   MACA Archive, SA/MAC/B.1/60, 'The MACA Annual Report 1948', p. 2.

29   MACA Archive, SA/MAC/B.1/66, 'The MACA Annual Report 1954', pp. 6–9.

30   For a brief overview of these changes, see Smith, 'Forging the "Missing Link"', 418–19; Strong, *Community Care in the Making*, pp. 50–60.

31 MACA Archive, SA/MAC/B.1/2, 'The MACA Annual Report 1888–88', Miss Davenport, p. 10.

32 MACA Archive, SA/MAC/A.1/2, H. Thornhill Roxby, 'The After Care Association for Poor Female Convalescents on Leaving Asylums for the Insane', unpublished paper, p. 1.

33 MACA Archive, SA/MAC/B.1/6, 'The MACA Annual Report 1892–93', p. 9.

34 J. Melling, '"Buried alive by her friends": asylum narratives and the English governess, 1845–1914', in J. Melling and P. Dale (eds), *Mental Illness and Learning Disability since 1845: Finding a Place for Mental Disorder in the United Kingdom* (Abingdon, 2006), pp. 65–90; p. 71. Melling identified a higher proportion of governesses amongst the admissions to the fee-paying Wonford House asylum in Exeter.

35 F. K. Prochaska, *Women and Philanthropy in Nineteenth-Century England* (Oxford, 1980), p. 3

36 K. Hughes, *The Victorian Governess* (London, 1993).

37 J. Melling, 'Sex and sensibility in cultural history: the English governess and the lunatic asylum, 1845–1914', in J. Andrews and A. Digby (eds), *Sex and Seclusion, Class and Custody: Perspectives on Gender and Class in the History of British and Irish Psychiatry* (Amsterdam, 2004), pp. 177–219.

38 See G. Stedman Jones, *Outcast London: A Study in the Relationship between Classes in Victorian Society* (1971: Harmondsworth, 1992), especially pp. 281–313.

39 See M. Jackson, *The Borderland of Imbecility: Medicine, Society and the Fabrication of the Feeble Mind in Late Victorian and Edwardian England* (Manchester, 2000), pp. 144–8.

40 MACA Archive, SA/MAC/B.1/1, 'The MACA Annual Report 1887–88', p. 7.

41 Ibid.

42 Thornhill Roxby, 'The After Care Association', pp. 1, 9.

43 80 per cent of men and 87.5 per cent of women were described as having obtained work.

44 'The MACA Annual Report 1888–89', p. 4.

45 Ibid., p. 10.

46 For an overview of Savage's career and his views on the causes of mental disorder and its treatment, see J. Andrews, 'Savage, Sir George Henry (1842–1921)', *Oxford Dictionary of National Biography*, Oxford University Press, 2004; online edition, May 2007: www.oxforddnb.com/view/article/38635.

47 'The MACA Annual Report 1887–88', pp. 10–15.

48 MACA Archive, SA/MAC/H.2/2, H. Thornhill Roxby cited in unknown paper, unknown date.

49 Lewis, *The Voluntary Sector*, pp. 33–44; Vincent, 'The Poor Law reports of 1909'.

50 SA/MAC/H.2/2, Thornhill Roxby cited in unknown paper.

51 SA/MAC/H.2/2, *Guardian* (12 February 1902).

52 'The MACA Annual Report 1887–88', p. 7.

53 MACA Archive, SA/MAC/B.1/30, 'The MACA Annual Report 1917', p. 7.

54 These are discussed in more detail in Long, 'The Mental After Care Association', pp. 43–51.

55 MACA Archive, SA/MAC/G.3/34, case notes – Alice T., 1915–24.

56 For a short overview of the main sectors of women's employment in this era, see S. Todd, *Young Women, Work, and Family in England 1918–1950* (Oxford, 2005), pp. 19–53. For a recent study on domestic service in the twentieth century, see L. Delap, *Knowing Their Place: Domestic Service in Twentieth-Century Britain* (Oxford, 2011).

57 See G. Braybon, *Women Workers in the First World War* (London and New York, 1981).

58 Soanes, 'Rest and Restitution', pp. 197–9.

59 P. Bartlett, 'The asylum and the Poor Law: the productive alliance', in J. Melling and B. Forsythe (eds), *Insanity, Institutions and Society, 1800–1914: A Social History of Madness in Comparative Perspective* (London, 1999), pp. 48–64.

60 MACA Archive, SA/MAC/B.1/1, 'The MACA Annual Report 1890–91', p. 6.

61 MACA Archive, SA/MAC/H.2/1, MACA pamphlet, early 1930s. Emphasis in original text.

62 On collaboration between statutory and voluntary sectors, see Harris, 'Voluntary action'.

63 The range of motivations and interests that inspired MACA workers is discussed in more detail in Long, 'The Mental After Care Association', pp. 5–21.

64 MACA Archive, SA/MAC/B.1/66, 'The MACA Annual Report 1954', pp. 7–8.

65 Although these services struggled to assist people with mental health problems: see V. Long, 'Rethinking post-war mental health care: industrial therapy and the chronic mental patient in Britain', *Social History of Medicine*, advance access, published online 10 March 2013.

66 'The MACA Annual Report 1954', pp. 7–8.

67 Soanes, 'Rest and Restitution', p. 251.

68 Ibid., pp. 214–18.

69 'The MACA Annual Report 1954', p. 9.

70 MACA Archive, SA/MAC/B.1/76, 'The MACA Annual Report 1964', p. 12.

71 MACA Archive, SA/MAC/F.1/9, 1948–62.

72 MACA Archive, SA/MAC/F.4/15, 1948–61.

73 These characteristics were critiqued in the 1960s by advocates of the therapeutic community and critics of the mental hospital; see discussion in Chapter 3.

74 These challenges are discussed in Chapter 4.

75 See J. K. Wing and G. W. Brown, *Institutionalism and Schizophrenia: A Comparative Study of Three Mental Hospitals 1960–1968* (Cambridge, 1970), pp. 161–4.

76 MACA Archive, SA/MAC/D.3/1/8. On the basis of the date of Annie's admission to the MACA home and the length of time she is said to have spent there, this interview was probably carried out as part of the appeal given on ITV London weekend television in 1979.

77 MACA Archive, SA/MAC/D.3/1/8, notes for ATV Appeal, '1 in 5', 7 April 1968.

78 'The MACA Annual Report 1954', pp. 6–7.

79 MACA Archive, SA/MAC/B.1/73, 'The MACA Annual Report 1961', p. 8. Warlingham Park Hospital featured in the BBC's documentary series 'The Hurt Mind', discussed in Chapter 6.

80 MACA Archive, SA/MAC/B.1/67, 'The MACA Annual Report 1955', p. 7.

81 MACA Archive, SA/MAC/B.1/74, 'The MACA Annual Report 1962', p. 8.

82 MACA Archive, SA/MAC/F.5/13/17, Mr Powell, speaking at the opening of a MACA hostel in Croydon, *Croydon Advertiser* (21 April 1961).

83 Ibid.

84 Wellcome Library, Robina Addis Archive, PP/ADD/D.14, 'National Association for Mental Health: Annual Report 1964–65', p. 13.

85 Ibid., inside cover.

86 Crossley, *Contesting Psychiatry*, p. 87.

87 Ibid., pp. 85–7.

88 PP/ADD/D.14, 'MIND, Annual Review 1970–71, incorporating the Annual Report', inside cover.

89 This series, 'The Hurt Mind', is discussed in the next chapter.

90 'MIND, Annual Review 1970–71', p. 2.

91 Crossley, *Contesting Psychiatry*, pp. 136–7. In the 1990s MIND dropped the capitalisation of its name to become Mind.

92 This paragraph draws upon ibid., pp. 126–43.

93 C. Jones, 'Raising the anti: Jan Foudraine, Ronald Laing and anti-psychiatry', in M. Gijswijt-Hofstra and R. Porter (eds), *Cultures of Psychiatry and Mental Health Care in Postwar Britain and the Netherlands* (Amsterdam, 1998), pp. 283–94.

94 See J. Toms, 'Mental Hygiene to Civil Rights: MIND and the Problematic of Personhood, c.1900–c.1980' (PhD thesis, University of London, 2005).

95 C. Mayhew, *Time to Explain: An Autobiography* (London, 1987), p. 192.

96 See H. Spandler, *Asylum to Action: Paddington Day Hospital, Therapeutic Communities and Beyond* (London, 2006), pp. 39–51.

97 Discussed in Crossley, *Contesting Psychiatry*, p. 149.

98 'The MACA Annual Report 1948', p. 1.

99 K. Laurie, *Employable or Unemployable? Report on Pioneer Experimental Work Covering the Period February 6 1939 – August 1 1940* (London, 1941), p. 2. Laurie's work is discussed at length in V. Long, '"A satisfactory job is the best psychotherapist": employment and mental health, 1939–1960', in Dale and Melling (eds), *Mental Illness and Learning Disability since 1850*, pp. 179–99.

100 See V. Long, *The Rise and Fall of the Healthy Factory: The Politics of Industrial Health in Britain, 1914–60* (Basingstoke, 2011), pp. 136–43.

101 This approach appears to have borrowed from the case histories undertaken by PSWs working in mental hospitals and child guidance clinics in the 1930s.

102 Laurie, *Employable or Unemployable?*, p. 20. Emphasis in original text.

103 MACA Archive, SA/MAC/B.1/65, 'The MACA Annual Report 1953', p. 5.

104 MACA Archive, SA/MAC/B.1/62, 'The MACA Annual Report 1950', p. 3.

105 MACA Archive, SA/MAC/B.1/71, 'The MACA Annual Report 1959', p. 7.
106 SA/MAC/F.1/9.
107 MACA Archive, SA/MAC/B.1/78, 'The MACA Annual Report 1966', pp. 6–7.
108 Ibid., pp. 8, 20.
109 MACA Archive, SA/MAC/F.5/13/17, Councillor Harry Anish and homeowner
     Doris Pargeter quoted in the *Isle of Thanet Gazette* (24 September 1976).
110 See D. H. Clarke, *The Story of a Mental Hospital: Fulbourn 1858–1983* (London,
     1996), pp. 190–1; 219–20.
111 MACA Archive, SA/MAC/B.1/81, 'The MACA Annual Report 1969', pp. 6–7.
112 'The MACA Annual Report 1946', p. 2.
113 BBC WAC, Caversham, BBC WAC S322/215/1, draft evidence to the Ministry
     of Health Joint Committee of the English and Scottish Health Services Councils,
     undated.
114 N. Crossley, 'Transforming the mental health field: the early history of the
     National Association for Mental Health', *Sociology of Health and Illness*, 20
     (1998), 458–88; 464.
115 MACA Archive, SA/MAC/C.4/4, Propaganda Committee Minute Book 31
     March 1921–25 February 1929.
116 Propaganda Committee minutes, 19 January 1927.
117 David Cantor's study of the Empire Research Council's fundraising and its per-
     ception of the public examines how the Association targeted large businesses in
     the 1930s, but had to appeal to broader groups of the public after the creation
     of the NHS, when sponsorship from industrialists dwindled. See D. Cantor,
     'Representing "the public": medicine, charity and emotion in twentieth-century
     Britain', in S. Sturdy (ed.), *Medicine, Health and the Public Sphere in Britain,
     1600–2000* (London, 2002), pp. 145–68.
118 MACA Archive, SA/MAC/H.2/, MACA eight-page pamphlet from the early
     1930s.
119 MACA Archive, SA/MAC/H.2/11, 'Extracts From Speeches At The AGM 1919',
     pamphlet.
120 MACA Archive, SA/MAC/D.3/1/1/6,unpublished letter to *The Times*, sent 7
     November 1938.
121 MACA Archive, SA/MAC/B.1/ 56, BBC Appeal Broadcast made on 6 August
     1944, cited in full in 'The MACA Annual Report 1944', p. 6, emphasis in original
     text.
122 On the provisions established for those disabled through war, see J. Anderson,
     War, Disability and Rehabilitation in Britain: 'Soul of a Nation' (Manchester,
     2011)
123 BBC Appeal, 8 May 1955, cited in 'The MACA Annual Report 1955', pp. 9–11.
124 MACA Archive, SA/MAC/D.3/1/7, appeals script for the Week's Good Cause,
     8 January 1961.
125 SA/MAC/D.3/1/8, ATV appeal, '1 in 5', 7 April 1968, flyer.
126 SA/MAC/D.3/1/8, notes for ATV Appeal, '1 in 5', 7 April 1968.

127   S. Sturdy, 'Introduction: medicine, health and the public sphere', in Sturdy (ed.), *Medicine, Health and the Public Sphere*, pp. 1–24; p. 12.

128   J. Habermas, *The Structural Transformation of the Public Sphere: An Inquiry into a Category of Bourgeois Society*, trans. T. Burger (1962; London, 1999).

129   H. McCarthy and P. Thane, 'The politics of association in industrial life', *Twentieth-Century British History*, 22 (2011), 217–29.

130   Finlayson, *Citizen, State, and Social Welfare*, see especially pp. 282–6, pp. 324–5 and pp. 401–3.

131   McCarthy and Thane, 'The politics of association'.

6

'THE PUBLIC MUST BE WOOED AND ENTICED WITH ENTERTAINMENT AND BUNS': HEALTHCARE PROFESSIONALS AND THE BBC

Anti-stigma campaigners frequently suggest that irresponsible broadcasting and newspaper coverage fuels stereotypes of the dangerous madman – a perception which Chapter 4 sought to nuance. This chapter develops these ideas, examining the role played by healthcare professionals in the production of BBC programming on mental health issues in the mid-twentieth century. The BBC's ethos of public service broadcasting enabled healthcare workers to secure a degree of influence, for the BBC sought to ensure that expert opinion informed its programmes. The records of the BBC thus provide an unparalleled opportunity to study how healthcare workers sought to destigmatise mental illness through the media, and whether these endeavours were characterised by a focus upon incipient and minor mental disturbance, at the expense of chronic mental health problems. These records also demonstrate that changes in government policy affected the BBC's willingness to cover the topic of mental illness, and that the power to shape broadcasting was distributed unevenly amongst the different interest groups within the field of mental health, with psychiatrists enjoying greater input into BBC programming.

The chapter commences by outlining debates regarding the factors which shape media coverage and the capacity of television to influence public opinion. It then turns to consider the BBC's growing interest in mental health issues, focusing on the first television show broadcast in Britain devoted to mental illness: the 1956 series 'The Hurt Mind'. This sought to reduce public fear surrounding mental illness by informing the audience of 'the facts', but in practice offered a rather one-dimensional analysis of the problems posed by mental illness which precluded debate and did little to alleviate public concerns regarding electroconvulsive therapy and psychosurgery.

Assessing contemporary media coverage, recent commentators argue that constraints within the media field militate against informative broadcasting.

Thus Pierre Bourdieu argued that demands for audience ratings, the pressure to dramatise events, time limitations and the internal circulation of information within the journalistic field all operated to stifle debate and information, transforming a potentially democratic sphere of debate and information into a site of entertainment.[1] Journalists, he complained, were not meeting public expectations; they were instead projecting 'their own inclinations and their own views'.[2] The work of the Glasgow media group suggests that such factors shaped media coverage of mental health issues.[3] Lesley Henderson, for example, argued that the constant pressure for audience ratings led many producers to prioritise entertainment over education. Seeking to depict events in a dramatic manner, documentaries on mental health issues either implied that people moved rapidly from illness to health or focused upon representing illness and crises. Networks pressurised producers to tell patients' stories through voiceover, giving the impression, as one producer grumbled, that 'these people couldn't speak for themselves'.[4]

In line with other sociological works that have stressed the capacity of audiences to resist media messages, researchers within the Glasgow media group found that on most subjects, 'personal experience was a much stronger influence on belief than media content'.[5] However, when examining media coverage of mental health issues, researchers found that this trend went into reverse: focus group respondents demonstrated an unerring capacity to reproduce media stories and frequently used the mass media as a reference point to justify or explain their opinions or beliefs.

Writing in the early and mid-1990s, the Glasgow media group believed that hostile public attitudes towards those with psychiatric disorders, arising from inaccurate media depictions linking violence and mental illness, threatened the integration of service users and the policy of community care.[6] Moreover, they argued, the stigma arising from negative portrayals of mental illness may have dissuaded people experiencing mental health problems from seeking help.[7] A similarly bleak conclusion could be drawn from Simon Cross's analysis of three television documentaries screened in the early 1990s following the transfer of responsibilities for community care to local authorities, each of which focused on schizophrenia. Cross, for example, examined how a Panorama programme on community supervision orders reinforced its message that individuals diagnosed with schizophrenia were dangerous by visualising sufferers of mental illness as dishevelled and easily identifiable madmen. In so doing, Cross argued, the programme called into question 'the wisdom of current British mental health policy in which potentially dangerous mental patients are living among us unsupervised'.[8] Similarly, 'A Place of Safety', a two-part documentary broadcast by ITV in 1993, sought to persuade viewers that hospital closures left potentially violent schizophrenics wandering round unsupervised.[9]

To what extent did the constraints of the journalistic field affect the press in earlier eras? Jürgen Habermas argued that the press evolved over the course of the eighteenth century into 'the public sphere's pre-eminent institution', facilitating rational-critical public debate which transcended commercial concerns.[10] Yet as greater political rights were enacted in the 1830s, the press relinquished its political stance to pursue commercial gains. Because technological and organisational advances in the printing of papers required more resources, papers became capitalist undertakings; 'the gate through which privileged private interests invaded the public sphere'.[11] Similarly, James Curran analysed how newspaper ownership and control fell out of the hands of the working classes as production costs rose in the 1860s and 1870s. Papers began to rely on money from advertisers for their revenue, and were in turn able to cut their cover prices. However, advertisers discriminated against left-wing publications in part because of political prejudice but also because they believed that the working classes were not sufficiently affluent to be good consumers. As newspaper ownership was conglomerated under the press barons in the 1920s and 1930s, the pressure to expand audiences led to an increase in human-interest stories believed to appeal to undifferentiated audiences, at the expense of coverage of public affairs and political events. Moreover, the framework within which most papers selected and represented stories served to depoliticise their readers. Thus Curran observed how most national newspapers portrayed the 1926 General Strike as 'a conflict between a minority and the majority', and thus 'detached strikers from their class base and obscured the true nature of the conflict'.[12]

The discussion thus far might lead to the conclusion that the pernicious characteristics of the media field identified by Bourdieu which militate against balanced coverage of mental health issues have operated consistently over a long period of time. Yet this interpretation overlooks the distinctions between different media forms or media organisations. Thus, Simon Cross has suggested that the work of the Glasgow media group tends to collapse 'all distinctions between factual and fictional representations', and thus fails to interrogate whether 'similarities in representations of mental illness are more significant than the differences arising from the particular genres and forms being employed'.[13] We should, therefore, consider the distinctiveness of the BBC. In its early years, Paddy Scannell has argued, the BBC was guided by the principle of broadcasting in the public interest and felt that it should focus on educating and enlightening the public, rather than entertaining its audience.[14] The first Director General, John Reith, hoped that the BBC might enrich democracy in Britain by offering its listeners more information from which to form their own opinion and make decisions.[15] Nevertheless, this vision of democracy was informed by certain assumptions which could conceivably inhibit its impact: namely the hope that BBC programming could improve the moral tone of its audience and bring together different classes. Moreover, the difficulties the BBC experienced in gaining independence from the government further impeded its mission. Thus in the field of health broadcasting the Ministry of Health and the Corporation were embroiled in a series of disputes in the 1930s and 1940s, as Anne Karpf has documented.[16]

Karpf suggested that programming in this period focused on health rather than medicine, pointing to the Ministry of Health's influence over BBC broadcasting. In the interwar years, the Ministry emphasised preventive health and downplayed the extent of morbidity in the population as it could not afford to implement extensive health services.[17] The BBC devoted little coverage to mental health issues in the 1930s and 1940s, in part because BBC staff believed that little effective treatment for mental illness was available. Following the general pattern of broadcasting on health issues, the few radio programmes on this subject dealt with topics relating to mental health rather than mental illness.

As the introduction to this book demonstrated, psychiatrists and other healthcare workers over the course of the nineteenth and early twentieth centuries tended to depict the public as an agglomerated mass which needed to be educated as to the correct views to hold so as to raise the status of psychiatry. In the eyes of many healthcare professionals, the malleable character of the public and its unfortunate predilection for sensationalist media coverage rendered this task virtually impossible. These frustrations surface, for example, in the presidential speech made in 1957 by R. W. Armstrong, Superintendent of Littlemore Hospital in Oxford, to the Royal Medico-Psychological Association, in which Armstrong reflected glumly on attempts to educate the public:

> All our conscientious efforts over a period of years to inform the public about our work and our psychiatric hospitals have been somewhat unrewarding. If we make painful progress with a series of carefully prepared television programmes it is only to slip further back into ignorance and prejudice as a couple of patients from Rampton make the headlines of the daily newspapers with their foolish exploits . . . The public must be wooed and enticed with entertainment and buns or they will stay away for the rather interesting reason that we have nothing very sensational in the line of padded cells or Snake Pits to show them.[18]

In many respects, Armstrong's views of the public strikingly echo similar speeches made by psychiatrists in the nineteenth century. However, by the

1950s, the impact of television and film on public opinion, alluded to here in references to the BBC series 'The Hurt Mind' (the 'series of carefully prepared television programmes') and the film *The Snakepit*, had become a matter of consideration. At the BBC, staff members began to consider whether the Corporation should begin to plan programming on mental health issues in the early 1950s, following a flood of applications from ex-patients wishing to broadcast their views. In a memorandum to colleagues, Isa Benzie, who had joined the BBC in 1927 and would later become a pivotal figure in the founding of the *Today* programme, raised the issue of how the BBC should handle programming about mental illness. 'From time to time', she noted,

> members of the medical profession let us know of their conviction that . . . we should put out talks about mental illness, particularly about the desirability of a change of attitude on the part of the public towards (a) mental illness in general and (b) voluntarily entering a mental hospital in particular . . . So far, to have not done much I think has been quite correct . . . but . . . the social climate is changing and therefore, I believe, the time has come to plan the inclusion . . . of material falling doubtless under the 'rubric' health education.[19]

The BBC's change of heart, evidenced here in Benzie's memorandum, can be attributed to the convergence of several factors: the desire of medical bodies to secure favourable publicity; an expansion of BBC programming on health issues; and recent developments in mental healthcare. We have seen throughout this book how mental healthcare workers expressed anxiety regarding their public image and sought to engender a change in attitudes. In the early to mid-1950s, the British Medical Association began to express similar anxieties. Keen to distance itself from the aura of medical politics which had coalesced in the debate over the NHS and to align itself with an image of progressive medical science, the Association began to re-orientate the function of its publicity.[20] Moreover, the recent formation of the NHS now enabled the BBC to depict a range of medical services which viewers were entitled to receive, and the Corporation consequently expanded its medical broadcasting, transmitting 'Matters of Life and Death' in 1951, 'Matters of Medicine' in 1952 and 'Thursday Clinic' in 1954 and 1956.[21] Nor did these developments exclude psychiatry. As we saw in Chapter 3, new treatment methods such as electroconvulsive therapy and lobotomy proved analogous to standard medical interventions, serving to reassert the somatic nature of mental illness. Moreover, the inclusion of mental hospitals within the NHS also promised to bring psychiatry within the rubric of general medicine.[22] Nevertheless, this was also an era in which overcrowding within psychiatric hospitals peaked, many mental hospital premises were outdated, and staff and facilities were in short supply.

Seeking a basis on which to plan future coverage, the BBC carried out audience research in 1956 to assess how receptive viewers would be to a television programme on mental illness. Three-quarters of the 180 viewers sampled distinguished between mental illness and insanity, believing the former to be caused by environmental factors and to be curable, and the latter to be the product of heredity, and to be more serious and incurable. More than half the people sampled claimed to know someone who was mentally ill while two in five had seen a film on mental illness. The sample provided a large mandate for a television programme on mental illness, although one in ten were opposed as they felt 'it would be too depressing or morbid' while another one in ten believed that such a programme 'might itself produce mental illness'.[23] These fears about the potential impact of such a programme point to a shared belief amongst medical and lay groups regarding the capacity of television to shape opinion: the psychiatrist William Sargant, for example, expressed his belief in 'the tremendous power of television for good or evil in matters of medicine'.[24] They echoed concerns surrounding the release of *The Snakepit* in British cinemas seven years earlier, when several national newspapers reported that a woman had been driven mad after seeing the film.[25]

The BBC's decision to incorporate mental illness programming into its schedules led staff members to question the purpose of such broadcasting. In general, staff felt that programming should aim to reassure the public about the treatment available within mental hospitals and destigmatise mental illness: to inform the public and correct misapprehensions, not to encourage debate. However, this position was not unproblematic. In her 1952 memo, Benzie noted that 'the branch of medicine dealing with deranged persons is in a fairly base and backward state, and I take it that it will be no part of our duty at any time to oblige persons outside by pretending things are better than they are'.[26]

Attempts to expose the 'real' conditions within mental hospitals – by implication failures and shortcomings – conflicted with the objective of destigmatising mental illness and reassuring the public. These tensions can be seen at work in the making of a regional programme on mental hospital services in Northern Ireland. Believing that conditions within mental hospitals in the region had improved significantly, the producer Diana Hyde submitted her proposal:

> One of the main problems now is the difficulty of educating the public in the matter of mental health. Ignorance on the subject is almost universal, and what knowledge there is, is largely distorted and unrelated to facts. Fears of being 'put away' and of the stigma attached to mental disorders and diseases prevent people from going forward in the early stages when cure is likely . . . films such as *The Snakepit* do great disservice by seeming to confirm the false ideas prevalent.[27]

Here we see familiar tropes: the public are portrayed as an undifferentiated mass, ignorant and unreasonably prejudiced against the mentally ill and
mental hospitals. Stigma needs to be broken down by correcting misapprehensions, and the objective is to persuade people suffering from incipient mental
disorder to seek treatment so as to prevent the onset of incurable insanity. The
difficulties facing people suffering from chronic mental health conditions, and
the challenges facing psychiatric hospitals, are not addressed. Initially, she
explained, 'I was quite convinced that the reasons for the fear and concealment
of mental illness were almost entirely due to ignorance of the facts'. However,
part way through her research for the programme, Hyde realised that people
concealed their experiences of mental illness for fear of adverse effects upon
their prospects of work, marriage and emigration. Public attitudes, she concluded, were 'not necessarily the result of ignorance, but also to a perfectly
reasonable fear of the consequences'.[28]

Yet in spite of her newly acquired appreciation of the complex factors
which shaped people's responses to mental distress, Hyde chose to produce
an unequivocal production designed to educate an imagined ignorant and
monolithic public, silencing any opposing ideas in the process. While carrying
out her interviews for the programme, Hyde also found that not all residents
of the hospital shared the views she sought to promote, and she appears to
have cut interviews to advance her chosen interpretation. This excerpt from an
interview was marked 'ok to leave':

D.H. – Are you happy here?
Woman – Oh, yes very.
D. H. – Do you feel you're getting better?
Woman – Oh definitely, decidedly.

However, written in the left-hand side of the next section of the interview was
'NO. NO'.

D. H. – Would you rather be here or anywhere else?
Woman – I think . . . (unintelligible, breaks down) . . . well I am very . . . I cer-
tainly would rather be out of it.
Dr – You would rather be home?
Woman – Yes, I think so.[29]

The records for programme suggestions reveal that BBC staff with prior
connections to mental illness initiated programmes. Hyde admitted that her
interest in the topic stemmed from her earlier work as a member of staff in a
mental home.[30] In 1959 the BBC employee David Gretton submitted suggestions for a programme on conditions in hospitals for the mentally defective,
explaining: 'We have a young studio manager who worked as a male nurse in

such a place . . . he is still on fire with the horror and disgrace of the conditions in which he found himself working'.[31] Other programme ideas came directly from healthcare workers. The BBC tended to privilege doctors' expertise when planning and producing mental health programming. Nevertheless, not all psychiatrists enjoyed the same reception.

We can begin to identify and analyse the factors which shaped the BBC's response to practitioners and influenced the direction of its programming if we examine Dr Joshua Bierer's repeated attempts to secure BBC coverage of his work. Bierer was the founder and Medical Director of the Institute of Social Psychiatry and worked at the Marlborough Day Hospital. He was a key figure in the social psychiatry movement which emphasised the role played by social factors in mental health and challenged the authority of the psychiatrist and the role of patient.[32] In 1956, he wrote to the BBC with a proposal for a programme entitled 'Are You Normal?' which would convey his view of mental illness:

> It is believed that everyone deep down within himself is afraid of becoming mentally deranged. This fear is likely to continue to influence everybody's thought and action as long as those of us who have not had to be treated for any disturbance believe we are *so* normal and that mental patients are *so* abnormal . . . Few points could be found so near to everyone's heart.[33]

Bierer's proposal encapsulated the belief that a continuum existed between mental health and illness, rather than a fixed divide. Emphasising that people who experienced mental illness were more alike than dissimilar to other people, he suggested, would allay fear and discrimination. He pitched a programme in which normal, neurotic and psychotic participants would hold discussions, and the public would be invited to adjudicate who was 'normal' and who was 'abnormal'. Bierer's talk of 'self-emancipation for the patient' who had previously been 'a tool in the well-meaning hands of his therapists' may have proved too controversial for BBC staff, who also expressed reservations on a separate occasion to providing any coverage of the Institute of Social Psychiatry because it was not part of the NHS.[34]

Medical politics and the basic premise of Bierer's proposal were by no means the only stumbling block. Isa Benzie, who met with Bierer, deemed his accent 'too thick to make him a desirable choice'.[35] Moreover, the BBC held deep reservations about the format Bierer suggested. BBC programming on healthcare issues tended to adopt the format of an authoritative doctor imparting his wisdom to the audience, and Benzie had expressed concerns about allowing ex-patients to broadcast their views five years earlier.[36] Bierer, however, wanted patients to demonstrate the normality of mental illness, and envisaged that the programme would entertain as well as educate; such a programme, he enthused, could be 'as interesting and thrilling to the masses as any other game'.[37] This format could be viewed as ideally suited to educating the public, given the belief, frequently voiced by psychiatrists, that the public were easily swayed by entertainment and sensationalism. Instead, BBC staff appear to have viewed this as a vulgar and distasteful suggestion which conflicted with their ethos of public duty and risked confusing the public. Intriguingly, Bierer appears to have been rather ahead of his time: clear parallels can be drawn between Bierer's proposed series and the 2008 BBC *Horizon* series, 'How Mad Are You', for which the premise was:

> Take ten volunteers [also termed 'contestants'] half have psychiatric disorders, the other half don't – but who is who?
>
> Over five days the group are put through a series of challenges – from performing stand-up comedy to mucking out cows. The events are designed to explore the character traits of mental illness and ask whether the symptoms might be within all of us.
>
> Three leading experts in mental health attempt to spot which volunteers have been diagnosed with a mental health condition. But will the individuals who have suffered from mental illness reveal themselves?[38]

Finally Bierer's interpretation of what mental illness was and how it should be treated counted against him in the eyes of the BBC. Bierer, who was committed to the development of social psychiatry, devoted his energies to extending psychotherapy, and developing therapeutic communities and day hospitals. Unlike many of his counterparts, Bierer focused his efforts on patients with severe and long-standing mental health problems.[39] As the example of 'The Hurt Mind' series demonstrates, the BBC tended to give greater credence to psychiatrists who ascribed to a physical illness interpretation of mental distress and sought to emphasise the curability of mental illness.

'The Hurt Mind'

Written records surrounding the production of radio and television programmes are sometimes rather scant. However, the making of 'The Hurt Mind', the first television series screened in Britain which examined mental illness, was richly documented, offering us an insight into the roles played by external organisations and medical bodies in the production of BBC programmes. The initial impetus for the series came from state bodies, medical professionals, and the NAMH, which sought to ensure that the BBC represented its interests by inviting BBC staff to sit on its committees. The appointment of the Royal Commission on the Law Relating to Mental Illness and

Mental Deficiency in 1954, which reported back in 1957, fuelled discussion of the treatment of mental illness, and the Board of Control and the Minister of Health urged the BBC to consider mental health as a programme subject. In November 1955, the psychiatrist Aubrey Lewis sent the BBC some pictorial representations of mental health statistics with the suggestion that they might be helpful in planning any television series. Mary Adams, an Assistant Controller at the BBC who was also involved in the NAMH, forwarded the figures to her colleagues.[40] The NAMH's newly formed Public Information Committee also felt it was time for the BBC to shed its earlier reticence with regard to mental illness, with the MP Kenneth Robinson suggesting that the focus should be on spreading knowledge of modern methods of treatment.[41]

The BBC enlisted Andrew Miller Jones – best known for his role as producer on *Muffin the Mule* and for helping to found *Panorama* – as producer, and issued a memorandum. This noted that the objectives of the series were:

1. To allay fear.
2. To encourage the sick to take advantage of available treatment in the early stages of disease.
3. To make known the latest advances of medical science and to increase the public's confidence in present-day medical science.[42]

It is worth noting that these objectives neither encouraged debate nor sought to raise awareness of poor conditions, and that the final objective also characterised other BBC programming on medical issues.[43] Around the same time that plans for 'The Hurt Mind' were under consideration, the Scottish Home Service was in the process of producing a documentary series at the request of the Scottish Department of Health with virtually identical objectives, covering the mental health of children; mental defect; alcoholism; work and mental health; physical and psychological causes and treatments of mental illness; and the effects of housing and the environment. This series followed in the wake of 'No Man an Island', a programme on depressive illness which combined dramatised sequences with excerpts of actuality footage.[44]

An examination of the professionals involved points to the predominance of doctors as experts. The BBC employed William Sargant, whom we met in Chapter 3, as the main consultant for 'The Hurt Mind'. Doubtless Sargant's reputation as a keen advocate of the new physical therapies and his position as Registrar of the Royal Medico-Psychological Association made him seem a desirable choice. Sargant also had a taste for public communication: *The Battle for the Mind*, Sargant's popular book on religious conversion and brainwashing techniques, was first published in 1954 and had sold over two hundred thousand copies by 1967.[45] The BBC paid Sargant 200 guineas for his advice on the content and policy of the programmes, and employed Dr Charles Fletcher, a general practitioner who subsequently presented the BBC series 'Your Life in Their Hands', to present the second, third and fourth programme for 150 guineas.[46] The decision to hire a general practitioner rather than a psychiatrist to front the programme suggests that presentation skills as much as expertise were a consideration. Expenses for nurses and patients involved in the film were far lower than those of the doctors involved. The BBC paid Dr M. A. Partridge 25 guineas to talk about leucotomy, but paid James P. only 3 guineas to appear as a patient in a demonstration of electroconvulsive therapy.[47]

The NAMH, which had urged the BBC to make the series, remained involved in the production. It supplied the BBC with background information and worked with the BBC to produce a leaflet about the programme. It also arranged with the BBC that letters received from the public in response to the series which had a casework content would be referred to the NAMH's casework department; subsequently, the NAMH drew upon these letters to publish the booklet 'Fifty Questions and Answers on Mental Illness'.[48]

The BBC paid the Labour MP Christopher Mayhew, who would later serve as chairman of the NAMH, £187 for presenting the first programme and acting as a chairman in the last. This was not Mayhew's first foray into television: in 1955, BBC's *Panorama* crew had filmed Mayhew taking mescaline in order to document the effects of the hallucinogenic drug. The programme was never aired, but Mayhew believed that the experience had given him an insight into the experiences of mental patients. Reasoning that the symptoms he exhibited upon ingesting mescaline could have been induced only by the drug as opposed to 'environmental stress, or genetic make-up, or some traumatic childhood experience', Mayhew concluded that mental illness must also 'surely have a simple physical origin'. 'All that was needed', he deduced, 'was to isolate and neutralize whatever chemical substance in the bloodstream of schizophrenics was distorting their perceptions, as mescaline had distorted mine'.[49] In his autobiography, Mayhew argued that most people in the 1950s viewed 'mental patients' as 'objects of fear and shame . . . they were widely seen as unpredictable and uncontrollable, at best embarrassing, at worst frightening'. He claimed that he 'thought television could be used to soften and civilize these attitudes, and persuaded the BBC and the Ministry of Health to allow, for the first time, a mental hospital to be filmed from the inside'.[50]

However, Warlingham Park Hospital, which featured in the first episode, was not just any mental hospital, and doubtless the BBC selected it for this very reason. Unlike most mental hospitals which had been constructed as asylums in the nineteenth century, it had been built at the start of the twentieth century. It was, moreover, a progressive mental hospital which specialised in treating alcoholic patients.[51] 'The chances are one in twenty that you or I will spend some part of our life as a patient in a mental hospital', began Mayhew, using a statistic to try and persuade his audience that mental illness concerned everyone: still a common tactic in campaigns seeking to destigmatise mental illness.[52] Eschewing a didactic authoritative tone, Mayhew adopted an inclusive approach which allowed viewers some grounds for their beliefs, while directing them towards a different view. He juxtaposed stigmatising stereotypes of mental illness with a reassuringly prosaic representation of Warlingham, depicting the hospital as a comfortable hotel replete with leisure facilities such as the shop, hairdressers, dances, films, magazines and chapel:

> This is a mental hospital here – does a sight like this fill you with foreboding? I know it did me. What is really going on inside there? Hopeless misery, raving, violence, weird uncanny behaviour? I thought I'd find out . . . here's the dormitory here – extremely civilised and pleasant, curtains between beds even . . . This was my cubicle – chest of drawers and reading light, perfectly comfortable . . . and this was the lounge of the ward, with the morning newspapers coming round. It wasn't bad at all, comfortable chairs, television, a warm fire and surprisingly quiet.

Mayhew also tried to alleviate fears by invoking a history of the mental hospital against which current practices could only favourably compare. Fifty years ago, he informed viewers, 'a mental hospital was a kind of prison. Treatment of insanity was widely thought to be a waste of time.' This approach allowed viewers a rational basis for their fears while implying that the situation had changed. It was a common strategy amongst mental health reformers, and bears the hallmarks of William Sargant who, as we saw in Chapter 3, conjured an eerie image of the gothic Victorian lock-up asylum and chronic lunatic in his memoir to serve as a foil for his portrayal of the modern treatment of mental illness. As Simon Cross has noted in his analysis of this episode, Mayhew contrasted the efficacy of modern treatments, 'personified by interviews with patients whom we are told are on the verge of discharge', with 'the human casualties of an older asylum system', via a visit to a ward which housed, in Mayhew's words, 'the hard core of chronic patients' who 'became ill before modern treatments became available'.[53]

The programme contained interviews with actual patients, although an examination of the script suggests that Mayhew controlled the direction of the conversation through a series of leading question, as in this extract of an interview with two alcoholics, Betty and Sybil.

> Mayhew – What did you feel when you came here, I mean, what did you expect a mental hospital would be like?

Betty or Sybil – Well, I expected locked doors for one thing, padded cells, I can't . . .
Mayhew – But weren't you a bit scared, I mean, you went into the canteen – did you?
Betty or Sybil – Yes, I was a bit frightened at first.
Mayhew – Mixing with the other patients mostly?
Betty or Sybil – Yes, but I found that most of them were quite friendly and . . .
Mayhew – More like a hotel, this place?
Betty or Sybil –Yes, it is.[54]

Mayhew used a similar tactic when interviewing a nurse, Mr Rowse. Mayhew had just asserted that 'emphasis on treatment has transformed this place from a prison to a hospital', and was using leading questions to get Rowse to admit that nurses in the bad old days had used violence to control patients.

Rowse – Well in 1933 when I came to the hospital it was like a prison . . .
Mayhew – And this made the patients frustrated I suppose and violent.
Rowse – Well naturally . . . they did tend to get irritable.
Mayhew – And then the nurses, I suppose, had to retaliate a bit?
Rowse – Well, on the whole they were a very tolerant staff . . .
Mayhew – You hit out because you were frightened? Was that it?
Rowse – Often in self-defence.

The programme consciously sought to stress the break with the past, as in this extract above, emphasising the modern treatment facilities on offer. However, it grappled with the paradox of attempting simultaneously to destigmatise mental illness and to persuade more people to seek early, voluntary treatment in mental hospitals, while admitting that the condition of many hospitals left much to be desired. Indeed, accompanying a sequence of footage shot at Cane Hill Hospital, Mayhew provided a commentary which emphasised how little things had changed in recent years at the vast majority of mental hospitals:

Out of over two hundred health service mental hospitals, only six have been built in the last forty years. These are ugly, oppressive, wretched places. You feel you're in a nineteenth-century prison or workhouse . . . staff shortage and overcrowding mean locked doors and gates – it's the only way hard working staff can manage. This gate locks patients into this exercise yard, or airing court as it's called. It's sunless, crowded, ugly, like a cage for wild animals.

The medical superintendent of the hospital used this opportunity to call for money, but also 'what's behind money. You see we need public opinion, public support', describing mental hospitals as the 'Cinderella' of the health services.

At this stage in the programme, Mayhew found himself having to balance the conflicting duties of BBC reporting:

Well that was a depressing film. We had to show it because it's the truth – more shame on all of us. But I know there'll be some people watching this tonight who feel responsible for some mentally ill person . . . or perhaps who are mentally ill themselves, who may feel put off from applying for treatment by the kind of thing we've just shown.

Mayhew then felt it necessary to reassure viewers that even in the older hospitals modern treatment was given to patients, who usually only required short stays in the more pleasant areas of the hospital; this detail may not have been so reassuring for those viewers who knew someone receiving care as a long-stay patient in a less pleasant area of a mental hospital. Mayhew's use of the pronoun 'us' sought to make viewers feel responsible for the state of the mental health services, and he used the documentary to attempt to boost nurse recruitment: 'This hospital, like most others, is badly short of female nurses. It seems a great pity – for people with imagination and compassion this is surely a fine job to do.'

'Mental diseases have almost certainly got physical causes, just like physical diseases', Mayhew informed viewers, 'and there's no real distinction to be made'. Given Sargant's role as consultant to the series this assertion is unsurprising – although, as we have seen, it was a view which Mayhew also shared. Intriguingly, however, the documentary made this point while showing a young woman visiting a general hospital in London to receive psychotherapeutic treatment for an anxiety state. 'Like most young and intelligent mental patients, this girl doesn't mind us filming her at all', commented Mayhew. 'She knows that she can't help her illness and it is nothing to be ashamed of, any more than any other illness.' An out-patients department was also shown, and the administration of treatments such as abreaction, modified insulin and electroconvulsive therapy. 'These patients will be back at home or at work later today', Mayhew announced, seeking to break the link in the public mind between mental disorder and a prolonged stay within a mental hospital.

No scripts survive for the subsequent programmes. The second programme dealt with different theories about the causes of mental disorder, and covered child guidance, Freudian ideas, heredity and chemical changes in the brain.[55] All the participants were doctors: this episode was later described by Leonard Miall, head of television talks, as 'terrible', although he had thought the first had been 'very good indeed'.[56] Indeed, summarising this programme for participants completing an audience questionnaire, the BBC was less than effusive, explaining that this episode was 'about the causes of mental illness. A lot of different people talked about the different causes . . . in fact the programme was mostly talk. You may remember being shown lots and lots of tins of salt. And there was a little girl who kept falling and would not respond to anyone.'[57] The third programme in the series dealt with psychotherapy and social therapy and depicted the different methods of treatment used for individuals and groups. Again, all participants were doctors.

The fourth programme examined physical methods of treatment, a topic close to Sargant's heart. Once again, the programme invoked a bleak history of bygone treatment methods to emphasise the progress that had been made. 'Twenty or thirty years ago it was no good even starting to open the doors of our mental hospitals, while there were so many mentally tortured persons only waiting for an opportunity to escape and perhaps to kill themselves', Sargant argued, warming to the topic. 'Fortunately these new physical methods of treatment have been found to help the sort of patient who is too depressed and agitated to be helped by psycho-therapeutic methods alone.'[58] This programme demonstrated electroconvulsive therapy and described insulin treatment, tranquillisers, abreaction and leucotomy; the efficacy of the latter demonstrated through a conversation with a compliant leucotomised patient. The doctors were quick to dismiss criticism of these treatments: Fletcher noted that, in spite of the positive review of electroconvulsive therapy given by the demonstration patient, 'there seems to be considerable fear of ECT, judging from letters sent in – even from patients who have *had* it and presumably not felt actual physical pain'. This telling comment demonstrated a refusal to acknowledge deviation from the sanctioned perspective of series and a denial of the validity of patients' perspectives. Meanwhile, Sargant dismissed the side effects of leucotomies: 'one must remember that the choice is *not* between what the person was before the illness and what they are after leucotomy, but between an utterly miserable and incapacitated patient and a normal or near normal person'.[59]

Within the BBC archives is a file of letters from people who had not been consulted by the BBC in the making of the programmes – psychiatrists, duly authorised officers, occupational therapists, charity workers, psychiatric nurses and PSWs – all seeking to ensure that their professions were adequately and accurately represented within the series. 'The going . . . has been pretty tough', admitted Miller Jones to a friend, 'as there is schism and faction throughout the field of psychiatry and psychology'.[60]

Some writers addressed the paradox that the programme makers had grappled with: how to emphasise the advances made in psychiatry and persuade more people to seek treatment, while acknowledging that conditions in many mental hospitals left much to be desired owing to lack of funding. This was voiced most strongly by Dr A. M. Spencer, the Medical Superintendent of Powick Hospital. While not denying the desirability of demonstrating to the public that mental hospitals 'have become places of treatment like other hospitals', he expressed his hope that 'the unsatisfactory features of so many hospitals will be spotlighted':

> We need, I think, not so much programmes which will allay people's fears but programmes which will stir the social conscience until something is done about the overcrowding, institutionalisation, poor feeding, poor clothing and general level of poverty to which so many of our patients are condemned.[61]

One may ask whether Dr Spencer came to regret these views some twelve years when the Granada documentary series *World in Action* exposed neglect of elderly patients in Powick Hospital, where he still served as Medical Superintendent.[62]

Other writers sought to correct errors in the programme which related to their work. Several duly authorised officers, for example, wrote in after the certification procedure was reported inaccurately and persuaded the BBC to correct this mistake in a subsequent programme. The MACA also wrote to Miller Jones hoping to get its work mentioned, only to find that it had been pipped to the post by the NAMH.[63] Yet, while enjoying a significant input into the series, the BBC did not appear to hold the NAMH in particularly high esteem. Isa Benzie, who sat on two of the NAMH's committees, rather scathingly described these as:

> the public relations committee which ought to be called the education of the public committee, and a committee originally set up to attempt some study of the influence upon the state of public knowledge of films which contain psychiatric material . . . This committee now serves no good purpose that I can see . . . But I still go to at least one meeting in every two . . . because the spectacle is most instructive, the spectacle, that is, of a somewhat undefined racket at work.[64]

Indeed, while the BBC eventually acceded to a request from the NAMH for a telerecording of the series, the initial response of BBC staff was rather hostile. 'I personally think that we should turn this request down completely', wrote the BBC talks organiser Cyril Jackson. 'We are making a pretty considerable contribution to the work of the Association by putting on these programmes and this should amply repay any co-operation we have had from them'.[65]

The occupational therapist Carol Henderson wrote in to express her belief that the public should be given an unambiguous account rather than being offered different explanations from which to form their opinions. On these grounds, she objected to the second programme in the series which covered different theories regarding the causation of mental illness:

> I look upon educating the public as one of the major tasks of any of us who work
> with mental patients . . . unfortunately . . . I didn't manage to see number one
> programme – but everyone I have discussed it with . . . all agree it was clear,
> constructive and instructive. Good television and good propaganda. I saw
> number two myself, and I'm afraid I didn't think it was up to the same standard.[66]

Henderson's primary agenda, however, was to ensure that her profession was
represented in a pleasing light. 'I wondered who has been advising you on the
OT side', she wrote. 'I can only hope they have persuaded you that it is not arts
and crafts, but that it is the organisation of the entire hospital into a therapeutic
community, with the aim of occupying every patient.'[67]

PSWs were also concerned that their profession had been neither consulted
nor recognised. Mary Lane, then Chairman of the APSW, wrote to Miller
Jones complaining that the programmes made no mention of the part played
by PSWs. Several letters were exchanged. 'I am sure that you will realise that
mental illness is far too big a subject to be covered in five short programmes',
wrote Miller Jones. 'I can only say that I was advised by most eminent members
of the medical profession, who were responsible for the content and emphasis
of the programmes',[68] he added, passing on Lane's letter and his response to
be vetted by his chief medical adviser, Dr Sargant. Sargant later responded to
Miller Jones: 'Dear Andrew, I have sent off your letter to Miss Lane. Actually
I think you have been much too polite, but I suppose you have to be.'[69] The
marginalisation of psychiatric social work from the programme is perhaps
not surprising. In 1949, Isa Benzie filed a report from a 1949 conference on
Mental Health in which she noted: 'I have by now looked in and out at a good
many conferences more or less of this sort, usually in the hope of collecting
new speakers, and usually one finds the same old drearies'. She reviewed PSWs
Marjorie Brown and May Irvine as 'either uninspiring or off-putting, or both.
Dreary.'[70] Moreover, Sargant's only reference to PSWs in his autobiography
was decidedly contemptuous, branding their activities as 'a waste of time'
which had been rendered obsolete by the advent of new physical therapies.[71]

BBC staff could thus be rather disrespectful towards healthcare workers,
aside from psychiatrists. They did, however, choose to retain their letters,
on the grounds that they might be worth referring to at a later stage. BBC
personnel were more dismissive of the 25,000 letters received from viewers
who lacked these professional credentials. These it deemed to be of 'no further
interest and could be thrown away as far as we're concerned'.[72] Consequently,
the BBC sent the letters to the NAMH and, owing to the current inaccessibility
of the NAMH archive, it is impossible to determine whether the letters have
survived. However, an analysis of a sample of three hundred letters undertaken
at the time by the NAMH suggests that most were sent by members of the

public with a prior connection to mental illness.[73] Thus, 237 dealt with obtaining treatment or advice; patients sent 102; and relatives and friends of patients wrote a further 135. According to the NAMH's analysis, many writers complained that their general practitioner was unsympathetic. Patients who had experienced shock treatment and found it frightening wrote in large numbers, expressing their determination to never submit to it again. This point of view had been swept over in the programme.

A BBC audience research report found that 15 per cent of the adult population of Britain – approximately five and a half million people – had seen the broadcasts, and the appreciation indices had been 80, 62, 70, 78 and 77 in order of transmission, which compared favourably against a mean appreciation index of all televised talks and discussions in the previous quarter of 64.[74] The report found that amongst those who had watched the series there was generally a slight reduction in the feeling that the mentally ill were different, accompanied by an increased insight into their condition and a more sympathetic attitude towards them. Viewers of the series were also more likely to believe that psychiatry had made great progress over the past twenty years – 58 per cent as opposed to 45 per cent who had not watched the programme.[75] Demonstrating the limitations of the didactic approach to public education favoured by many healthcare professionals, the researchers found that changes in attitude or knowledge tended not to occur when a point had been conveyed by a statement; confronting viewers with patients, or making the point in concrete terms, proved more efficacious.[76] The programme did fail to alter some beliefs: 90 per cent of viewers and non-viewers alike still believed that there was a difference between mental illness and insanity (the former regarded as more curable than the latter), while viewers of the series continued to underestimate the percentage of hospital beds used by the mental health services. Despite Sargant's brisk assurances about the efficacy of leucotomy, viewers also remained unconvinced that the operation would leave the patient's personality unaltered: 46 per cent of both viewers and non-viewers believed that the personality could change, while a further 40 per cent remained uncertain.[77]

Conclusion

Recent commentators have blamed the media for the stigma surrounding mental illness, pointing to pressures operating on media coverage which distorts coverage. In the 1950s, however, the BBC perceived educational broadcasting to be its duty. Seeking political autonomy from the government, the BBC was unsure if it should be supporting government health services, or drawing public attention to their shortcomings. This dilemma was clearly

reflected in BBC programming on mental health. By acknowledging that problems existed in the mental health services, programmes provided viewers with
different ways of perceiving the situation. However, the BBC's paternalistic
attitude and its belief that it should be enlightening an ignorant public and
destigmatising mental illness, beliefs shared by the mental healthcare professionals and organisations it worked with, often led the Corporation to portray
the problems posed by mental illness in a rather one-dimensional fashion, pre-
cluding debate. Such problems do not appear to be confined to programming
on mental health, or indeed coverage from the 1950s. Reviewing more recent
media coverage, Ann Karpf observed that 'medical definitions and perceptions
still prevail and squeeze out more contentious, oppositional viewpoints which
take an environmental approach and look at the politics of health'. 'By exclud-
ing or marginalising other perspectives – notably, a more explicitly political
analysis of the origins of illness', Karpf argued, 'the media play a significant part
in narrowing public debate about health, illness and medicine'.[78]

With 'The Hurt Mind', the BBC seems to have missed an opportunity.
The series sought to convey a narrow perspective of what mental illness was,
marginalising the perspectives of many healthcare professionals and silencing
patients' experiences: a pattern which the Glasgow media group has identified in more recent coverage. However, these traits also bear the distinctive
hallmark of William Sargant, the main consultant for the series. Sargant, for
example, brought his rather one-dimensional perspective on mental illness
to bear on the programme. Thus, the series implied that mental illness had
biological causes, and illustrated the progress made in mental healthcare by
reinforcing the sense of despondency attached to chronic mental illness. One
might query whether Sargant was the right candidate to reassure the public: it
was Sargant who first gained a public profile by authoring a book on brainwashing; who, as we saw in Chapter 3, recounted undertaking surgery while drunk
as an amusing anecdote in his autobiography; and who adopted a rather blasé
approach to treatments, as recent testimony from former patients and colleagues involved in his deep sleep treatments illustrates.[79] In a highly revealing
statement which certainly helps explain why patient perspectives were given so
little credence in the series, June, one of Sargant's former patients, described his
'very, very arrogant manner'. 'He didn't discuss things with you', June recalled
'he told you, he talked at you, but he didn't really listen to what you might have
to say, in fact I can't ever remember saying anything to him much'.[80]

Looking beyond the BBC, the correspondence sent in by disgruntled
healthcare workers who were not consulted by the programme makers indicates that the BBC would have struggled to incorporate all views within the
programme. While virtually all correspondents concurred on the need to

educate the public – envisaged as a homogeneous mass, easily swayed by padded cells and buns – consensus as to what message should be conveyed to the public was demonstrably lacking. Some hoped to engender a greater willingness to seek treatment by promoting the image of modern and well-equipped mental health services, while others hoped to cast the spotlight on the inadequacies of existing provisions so as to demand improvements. Many hoped that the series would help raise the status of their profession. Moreover, given the range of occupational groups involved in the care and treatment of people who experienced mental distress, each holding a distinctive view of what mental illness was, how it should be treated and what the priorities were within the field of mental health, the frequently expressed assumption that there was a 'correct' view of mental illness and its treatment with which the public could be inculcated through didactic propaganda appears rather naive. In practice, analysis of 'The Hurt Mind' illustrates how the relative power of different organisations in the field of mental health affected their capacity to influence the media.

Notes

1 P. Bourdieu, *On Television and Journalism* (London, 1998), p. 10.
2 Ibid., p. 3.
3 See, for example, G. Philo (ed.), *Message Received: Glasgow Media Group Research 1993–1998* (Harlow, 1999), and G. Philo (ed.), *Media and Mental Distress* (Harlow, 1996).
4 L. Henderson, 'Selling suffering: mental illness and media values', in Philo (ed.), *Media and Mental Distress*, pp. 18–36.
5 G. Philo, 'The media and public belief', in Philo (ed.), *Media and Mental Distress*, pp. 82–104; p. 103.
6 This is discussed in more detail in Chapter 4.
7 G. Philo, 'Users of services, carers and families', in Philo (ed.), *Media and Mental Distress*, pp. 105–14.
8 S. Cross, 'Visualizing madness: mental illness and public representation', *Television & New Media*, 5 (2004), 197–216; 207. Cross analysed the *Panorama* programme 'Whose Mind Is It Anyway?', produced by Andrew Williams and broadcast by the BBC on 1 March 1993.
9 Ibid. 'A Place of Safety', produced by Mike Beckham and broadcast by ITV on 25 February and 4 March 1993.
10 J. Habermas, *The Structural Transformation of the Public Sphere: An Inquiry into a Category of Bourgeois Society*, trans. T. Burger (1962; Cambridge, 1999), p. 181.
11 Ibid., p. 185.
12 J. Curran and J. Seaton, *Power Without Responsibility: The Press and Broadcasting in Britain* (London, 1997), pp. 52–3.

13 Cross, 'Visualizing madness', 202.
14 P. Scannell, 'Public service broadcasting: the history of a concept', in A. Goodwin and G. Whannel (eds), *Understanding Television* (London, 1990), pp. 11–29.
15 Ibid., p. 14.
16 A. Karpf, *Doctoring the Media: The Reporting of Health and Medicine* (London, 1988), pp. 38–43.
17 See C. Webster, 'Healthy or hungry thirties?', *History Workshop Journal*, 13 (1982), 110–29; S. Sturdy, 'Hippocrates and state medicine: George Newman outlines the funding policy of the Ministry of Health', in C. Lawrence (ed.), *Greater than the Parts: Holism in Biomedicine, 1920–1950* (Oxford, 1998), pp. 112–34.
18 R. W. Armstrong, 'Education in psychiatry: presidential address', *JMS*, 103 (1957), 691–8; 695.
19 BBC WAC, R51/219, letter from Miss I. D. Benzie to chief assistants D. Boyd, J. Green, the editor of *Woman's Hour* and Mr Thornton, 27 November 1952.
20 See K. Loughlin, '"Your Life in Their Hands": the context of a medical-media controversy', *Media History*, 6 (2000), 177–88.
21 Ibid.
22 See J. V. Pickstone, 'Psychiatry in general hospitals: history, contingency and local innovation in the early years of the National Health Service', in J. V. Pickstone (ed.), *Medical Innovations in Historical Perspective* (Houndmills, 1992), pp. 185–99, and S. Cherry, *Mental Health Care in Modern England: The Norfolk Lunatic Asylum / St Andrew's Hospital c.1810–1998* (Woodbridge, 2003), pp. 231–40.
23 BBC WAC, S322/117/3, BBC audience research report, 12 November 1956, p. 5.
24 W. Sargant, 'The Hurt Mind', *British Medical Journal*, 1:5096 (1958), 517.
25 M. Shortland, 'Screen memories: towards a history of psychiatry and psychoanalysis in the movies', *British Journal for the History of Science*, 20 (1987), 421–52.
26 Letter from Miss I. D. Benzie to chief assistants D. Boyd, J. Green, the editor of *Woman's Hour* and Mr Thornton, 27 November 1952.
27 BBC WAC, N14/6/7/1, memo from D. Hyde, 15 August 1955, for programme suggestion, 'Within Our Province'. Hyde's programme, 'Within our Province: The Sick Mind', was aired on 11 December 1956 on the Northern Ireland Home Service.
28 Ibid., report on visit by D. Hyde, 1 May 1956, 'Within Our Province'.
29 Ibid., transcript of interviews, tape two, 'Within Our Province'. The first 'NO' written in the margins was underlined twice.
30 Ibid., memo from D. Hyde, 25 August 1955, 'Within Our Province'.
31 BBC WAC, R51/844/1, memo from D. Gretton to Miss I. D. Benzie, 30 October 1959.
32 For an overview of Bierer's career, see L. Clarke, 'Joshua Bierer: striving for power', *History of Psychiatry*, 8 (1997), 319–32.
33 BBC WAC, R51/845/1, letter from J. Bierer to the BBC, 15 October 1956, typed underlining in text.
34 BBC WAC, R51/222, memo from Miss I. D. Benzie to R. Lewin, March 1949.

35 BBC WAC, R51/845/1, memo from Miss I. D. Benzie to Miss Quigley and Mr Newby, 8 February 1957.

36 Letter from Miss I. D. Benzie to chief assistants D. Boyd, J. Green, the editor of *Woman's Hour* and Mr Thornton, 27 November 1952.

37 Letter from J. Bierer to the BBC, 15 October 1956. Underlining in pencil, probably by BBC staff.

38 The synopsis of this series is no longer available on the BBC website. A summary can be viewed at http://topdocumentaryfilms.com/how-mad-are-you/, consulted 17 February 2013.

39 See Clarke, 'Joshua Bierer'. These themes are examined in more detail in Chapter 3.

40 BBC WAC, S322/117/2, memo from Mrs M. Adams to C.P. Tel, H.T. Tel., editor, women's programmes Tel. and J. McCloy, 16 November 1955. Adams enclosed Lewis's letter and referred to approaches from the Ministry of Health and the Board of Control in her memorandum.

41 Ibid., NAMH Public Information Committee, 19 April 1956.

42 BBC WAC, R19/1759/1, memo from L. Miall, Head of Talks, television, 25 May 1956.

43 See Loughlin, '"Your Life in Their Hands"'.

44 BBC WAC, R19/1759/1, memo from Archie Lee, Features Producer Glasgow, 12 January 1956.

45 W. Sargant, *The Unquiet Mind: The Autobiography of a Physician in Psychological Medicine* (London, 1967). Figures given for the distribution of *The Battle for the Mind* on p. 175.

46 BBC WAC, T32/845/1. Dr E. D. Barlow was also paid 200 guineas for research and assistance in writing the script and appearing in one of the programmes.

47 BBC WAC, T32/846/1, expenses for 'The Hurt Mind'.

48 BBC WAC, S322/215/1, draft evidence to the Ministry of Health Joint Committee of the English and Scottish Health Services Councils.

49 C. Mayhew, *Time to Explain: An Autobiography* (London, 1987), pp. 149–55; p. 154.

50 Ibid., p. 154. The surviving BBC files give little indication as to Mayhew's role in determining the nature of the programmes.

51 See B. Thom, *Dealing with Drink: Alcohol and Social Policy from Treatment to Management* (London, 1999), pp. 36–9.

52 BBC WAC, S322/117/1, transcription of programme, 'Put Away', shown 1 January 1957.

53 S. Cross, *Mediating Madness: Mental Distress and Cultural Representation* (Houndmills, 2010), p. 84.

54 'Put Away'.

55 BBC WAC, S322/117/1, outline of programme two.

56 BBC WAC, T32/845/1, memo from Head of Talks L. Miall, 30 January 1957.

57 Wellcome Library, William Sargant Archive, PP/WWS/J.1/5, questionnaire, 'The Hurt Mind: Effects'.

58 BBC WAC, S322/117/1, outline of programme four.
59 Ibid. Underlining in original text.
60 BBC WAC, T32/200, letter from A. Miller Jones to T. Barnett, 4 February 1957.
61 BBC WAC, T32/200, letter from Dr A. M. Spencer to the BBC, 19 December 1956.
62 'This week in . . .', *Worcester News* (18 August 2008), accessed online at www.worcesternews.co.uk/news/nostalgia/thisweekin/3601926.AUGUST_16_23/.
63 BBC WAC, T32/200, letter from D. Meier to W. P. King, 12 February 1957.
64 BBC WAC, R51/219, memo from Miss I. D. Benzie, 25 March 1949.
65 BBC WAC, T32/845/1, memo from C. Jackson to head of talks, television, 19 December 1956.
66 BBC WAC, T32/200, letter from C. Henderson to A. Miller Jones, 10 January 1957.
67 Ibid.
68 BBC WAC, T32/200, letter from A. Miller Jones to M. A. Lane, copied to Dr W. Sargant, 25 February 1957.
69 BBC WAC, T32/200, letter from Dr W. Sargant to A. Miller Jones, 26 February 1957.
70 BBC WAC, RIS/219, memo from I.D. Benzie to A.C.T., A.H.T.D., 26 March 1949.
71 Sargant, *The Unquiet Mind*, p. 36.
72 BBC WAC, T32/200, letter from Daphne Meier to the BBC Registry, undated.
73 BBC WAC, S322/117/3, NAMH Public Information Committee minutes, 26 April 1957.
74 BBC WAC, T32/846/1, BBC, 'An Audience Research Report. "The Hurt Mind" – An Enquiry into Some of the Effects of the Series of Five television Broadcasts about Mental Illness and its Treatment' (1957).
75 Ibid., p. 9.
76 Ibid., p. 17.
77 Ibid., p. 7.
78 Karpf, *Doctoring the Media*, p. 2.
79 J. Maw, 'Revealing the Mind Bender General', BBC documentary, broadcast on Radio 4 on 17 March 2009.
80 June, in ibid.

CONCLUSION: IS IT TIME TO CHANGE OUR APPROACH TO ANTI-STIGMA CAMPAIGNS?

Myth: Mental health problems are very rare
Fact: Mental health problems affect one in four people
Myth: People with mental illness can't work.
Fact: You probably work with someone with mental illness.
Myth: People with mental illness never recover.
Fact: People with mental illness can and do recover.[1]

Time to Change, 2009

Imagine a campaign by a cancer charity, which gave the impression that everyone survives, picks up their lives where they left off, no worries about whether the cancer returns, no scars. . .It wouldn't be believable would it? This is what's being presented as what happens if you have a mental illness.[2]

'JM', 2010

For many campaigners, the stigma attached to mental illness often appears to be consistent: emanating from public fear and ignorance, and evident in every historical era. Thus psychologist Stephen Hinshaw, for example, acknowledges that understandings of and treatment for mental disorder changed over time, but suggests that the stigmatisation and exclusion of people with mental disorders has persisted 'across the millennia'.[3] This point is reinforced by the image on the cover of Hinshaw's book: *Removing the Stone of Folly*, a fifteenth-century painting by Hieronymus Bosch used in this instance to represent trepanning and thus encapsulating Hinshaw's assertion that people with mental disorders have been subjected to centuries of brutalisation. Such a perception simultaneously risks generating a sense of inevitability by implying that changing public attitudes is insurmountable, while implying that the solution is straightforward: effective education of the public so as to counter prejudice founded upon ignorance.

This book has sought to destabilise such assumptions by denaturalising 'the stigma of mental illness', arguing that the records of mental health groups researched for this book rarely defined what they meant by public opinion or stigma. While healthcare workers frequently bemoaned public ignorance or prejudice, they made no systematic attempt to gauge the extent of such beliefs. At times, indeed, those active in the field of mental health were forced to concede that their preconceptions regarding public prejudice required modification. As we saw in the previous chapter the radio producer Diana Hyde rescinded her view that the stigma attached to mental illness emanated from ignorance and fear and could be removed by public education. Hyde conceded in a report that people feared mental distress because they recognised that sufferers experienced discrimination in their relationships and careers.[4]

What is curious about Hyde's epiphany is that she chose not to act upon it. Rather than address the distress and discrimination experienced by people diagnosed with a mental illness, Hyde produced a programme designed to educate an imagined ignorant and monolithic public.[5] These traits are evident in contemporary anti-stigma campaigns, which seek to correct perceived public ignorance and misconceptions with facts. In 2009, the campaigner and activist Dawn Willis was filmed on a Sheffield tram which had been converted into a padded cell, an event orchestrated by Time to Change to convey the message that mental health problems were common and that those affected got on with their lives like everyone else. Willis explained that she was motivated in part by defiance, 'as if I was saying to the world, to the people in my family who were ashamed of my mental illness "Bring it on, I challenge you to tell me that I'm lesser than YOU."' However, as she reflected, 'I didn't encounter that response'. Instead, she described how the people she met on the tram

> Weren't all the ignorant, ill-informed bigots I was expecting, they were people just like me, people who were scared by the prospect of suffering mental illness, fearful of it happening to someone in their families, aware that they or the people they knew were affected and concerned not only by discrimination and stigma, but by the treatments available to them.[6]

It dawned on Willis that the discrimination experienced by people suffering from mental distress stemmed not from public ignorance, but from public knowledge that mental health problems could inflict profound distress on sufferers, whose difficulties were further compounded by structural discrimination. In conversation with a friend, Willis began to wonder whether Time to Change had adopted an accusatory tone, implying that the public should be blamed for stigmatising mental illness. Similarly, the activist and service user Dave Neenan felt that Time to Change had 'not so much been engaging the public as blaming the public' for causing the difficulties that people with mental health issues face.[7]

This book has interrogated the role of healthcare professionals who purportedly sought to tackle 'public ignorance' in the period 1870 to 1970, examining the disjuncture between their expressed desire to educate the public and the ways in which they inadvertently (and at times deliberately) stigmatised some of their patients. Most healthcare workers appeared to believe that destigmatising mental illness was a black and white issue: stigma arose from public ignorance as to the true nature of mental illness and its treatment, and could be overcome if healthcare professionals supplied this missing knowledge through didactic propaganda. However, the fallacy of this interpretation rapidly becomes apparent when workers' efforts to educate the public are examined, for amongst healthcare workers there was no consensus as to what they were trying to mobilise public opinion for. Were they hoping to engender a greater willingness to seek treatment; to destigmatise mental illness; to draw attention to innovations; to highlight deficiencies in provisions and demand improvements in services; to raise the status of their profession, or to emphasise the unappealing aspects of their work as a means of securing higher wages? Some of these objectives complemented one another but others conflicted.

Moreover, the range of occupational groups involved in the care and treatment of people who experienced mental illness increased over the course of the twentieth century, with each holding a distinctive view of what mental illness was, how it should be treated and where it should be treated. Indeed, there could be considerable variation within each profession at any given moment – take, for example, the divisions between psychiatrists who adopted a biomedical approach to the causes of mental disorder and its treatment and those who believed that mental disturbance had complex psycho-social causes. Gender fuelled the divisions within and between occupational groups, influencing representations of mental illness. Its impact was most marked within the field of psychiatric nursing, polarising representations of both nurses and patients. Throughout the twentieth century, the image of the nurse exercising her medical training to care for sick patients within a hospital oscillated with the image of the attendant, who used physical force to restrain violent, deviant inmates. The relative power of different organisations in the field of mental healthcare determined their capacity to influence the media, and, while it is not my intention to suggest that the media play no role in generating stigmatising images of mental distress, in some instances one can trace stigmatising media coverage back to healthcare professionals.

Rather than moralise about the strategies adopted by healthcare workers, this book has situated their debates within the field of mental healthcare, tracing the interconnections of agents and groups within a hierarchical field that was buffeted by cultural trends, economic considerations, the trajectory of general medicine and political shifts. The agency of insecure professional groups in particular was circumscribed by the forces of this field: their strategies were shaped by the aspirations and relative power of other healthcare workers, informed by the pattern of healthcare policy, and subject to broader structural forces. Some occupational groups believed they needed to advance their own professional interests before they could advance the interests of those who suffered from mental illness. Stigma, however, could not be contained within the interconnected field of mental healthcare, for the reputation of healthcare workers was intimately bound up with perceptions of their patients and of the mental hospitals in which many worked.

Fundamental to this analysis has been the contention that 'mental illness' is best viewed as a concept to be analysed, rather than a category of analysis. One of the problems of the term is its capacity to conceal disparate experiences of mental distress, and differing levels of stigma. As this historical study has repeatedly demonstrated, most healthcare workers sought to distinguish between acute, treatable mental disorders, and chronic psychotic disorders. Time and time again, efforts to destigmatise mental illness focused on 'promising' patients, at the expense of 'chronic' patients. Thus, the new therapeutic optimism embodied by physical treatment methods, for example, was achieved in part by segregating those whose illnesses were more long standing and less amenable to somatic treatment methods, while the appeal of admissions wards was enhanced by removing chronic patients to segregated wards. My concern is that current anti-stigma campaigns also focus upon acute, minor and transient experiences of mental disorder, and similarly risk worsening the discrimination experienced by people with enduring mental health conditions.

As noted in the introduction, 'mental illness' is a time-bound concept; one, indeed, which is now coming under attack from different quarters. Consciously or unconsciously channelling the spirit of William Sargant, Mary Barker, President of the European Parkinson's Disease Association, and Matthew Menken of the World Federation of Neurology urged medical colleagues to discard the term 'mental illness' in favour of 'brain illness' on the grounds that the '"mental" paradigm' was ambiguous, helped perpetuate stigma and conveyed the impression that 'some brain disorders are not physical ailments'.[8] In short, Barker and Menken felt the term 'mental illness' failed to effectively convey the centrality of 'illness'. Conversely, a more prevalent trend is the growing willingness to discard the term mental illness in favour of the term mental health, or mental health problems. Mind, for example, vacillates between 'mental health problems' and 'mental illness',[9] while Time to Change avoids the term 'mental illness' and refers only to 'mental health problems'.[10]

Such sentiments similarly inform the current enthusiasm to place mental well-being or mental flourishing at the heart of destigmatisation campaigns and policies, such as the Scottish government's 2009 report, *Towards a Mentally Flourishing Scotland*.[11] This document borrows loosely from the idea of the mental health/illness continuum and asserts that mental health concerns us all. 'Our immediate aim is to help everyone to understand how their own and other's mental health can be improved', explained Shona Robison in the Ministerial Foreword.[12] Most of the document focuses on improving mental well-being in the community at large and preventing mental health problems; only the sixth – and final – priority addresses how the 'quality of life of those experiencing mental health problems and mental illness' might be improved.[13] The Future Vision Coalition demonstrates how professional, voluntary and statutory bodies continue to collaborate in the design and delivery of services, for it represents the views of the Association of Directors of Adult Social Services; the Association of Directors of Children's Services; the Local Government Association; the Mental Health Foundation; the Mental Health Providers Forum; Mind; NHS Confederation – Mental Health Network; Rethink Mental Illness; the Royal College of Psychiatrists; the Sainsbury Centre for Mental Health and Together. It insisted in its 2009 report, *A Future Vision for Mental Health*, that 'prevention and treatment of mental ill health are complementary endeavours, and should not compete for funding'. Nevertheless, the Coalition also emphasised the model of recovery, arguing that 'focusing more attention "upstream" into promotion, education, prevention and early intervention has a strong moral case (to avert avoidable suffering) and makes sound economic sense'.[14]

A number of anti-stigma campaigns thus appear to be discarding the concept of 'mental illness' in favour of 'mental health' or 'mental health problems'. These more fashionable terms succeed in broadening out the object under consideration. They convey the idea that a continuum exists between mental health and illness, emphasising the possibility of recovery and avoiding the kind of pessimism and despondency which fuelled the image of the chronic, burnt-out psychotic; an individual whose status as a citizen had been subsumed and eroded by their diagnosis and for whom relocation from the hospital to the community, as Peter Barham has so eloquently demonstrated through interviews with service users, often seemed to involve little more than the substitution of the label 'mental hospital patient' with the new identity of 'community mental patient'.[15] One might, however, query the novelty of such an approach, echoing as it does the discourse of the mental hygiene movement of the interwar years, discussed in Chapter 3. As my analysis of this movement revealed, destigmatising incipient mental distress and promoting mental health were accomplished by reinforcing the stigma attached to severe and enduring mental disorders. In turn, the resources available to support such people were cut back. Subsuming discussion of the needs of people experiencing mental health problems as a small facet of a larger document which focuses primarily on mental well-being could have a similar consequences. In this connection, it is striking that of the major mental health charities it is Rethink Mental Illness, the charity founded in 1970 as the National Schizophrenia Fellowship, which continues to refer on its website primarily to mental illness. Indeed, the charity lengthened its name in 2011 from Rethink to Rethink Mental Illness, hoping this would clarify its purpose.[16]

However the concept of mental illness, which encapsulates and conflates the differing experiences of people who experience mental distress, may also lead to the neglect of the needs of people who experience enduring and/or severe mental health problems. Proponents of a medicalised model argue that representing mental illness as an illness like any other helps remove stigma by reframing sufferers as innocent victims of their own biology. Yet the illness model, with its emphasis on cure and recovery, does not serve the needs of people who experience enduring mental distress. It is difficult, as Helen Spandler has observed, to challenge concepts such as recovery or social inclusion, because they are presented as 'self evidently desirable and unquestionable'.[17] Rethink Mental Illness attempts to surmount the dilemma of perpetuating pessimism on the one hand, and creating models of recovery which may be unobtainable for some on the other. It distinguishes between clinical recovery, 'an idea that has emerged from the expertise of mental health professionals, and involves getting rid of symptoms, restoring social functioning, and in other ways *"getting back to normal"'*, and personal recovery; the latter defined as helping people to build a meaningful life in their own terms, irrespective of any ongoing clinical symptoms.[18] Social inclusion, Spandler suggests, envisages that service users should aspire to conform to the norms of social and economic life, and thus insidiously imposes a regulatory framework upon service users.[19] Equally, 'recovery', as Barbara Taylor observes, all too often conveys the expectation that service users should aspire to self-reliance and independence, rather than burden the state by requiring financial, medical or emotional support.[20]

Another approach which may help alleviate the discrimination experienced by people with enduring mental health problems would be to apply the principles of the social model of disability. Liz Sayce, for example, suggests that this would provide the grounds to demand that society should make adjustments to enable people who experience mental distress to function. It acknowledges the reality of recurrent episodes of severe mental disturbance, but is underpinned by a rights agenda.[21] Conversely, the concept of mental illness situates the root of the problem within the biology of the individual sufferer, lifting the onus of responsibility from society. By no means all service users favour such an approach. Anne Plumb, for example, believes that including people who experience mental distress within the social disability movement on the grounds that they have a 'hidden impairment' reinforces the medicalisation of mental distress and risks subsuming the distinctive interests and needs of service users or psychiatric system survivors.[22] Recent critiques of the social model of disability also challenge Sayce's views. Thus Tom Shakespeare and Nicholas Watson urge discarding the social model in favour of an embodied ontology which situates disability within a spectrum of impairment inherent in the human condition. They argue that this would surmount discrimination by revealing how fallacious the dichotomy between the able-bodied and the disabled is in practice.[23]

We could invert Shakespeare and Watson's logic on the grounds that the idea of a continuum between mental health and illness has led to a neglect of the needs of people living with enduring and severe mental distress. Moreover, the biological model has embedded mental disorder within the body of the sufferer, militating against social adjustment to meet the needs of the individual. Shakespeare and Watson's assertion that the social model is too narrow to effectively advance disability rights may well be astute in many ways. However, the social model may yet prove beneficial as a means of countering the discrimination facing individuals who experience severe and enduring mental distress, whose difficulties have tended hitherto to be interpreted via the medical model, and who have arguably been positioned at or near the bottom of the hierarchy of disability.[24] These debates point to the difficulty of advocating a single approach to meet the needs of disparate groups facing discrimination.

Few have openly criticised Time to Change, in part because its stated objectives are (to borrow once more the words of Helen Spandler) 'self evidently desirable and unquestionable'.[25] However, some service users, including individuals recruited to the Campaign's Lived Experience Advisory Panel which ostensibly drove the Campaign's strategy, reported that Time to Change offered them only limited input and sought to co-opt, and take credit for, the activities of other service-user-led groups.[26] Dawn Willis had been involved in the first wave of the Time to Change campaign, and recalled on her blog her excitement that it might herald 'the beginning of a revolution in the perception of mental illness and more importantly for me, the promotion of the reality that whilst having a mental illness is sometimes quite scary, it doesn't make me a "freak", it doesn't mean I'm "bad" or "stupid" or incapable of being a success, or that I possess [sic] a "threat" to the general public (whoever they may be)'. As time went on however, Willis's unabashed enthusiasm gave way to ambivalence as she encountered sceptical service users, frustrated that the only people featured in Time to Change campaigns were 'successful people with a diagnosis, or well-maintained celebrities' who had recovered from their distress. The people Willis spoke to expressed their concerns that Time to Change would erode public sympathy for individuals with severe mental health issues, some describing how their offer to help with the campaign had been ignored because 'my meds make me walk differently and talk differently, but without them I would be psychotic'; 'it's obvious that I have schizophrenia'; 'I was too unwell'.[27] Many of those who responded to Willis's post corroborated these sentiments. Dave Neenan expressed his frustrations with 'remote and uncommunicative mental health charity professionals trying to stage manage representation and bulldoze through their notions of our concerns, needs and aspirations in a top down way'.[28] 'Who is talking about the people who are so damaged by old types of meds, that their recovery is limited?' asked Jane. 'Not TTC [Time to Change], they are too busy telling us how celebs recovered . . . I look out my window onto a car park, live off £65 a week benefit and am still waiting for talking therapy for depression.'[29] The tensions between the objectives of Time to Change and the perception of service users who live with chronic mental health conditions are reflected in the epigraphs which open this conclusion.

The seeming unwillingness of Time to Change to allow service users to lead anti-stigma campaigns reflects the paternalistic approach adopted by the MACA towards its clients, examined in Chapter 5. Potentially the Time to Change grants fund, launched in May 2012 and running until March 2015, could diversify the Campaign's messages and image, as it will support up to seventy-five community projects. However, the £2.7 million allocated to this fund constitutes less than 15 per cent of the funding allocated by the government to Time to Change for this period.[30] Expressing his concern that resources had been unfairly distributed amongst different mental health 'diagnosis and need groups', Dave Neenan blamed Time to Change and other recent campaigns for creating the false impression 'that people with mental health issues are a homogenous group'.[31]

Do campaigns informed by broadly conceived concepts of 'mental health' or 'mental illness' give sufficient consideration to the needs of individuals with enduring mental health problems, and do they convince their audience? Only 16 per cent of the people polled by the Office of National Statistics in 2010 believed that one in four people would experience a mental health problem at some point in their lives.[32] Similarly, a survey undertaken by the Health Education Authority in 1997 found that statistics regarding the prevalence of mental illness were given little credence.[33] When presented with this statistic, one interviewee responded, 'don't believe it. No one I know is mental. How can it be one in four.'[34] We could interpret this response as evidence of the need to educate the public about the prevalence of mental disorder and to remind people that those close to them might suffer from mental health problems. However, another interpretation presents itself: that the respondent associated mental illness with schizophrenia, and did not view depression and anxiety as mental disorders. In this connection, we might recall the findings of the BBC's audience report into the screening of the 'Hurt Mind' series, in which 90 per cent of those surveyed distinguished between mental illness and insanity.[35] Indeed, such distinctions were sometimes drawn by former patients. Thus in her autobiographical account, Marcia Hamilcar acknowledged that she had been suffering from 'simple mental depression', but insisted, 'I was never insane'.[36]

It is helpful, at this point, to turn back to an observation made by Joan Busfield which we considered in Chapter 4. In the course of dismantling the argument that women are disproportionately diagnosed with mental illnesses, Busfield reminded her readers that such claims were dependent upon how one defines what constitutes mental illness. 'It is less "madness" that is identified as the female malady', she concluded, 'than the broader territory of more "minor" psychiatric conditions'.[37] The 'one in four' statistic which has featured in so many anti-stigma campaigns relies upon a concept of mental illness which incorporates a broad and diverse range of mental disturbances – what Busfield terms the 'minor' psychiatric conditions. If we remove such conditions from the equation, the 'one in four' statistic loses its credence, and the gender of the mentally disturbed individual shifts from female to male. Indeed, while Elaine Showalter identified a 'pervasive cultural association of women and madness' over the course the twentieth century,[38] this book reveals how representations of mental illness in twentieth-century Britain were shaped by the image of the violent male patient.

Most cases of mental disturbance have traditionally been divided into two loose clinical groupings, the neuroses and the psychoses. In the words of the Mental Health Foundation, the neuroses are now more commonly described as 'common mental health problems', and neurotic symptoms 'can be regarded as severe forms of "normal" emotional experiences such as depression, anxiety or panic'. Psychotic symptoms, the Foundation explains, 'interfere with a person's perception of reality, and may include hallucinations such as seeing, hearing, smelling or feeling things that no one else can'.[39] Half a century ago, Henry Yellowlees similarly distinguished between the neuroses – 'the functional nervous disorders' – and the psychoses: 'the insanities'.[40] In so doing, Yellowlees sought to 'enlighten the public' who, he sneered, viewed the neuroses as 'just nerves, Doctor, nothing wrong with him, really' and the psychoses as 'going mental'.[41] Yet this demonstrates that medical and lay beliefs converged, rather than diverged. Far from pointing to the inability of the public to grasp medical ideas, the respondents' seeming intransigence and obtuseness when presented with campaigns which bracket together the neuroses and psychoses and seek to persuade the reader that one in four people will suffer from a mental health problem demonstrates shared lay and medical understandings. No wonder anti-stigma campaigns which have sought to counter prejudice by emphasising the prevalence of mental disturbance, equating an episode of depression or anxiety with a diagnosis of schizophrenia, have proved so ineffectual. This point has been made by service users who are sceptical of the Time to Change campaign, as the opening epigraph by JM illustrates. Noting that the main messages of the campaign were 'that mental illness is common ("One in Four") and no barrier to success (Ruby Wax), in other words, that it is no big deal', 'Neuroskeptic' similarly observed that, unfortunately for some, mental illness 'is a big deal . . . and to pretend otherwise is insulting to service users who aren't currently living the TTC [Time to Change] dream, and to the public (who aren't stupid)'.[42]

Considering these findings alongside the inability of anti-stigma campaigns to make any inroads into perceptions that mental disturbance is accompanied by violence, it appears that the stigma attached to mental distress is most entrenched in the area of enduring mental health problems, particularly surrounding the psychoses rather than the neuroses. This is an observation which healthcare workers sometimes make, pointing to more nuanced attempts to engage with the problems of stigma. Thus in a book documenting a global anti-stigma programme established by the World Psychiatric Association, Norman Sartorius and Hugh Schulze recount how the Association opted to focus on schizophrenia rather than all mental illnesses. While a broader campaign would potentially engage a larger number of patients, the Association felt that the stigma attached to schizophrenia was more pronounced than the stigma attached to anxiety states. The public, Sartorius and Schulze note, tend to enumerate the symptoms of schizophrenia when asked to describe a mentally ill person.[43] Despite the focus of the campaign, Satorius and Schulze nevertheless entitled their book *Reducing the Stigma of Mental Illness*, camouflaging the focus of their work. Similarly, the psychiatrist Patrick W. Corrigan described his frustration when the people he helped 'with serious mental illness' subsequently encountered prejudice when searching for housing and employment, and outlined how perceptions that mental illness was accompanied by violence fuelled stigma. Yet Corrigan's book once more conceals how discrimination was disproportionately linked to serious mental illness, referring throughout simply to 'the stigma of mental illness'.[44] The emphasis placed by Time to Change on recovery has been justified by some on the grounds that campaigning on mental health issues is in its infancy, and should therefore project positive and unthreatening messages to an uniformed public.[45] Participants acknowledge that the campaign paints an incomplete picture which camouflages the discrimination encountered by people who experience serious and enduring mental health problems, but do not feel that this should be publicised. One member of the campaign's Lived Experience Advisory Panel admitted that 'I can't say I have personally agreed with it all', but felt that the campaign was justified on the grounds that it targeted the general public, not service users.[46]

To what extent have the efforts made by healthcare professionals over the course of the twentieth century to destigmatise treatment for incipient cases helped embed the stigma attached to enduring or chronic mental disorder? To hold healthcare workers accountable for failing to alleviate the discrimination experienced by mental health service users would arguably be to overstate the power wielded by healthcare workers and to overlook the constraints they operated under, the role of other groups and the impact of government policy. While this book has demonstrated why the permeation of professional aspirations into anti-stigma campaigns could be problematic, it has also demonstrated why this occurred: mental healthcare workers to some extent shared the stigma attached to their patients and tended to be positioned as a less prestigious branch of a broader medical profession. Indeed, the credentials of these workers as medical professionals providing treatment to sick patients was frequently called into question by the broader medical profession, which in turn partially explains why health workers' attempts to alleviate the stigma of mental distress tended to be grounded on the premise that mental illness was a biological illness like any other.[47] This also helps explain why many healthcare workers sought to draw public attention to those patients whose conditions were amenable to biomedical therapies, while concealing the plight of long-stay patients suffering from chronic conditions. It would be unrealistic to expect psychiatric nurses to have campaigned voraciously on behalf of their patients in the early 1960s, when the changing structure of mental health services appeared poised to render their profession obsolete. Similarly, we might well ask how charities could be expected to improve public attitudes and provide community services to fill the gap left by disappearing state services, at a time when the government cut the funding it provided to them.

Responding to government proposals to close down mental hospitals in 1961, Richard Titmuss observed how 'statutory magic' and 'comforting appellation' could transform 'wild and unlovely weeds . . . into attractive and domesticated flowers'. 'Community Care', he ventured, conjured 'a sense of warmth and human kindness', yet in the absence of services or funding, it remained an attractive but hollow phrase.[48] Did discussion of the need to educate the public so as to alleviate the stigma of mental illness serve to divert attention from inadequate government funding and resources, leaving mental healthcare professionals and the voluntary sector to operate as best they could in often difficult circumstances? In a paper prepared for the Standing Mental Health Advisory Committee in 1960 which projected a declining need for beds in mental hospitals, the Ministry of Health acknowledged that 'there is no guarantee that the social atmosphere that tolerates eccentrics and an economy that enabled them to be largely self-supporting will continue'.[49] By the mid-1980s, a report into community care undertaken by the Social Services Committee asserted that the term *community care* was 'virtually meaningless', reiterating the view of the National Council for Voluntary Organisations that 'the pleasant connotations of the phrase can be misleading'. The authors of the report cautioned against using the phrase to connote voluntary or familial as opposed to statutory care, or a means of saving money on the costs of hospital care.[50] The Committee expressed concerns that hospital services were being closed down before adequate extra-mural facilities had been established to fill their space, yet they urged the government to 'promote a positive programme designed to procure a greater degree of community acceptance of community care policies', encouraging voluntary groups to 'follow up the Minister's invitation to apply for funds for such purposes'.[51]

Ostensibly, campaigns such as See Me and Time to Change aim to erode the stigma of mental distress, and have not been initiated to engender public support for government mental health policy. Nevertheless, the image of recovery and autonomy which lies at the heart of such campaigns echoes the message at the heart of *Towards a Mentally Flourishing Scotland* and *A Future Vision for Mental Health*, and can be used to legitimate a reduction in community-based provisions, as Barbara Taylor has observed.[52] The apparent symbiosis between Time to Change, which has represented those suffering from mental health problems as successful employees, and welfare reform, which is underpinned by the principle that many current benefit claimants are capable of work, has generated even more anxiety. Mind and Rethink Mental Illness, the two mental health charities leading Time to Change, have fervently attacked welfare reform, expressing concerns that the campaign to enact policy stigmatised benefit claimants as scroungers, and that the new system would have a detrimental impact upon sufferers of mental distress who relied upon benefits.[53] One poster on the Mental Health Forum commented that s/he had become wary of the Time to Change campaign after seeing 'various politicians who are intent on frightening the mentally ill with the welfare reform changes giving their support to it'. In a memorable analogy, s/he explained, 'that is like Jack the Ripper lending his support to a campaign to safeguard the lives of Whitechapel prostitutes'.[54] Peter Beresford, Professor of Social Policy at Brunel University and a self-identified long-term user of mental health services, asked 'why is the government supporting an anti-discrimination campaign when its rhetoric in relation to welfare reform is saying something very different'. 'Is a public education campaign really what is needed', Beresford wondered, 'when the principle [sic] shapers of negative public opinion actually seem to be the government ... Challenging mental health stigma and discrimination is one policy that needs to come from the top down, rather than the bottom up.'[55]

Anti-stigma campaigns have shied away from depicting the discrimination experienced by individuals who suffer from serious and enduring mental health problems. Instead, campaigns assert that mental ill-health is common, not serious, and no barrier to success. These campaigns conceptualise stigma in much the same way as Erving Goffman did;[56] they focus on interpersonal interactions and assert that stigma emanates from the behaviour and attitudes of the public. In turn, these supposed public attitudes are mocked, as (according to campaigns) mental ill-health is an inconsequential matter which would have little impact on the lived experience of individuals, were they not also the victim of public prejudice. Such an approach conveniently overlooks how social, political and economic factors foster discrimination,[57] and threaten to trivialise severe mental distress. Elizabeth Toon has observed that in the 1950s, when cancer sufferers 'all too frequently died painful and lonely deaths', the problem facing health educators was not, as health educators frequently claimed, public ignorance of cancer but 'the public's knowledge of the disease's all-too-frequent consequences'.[58] As JM's observation at the start of this conclusion demonstrates, this diagnosis could well be applied to contemporary anti-stigma campaigns. If the objective is to end the discrimination encountered by service users, we need campaigns led by grassroots groups and supported by the major voluntary sector groups which depict the experiences of individuals who live with serious mental health issues, highlighting how their lives are made more difficult by forms of structural discrimination and challenging government policies which perpetuate such discrimination. Instead of rehashing the idea of the continuum in the hope of eliciting greater public sympathy for sufferers of severe mental distress by portraying individuals with minor mental health issues – an unconvincing strategy which compounds the stigma surrounding enduring mental health problems and reduces the resources available to support such individuals – perhaps contemporary campaigners should consider revisiting some of the more unflinching accounts of psychoses and schizophrenia from the 1960s and 1970s. Mary Barnes and R. D. Laing, for example, depicted severe mental disturbances as profoundly distressing experiences which nevertheless did not erode personhood, and could be understood in the context of an individual's life.[59]

Notes

1   Time to Change, 'Is your mind made up about mental illness?', poster displayed on the London Underground, 2009. Poster available online from Time to Change, 'Launch Campaign – January 2009': www.time-to-change.org.uk/about/about-our-campaign/launch-campaign-%E2%80%93-january-2009, consulted 18 February 2013.

2   Response by 'JM' on 3 October 2010 to D. Willis, 'Shiny happy service users – is the TTC campaign about to become counterproductive?', 18 September 2010: www.dawnwillis.wordpress.com/2010/09/18/shiny-happy-service-users-%E2%80%93-is-the-ttc-campaign-about-to-become-counter-productive/. Ellipsis in original text.

3   S. P. Hinshaw, *The Mark of Shame: Stigma of Mental Illness and an Agenda for Change* (Oxford, 2007), p. 71.

4   BBC WAC, N14/6/7/1, memo from D. Hyde, 15 August 1955, for programme suggestion, 'Within Our Province', and report on visit by D. Hyde, 1 May 1956.

5   Hyde's programme is discussed in Chapter 6.

6   Willis, 'Shiny happy service users'.

7   D. Willis, follow up to 'Shiny happy service users', 4 October 2010, and Dave Neenan, response to 'Shiny happy service users', 22 September 2010.

8   M. Barker and M. Menken, 'Time to abandon the term mental illness', *British Medical Journal*, 322:7291 (2001), 937.

9   Mind, 'Understanding mental health problems', www.mind.org.uk/help/diagnoses_and_conditions/mental_illness, accessed 4 April 2012.

10 Time to Change, 'About us', www.time-to-change.org.uk/about (2008).

11 The Scottish Government, *Towards a Mentally Flourishing Scotland: Policy and Action Plan, 2009–2011* (Edinburgh, 2009).

12 Ibid., p. 3.

13 Ibid., pp. 41–5.

14 The Future Vision Coalition, *A Future Vision for Mental Health* (2009), p. 15.

15 See P. Barham, *Closing the Asylum: The Mental Patient in Modern Society* (Harmondsworth, 1997).

16 See Rethink Mental Illness, 'About our new look', 25 November 2011, www. rethink.org/about_us/about_our_new_look.html.

17 H. Spandler, 'From social exclusion to inclusion? A critique of the inclusion imperative in mental health', *Medical Sociology Online*, 2:2 (2007), 3–16; 3.

18 Rethink, 'What is Recovery?', www.rethink.org/living_with_mental_illness/ what_is_recovery/index.html, updated 19 September 2011. Bold type in original text.

19 Spandler, 'From social exclusion to inclusion'.

20 B. Taylor, 'The demise of the asylum in late twentieth-century Britain: a personal history', *Transactions of the Royal Historical Society*, 21 (2011), 193–215.

21 L. Sayce, *From Psychiatric Patient to Citizen: Overcoming Discrimination and Social Exclusion* (Houndmills, 2000).

22 A. Plumb, '. . . Distress or disability?' (1994), reproduced in J. Anderson, B. Sapey and H. Spandler (eds), *Distress or Disability? Proceedings of a Symposium Held at Lancaster University, 15–16 November 2011* (Bowland North, 2012), pp. 4–12.

23 T. Shakespeare and N. Watson, 'The social model of disability: an outdated ideology?', *Research in Social Science and Disability*, 2 (2002), 9–28.

24 J. L. Tringo, 'The hierarchy of preference towards disability groups', *Journal of Special Education*, 4 (1970), 295–30.

25 Spandler, 'From social exclusion to inclusion', p. 3.

26 R. Griffiths, 'The bigger picture', *Mental Health Today* (January/February, 2012), 20. I am very grateful to Alasdair Cameron for sharing this article with me and for his observations on some of these issues.

27 Willis, 'Shiny happy service users'.

28 Response by Dave Neenan to Willis's post, 'Shiny happy service users', 19 September 2010.

29 Response by 'Jane' to Willis's post, 'Shiny happy service users', 19 September 2010.

30 For figures on funding for the Time to Change grants scheme, see Time to Change, 'Time to Change grants fund – open for applications', http://time-to-change.org.uk/grants/landing, consulted 27 August 2012. On funding for Time to Change as a whole, see Department of Health, '£20 million to knock down mental health stigma', 10 October 2011: http://mediacentre.dh.gov.uk/2011/10/10/20-million-to-knock-down-mental-health-stigma/.

31 Response by Dave Neenan to Willis's post, 'Shiny happy service users', 19 September 2010.

32 J. Tudor, 'Public attitudes slowly heading in the right direction', 31 March 2010: www.time-to-change.org.uk/news/public-attitudes-heading-slowly-right-direction.

33 Sayce, *From Psychiatric Patient to Citizen*, p. 208.

34 Ibid., p. 208.

35 BBC Written Archives Centre Caversham, T32/846/1, BBC, 'An Audience Research Report – 'The Hurt Mind' – An Enquiry into Some of the Effects of

the Series of Five television Broadcasts about Mental Illness and Its Treatment' (1957).

36   M. Hamilcar, *Legally Dead: Experiences during Seventeen Weeks' Detention in a Private Asylum with an Introduction by Dr. Forbes Winslow* (London, 1910), pp. 67–8.

37   J. Busfield, *Men, Women and Madness: Understanding Gender and Mental Disorder* (Houndmills, 1996), pp. 13–30; p. 19.

38   E. Showalter, *The Female Malady: Women, Madness and English Culture, 1830–1980* (1987; London, 2001), p. 4.

39   Mental Health Foundation, 'What are mental health problems?' www.mentalhealth.org.uk/help-information/an-introduction-to-mental-health/what-are-mental-health-problems/?view=Standard, accessed 30 January 2012.

40   H. Yellowlees, *To Define True Madness: Commonsense Psychiatry for Lay People* (1953; Harmondsworth, 1955), p. 10.

41   Ibid., p. x.

42   Response by 'Neuroskeptic' to Willis's post, 'Shiny happy service users', 19 September 2010.

43   N. Sartorius and H. Schulze, *Reducing the Stigma of Mental Illness: A Report from a Global Programme of the World Psychiatric Association* (Cambridge, 2005), p. 6.

44   P. W. Corrigan 'Introduction', in P. W. Corrigan (ed.), *On the Stigma of Mental Illness: Practical Strategies for Research and Social Change* (Washington, DC, 2005), pp. 3–7; p. 3.

45   Responses by 'Oz' to Willis's post, 'Shiny happy service users', 20 September and 27 September 2010.

46   Response by 'KM' to Willis's post, 'Shiny happy service users', 26 September 2010.

47   A point also made by Duncan Mitchell in relation to learning disability nursing: see D. Mitchell, 'Parallel stigma? Nurses and people with learning disabilities', *British Journal of Learning Disabilities*, 28 (2000), 78–81.

48   Titmuss is cited in C. Ungerson, *Policy Is Political: Sex, Gender and Informal Care* (London, 1987), pp. 6–7.

49   TNA, MH 133/424, Ministry of Health, 'Trends in the mental hospital population and their effects on future planning', 2 December 1960.

50   *Second Report from the Social Services Committee Session 1984–85: Community Care with Special Reference to Adult Mentally Ill and Mentally Handicapped People* (London, 1985), p. x.

51   Ibid., p. lxviii.

52   Taylor, 'The demise of the asylum'.

53   See Rethink, 'Welfare Reform Act 2012', www.rethink.org/how_we_can_help/our_campaigns/stigma_and_discrimination/welfare_reform_act_2.html, last updated 17 May 2012, and T. Pollard, 'Welfare: where to from here?', http://www.mind.org.uk/blog/6853_welfare_where_to_from_here, 17 May 2012. The latter post by Mind's senior policy officer generated some rather critical comments in response, which can be viewed at the webpage above.

54 Firemonkee, 'Time to Change', www.mentalhealthforum.net/forum/thread4637. html, 10 May 2011.

55 P. Beresford, 'Mental health discrimination is coming from the top, not the public', *The Guardian* (30 November 2011), www.guardian.co.uk/society/joepublic/ 2011/nov/30/mental-health-discrimination-campaign.

56 E. Goffman, *Stigma: Notes on the Management of a Spoiled Identity* (1963; Harmondsworth, 1968).

57 Critics of Goffman's work argue that such structural factors are intrinsic in the stigmatisation of individuals, and fuel discrimination. See B. G. Link and J. C. Phelan, 'Conceptualizing stigma', *Annual Review of Sociology*, 27 (2001), 363–84.

58 E. Toon, '"Cancer as the general population knows it": knowledge, fear, and lay education in 1950s Britain', *Bulletin of the History of Medicine*, 81 (2007), 116–48; 138, 132.

59 M. Barnes and J. Berke, *Mary Barnes: Two Accounts of a Journey through Madness* (London, 1971); R. D. Laing, *The Divided Self* (London, 1959).

Timeline: key dates

1808 County Asylums Act (Wynn's Act): this legislation empowered justices of the peace to establish asylums in English counties for the care of pauper and criminal lunatics, and to raise local funds for this purpose.

1841: Asylum superintendents established the Association of Medical Officers of Asylums for the Insane.

1845 Lunacy Act: this legislation established the Lunacy Commission, which was responsible for inspecting and regulating all asylums in England and Wales, and for overseeing the rights of people certified as insane.

1845 County Asylums Act: this Act compelled all counties in England and Wales to construct asylums for pauper lunatics.

1857 Lunacy (Scotland) Act: this legislation compelled Scottish districts to construct asylums for pauper lunatics, and established the Board of Commissioners in Lunacy for Scotland, which exerted similar powers to the Lunacy Commission in England and Wales.

1865: The Association of Medical Officers of Asylums for the Insane renames itself the Medico-Psychological Association.

1879: Establishment of the After-care Association for Poor and Friendless Female Convalescents on Leaving Asylums for the Insane (later renamed the Mental After Care Association).

1890 Lunacy Act: This Act sought to prevent wrongful confinement and abuses within asylums. It elaborated and formalised arrangements with regards to administration; admission of patients to asylums or licensed houses; inspection of asylums and licensed houses by the Lunacy Commissioners; patients' rights to correspond with the authorities and discharge arrangements.

1908 Report of the Royal Commission on the Care and Control of the Feeble-Minded: this Report advocated a specialised system of care for people diagnosed as mentally defective.

1910: Establishment of the National Asylum Workers' Union.

1913 Mental Deficiency Act: this legislation required county and borough authorities in England and Wales to ascertain defectives and to provide community supervision, guardianship and institutional care. The Board of Control replaced the Lunacy Commission and assumed responsibility for administering the lunacy and mental deficiency systems.

1926: Publication of the Report of the Royal Commission on Mental Illness. Viewing mental illness as a form of physical illness, this Report urged that older terminology should be replaced with medical terminology. It believed that allowing patients to enter mental hospitals voluntarily would aid treatment and prevention, and it sought to abolish the distinction between private and pauper patients. It also urged local authorities to establish out-patient clinics.

1926: The Medico-Psychological Association becomes the Royal Medico-Psychological Association.

1929 Local Government Act: this legislation abolished Poor Law unions and boards of guardians, transferring their powers to local authorities.

1929: Establishment of the Association of Psychiatric Social Work.

1930 Mental Treatment Act: this legislation enacted many of the recommendations of the 1926 Royal Commission Report. Notably, it enabled patients to seek admission as voluntary patients, and retitled asylums as mental hospitals.

1930: The National Asylum Workers' Union renamed itself the Mental Hospital and Institutional Workers' Union.

1946: The Central Association for Mental Welfare (founded 1913), the National Council for Mental Hygiene (established 1922) and the Child Guidance Council (formed 1927) amalgamate to form the National Association for Mental Health.

1946 National Health Service Act: this legislation brought mental health services within the new National Health Service. The Ministry of Health assumed authority over county mental hospitals in 1948 as the National Health Service came into operation.

1946: The Mental Hospital and Institutional Workers' Union federates with the Hospital and Welfare Services Union to form the Confederation of Health Service Employees.

1956: The BBC broadcasts 'The Hurt Mind' – the first British television series on mental illness.

1957: Publication of the Report of the Royal Commission on the Law Relating to Mental Illness and Mental Deficiency. This urged relocating mental healthcare from hospitals to community settings.

1959: Publication of the Report of the Working Party on Social Workers in Local Authority Health and Welfare Services. Also known as the Younghusband Report, this stressed the need for professionally trained and experienced social workers and identified a shortfall in the number of psychiatric social workers required to adequately staff local authority services.

1959 Mental Health Act: repealing earlier legislation, this Act provided a single legal code for all types of mental disorder and enabled local authorities to provide a range of community-based services. It also allowed people to seek treatment without formalities. The Act abolished the Board of Control and transferred its powers of inspection to local authorities. A new independent body, the Mental Health Review Tribunal, was established to monitor patients' rights. Psychopathy was defined as a condition which fell within the category of mental disorder.

1960 Mental Health (Scotland) Act: this Act in many respects mirrored the 1959 Mental Health Act, but established the Scottish Mental Welfare Commission to oversee the liberty of psychiatric patients.

1961: Health Minister Enoch Powell announces plans to incrementally close down Britain's psychiatric hospitals in a speech to the National Association for Mental Health.

1970: The Association of Psychiatric Social Work and its members were absorbed into the British Association of Social Workers. New generic training for all social workers replaced the specialist university courses which had previously trained psychiatric social workers.

1971: The Royal Medico-Psychological Association is renamed the Royal College of Psychiatrists.

1972: The National Association for Mental Health is rebranded MIND.

1973: Foundation of the Mental Patients' Union.

Bibliography

Primary sources

Archival collections

BBC Written Archives Centre, Peppard Road, Caversham Park, Reading.

Lothian Health Services Archive, University of Edinburgh Centre for Research Collections, Main Library, George Square, Edinburgh:
- Royal Edinburgh Hospital Archive

Modern Records Centre, University Library, University of Warwick, Coventry:
- Association of Psychiatric Social Work Archive
- Confederation of Health Service Employees Archive
- National Asylum Workers' Union / Mental Hospital and Institutional Workers' Union Archive

The National Archives, Kew, Richmond, Surrey:
- Ministry of Health Records

NHS Greater Glasgow and Clyde Archives, the Mitchell Library, Glasgow:
- Gartnavel Royal Hospital Archives

Wellcome Library, London:
- Mental After Care Association Archives
- Robina Addis Archive
- William Sargant Collection

Published sources

Allen, H., 'A narrative of God's gracious dealings with that choice Christian Mrs. Hannah Allen' (1683), in A. Ingram (ed.) *Voices of Madness: Four Pamphlets, 1683–1796* (Stroud, 1997), pp. 1–22.

Altschul, A., 'The role of the psychiatric nurse in the community', in Association of Psychiatric Social Workers, *New Developments in Psychiatry and the Implications for the Social Worker* (London, 1969), pp. 37–9.

Anonymous, 'They said I was mad', *Forum and Century*, 100 (1938), 231–7.

Anonymous, *The Autobiography of David, edited by Ernest Raymond* (London, 1946).

Barnes, M. and Berke, J., *Two Accounts of a Journey through Madness* (London, 1971).

Beers, C., *A Mind that Found Itself: An Autobiography* (London, 1908).

Belcher, W., 'Address to humanity: containing, a letter to Dr. Monro; a receipt to make a lunatic, and seize his estate; and a sketch of a true smiling hyena' (1796), in A. Ingram (ed.) *Voices of Madness: Four Pamphlets, 1683–1796* (Stroud, 1997), pp. 127–36.

Brown, G. W., Bone, M., Dalison, B. and Wing, J. K., *Schizophrenia and Social Care: A Comparative Follow-Up Study of 339 Schizophrenic Patients* (London, 1966).

Bruckshaw, S., 'One more proof of the iniquitous abuse of private madhouses' (1774), in A. Ingram (ed.) *Voices of Madness: Four Pamphlets, 1683–1796* (Stroud, 1997), pp. 75–126.

Clarke, D. H., *The Story of a Mental Hospital: Fulbourn 1858–1983* (London, 1996).

Clouston, T., *The Hygiene of the Mind* (London, 1906).

Crichton-Browne, J., *Burns, From a New Point of View* (London, 1926).

Crichton-Browne, J., *The Doctor's Second Thoughts* (London, 1931).

Crichton-Browne, J., *The Doctor Remembers* (1932; London, 1938).

Crichton-Browne, J., *From the Doctor's Notebook* (London, 1937).

Crichton-Browne, J., *Stray Leaves from a Physician's Portfolio* (London, 1938).

Cruden, A., 'The London-citizen exceedingly injured' (1739), in A. Ingram (ed.) *Voices of Madness: Four Pamphlets, 1683–1796* (Stroud, 1997), pp. 23–74.

Gibson, G., edited by W. Gibson, *Reminiscences* (Eastbourne, 2004).

Grant-Smith, R., *The Experiences of an Asylum Patient with an Introduction and Notes by Montagu Lomax M.R.C.S.* (London, 1922).

Hamilcar, M., *Legally Dead: Experiences during Seventeen Weeks' Detention in a Private Asylum with an Introduction by Dr. Forbes Winslow* (London, 1910).

Irwin, E., Mitchell, L., Durkin, L. and Douieb, B., 'The need for a mental patients' union' (1972). Reproduced on the webpage: http://studymore.org.uk/mpu. htm#FishPamphlet.

Laing, R. D., *The Divided Self: An Existential Study in Sanity and Madness* (1959; Harmondsworth, 1965).

Laing, R. D., *Wisdom, Madness and Folly: The Making of a Psychiatrist 1927–1957* (1985; London, 1986).

Laurie, K., *Employable or Unemployable? Report on Pioneer Experimental Work Covering the Period February 6 1939 – August 1 1940* (London, 1941).

Lomax, M., *The Experiences of an Asylum Doctor with Suggestions for Asylum and Lunacy Law Reform* (London, 1921).

Martin, D. V., *Adventure in Psychiatry: Social Change in a Mental Hospital* (Oxford, 1962).

Maudsley, H., *The Physiology and Pathology of the Mind* (London, 1867).

Mayhew, C., *Time to Explain: An Autobiography* (London, 1987).

McDougall, K. F., 'Chairman's introduction', in E. M. Goldberg, E. E. Irvine, A. B. Lloyd Davies and K. F. McDougall (eds), *The Boundaries of Casework: A Report on a Residential Refresher Course Held by the Association of Psychiatric Social Work* (London, 1959), p. 8.

Medico-Psychological Association, *Handbook for Attendants on the Insane* (London, 1908).

Ministry of Health, *Report of the Committee on Administration of Public Mental Hospitals*, Cmd. 1730 (London, 1922).

Ministry of Health, *Report of the Departmental Committee on Sterilisation*, Cmnd. 4485 (London, 1934).

Ministry of Health, *Report of the Working Party on Social Workers in Local Authority Health and Welfare Services* (London, 1959).

Osbaldeston, M., 'Nobody wants to know', in B. Robb, *Sans Everything: A Case to Answer* (London, 1967), pp. 13–18.

Report of the Committee on Medical Auxiliaries, Cmd. 8188 (London, 1951).

Report of the Interdepartmental Committee on Mental Deficiency, 1925–1929 (London, 1929).

Report of the Royal Commission on the Law Relating to Mental Illness and Mental Deficiency, Cmnd. 169 (London, 1957).

Report of the Tribunal Appointed to Inquire into Allegations Reflecting on the Official Conduct of Ministers of the Crown and Other Public Servants, Cmd. 7617 (1949).

Robb, B., *Sans Everything: A Case to Answer* (London, 1967).

Robinson, P. (director), *Asylum* (film, 1971).

Rolph, C. H., 'Cruelty in the old people's ward', in B. Robb, *Sans Everything: A Case to Answer* (London, 1967), pp. 3–7.

Sargant, W., *The Unquiet Mind: The Autobiography of a Physician in Psychological Medicine* (London, 1967).

Sargant, W. and Slater, E., *An Introduction to Physical Methods of Treatment in Psychiatry* (Edinburgh, 1948).

Second Report from the Social Services Committee Session 1984–85: Community Care with Special Reference to Adult Mentally Ill and Mentally Handicapped People (London, 1985).

Smith, T., 'The role of the psychiatric nurse in the community', in Association of Psychiatric Social Workers, *New Developments in Psychiatry and the Implications for the Social Worker* (London, 1969), pp. 40–6.

Stafford-Clarke, D., *Psychiatry To-day* (1952; London, 1963).

Timms, N., *Psychiatric Social Work in Britain, 1939–1962* (London, 1964).

Vincent, J., *Inside the Asylum* (London, 1948).

Wing, J. K., 'Trends in the care of the chronically mentally disabled', in J. Wing and R. Olsen (eds), *Community Care for the Mentally Disabled* (Oxford, 1979), pp. 1–13.

Wing, J. K., Bennett, D. H. and Denham, J., *The Industrial Rehabilitation of Long-Stay Schizophrenic Patients: A Study of 45 Patients at an Industrial Rehabilitation Unit: MRC Memorandum No. 42* (London, 1964).

Wing, J. K. and Brown, G. W., *Institutionalism and Schizophrenia: A Comparative Study of Three Mental Hospitals 1960–1968* (Cambridge, 1970).

Wootton, B., *Social Science and Social Pathology* (1959; London, 1963).

Yellowlees, H., *To Define True Madness: Commensense Psychiatry for Lay People* (1953; Harmondsworth, 1955).

Newspapers and periodicals

British Journal of Psychiatric Social Work
British Medical Journal
Daily Record

Daily Telegraph and Morning Post
Health Services Journal
Journal of Applied Behavior Analysis
Journal of Mental Science
Lancet
Mental Hospital and Institutional Workers' Union Journal
National Asylum Workers' Union Magazine
Pall Mall Gazette
The Times
Truth

Secondary sources

Printed sources

Anderson, J., *War, Disability and Rehabilitation in Britain: 'Soul of a Nation'* (Manchester, 2011).

Andrews, J., 'R. D. Laing in Scotland: facts and fictions of the "rumpus room" and interpersonal psychiatry', in M. Gijswijt-Hofstra and R. Porter (eds), *Cultures of Psychiatry and Mental Health Care in Postwar Britain and the Netherlands* (Amsterdam, 1998), pp. 121–40.

Andrews, J. and Digby, A., 'Introduction', in J. Andrews and A. Digby (eds), *Sex and Seclusion, Class and Custody: Perspectives on Gender and Class in the History of British and Irish Psychiatry* (Amsterdam and New York, 2004), pp. 7–44.

Andrews, J. and Scull, A., *Customers and Patrons of the Mad-Trade: The Management of Lunacy in Eighteenth-Century London with the Complete Text of John Monro's 1766 Case Book* (London, 2003).

Appignanesi, L., *Mad, Bad and Sad: A History of Women and the Mind Doctors since 1800* (London, 2008).

Barfoot, M. and Beveridge, A., 'Madness at the crossroads: John Home's letters from the Royal Edinburgh Asylum, 1886–87', *Psychological Medicine*, 20 (1990), 263–84.

Barham, P., *Closing the Asylum: The Mental Patient in Modern Society* (Harmondsworth, 1997).

Barham, P., *Forgotten Lunatics of the Great War* (London, 2004).

Barham, P. and Hayward, R., *Relocating Madness: From the Mental Patient to the Person* (London, 1995).

Bartlett, P., 'The asylum and the Poor Law: the productive alliance', in J. Melling and B. Forsythe (eds), *Insanity, Institutions and Society, 1800–1914: A Social History of Madness in Comparative Perspective* (London, 1999), pp. 48–64.

Bartlett, P. and Wright, D. (eds), *Outside the Walls of the Asylum: The History of Care in the Community 1750–2000* (London and New Brunswick, 1999).

Berridge, V., 'Medicine and the public: the 1962 Report of the Royal College of Physicians and the new public health', *Bulletin of the History of Medicine*, 81 (2007), 286–311.

Berridge, V., 'Medicine, public health and the media in Britain from the nineteen-fifties to the nineteen-seventies', *Historical Research*, 82 (2009), 360–73.

Beveridge, A., 'Voices of the mad: patients' letters from the Royal Edinburgh Asylum, 1873–1908', *Psychological Medicine*, 27 (1997), 899–908.

Beveridge, A., 'Life in the asylum: patients' letters from Morningside, 1873–1908', *History of Psychiatry*, 9 (1998), 431–69.

Beveridge, A., *Portrait of the Psychiatrist as a Young Man: The Early Writing and Work of R. D. Laing, 1927–1960* (Oxford, 2011).

Boston, S., *Women Workers and the Trade Unions* (London, 1980).

Bourdieu, P., *Distinction: A Social Critique of the Judgement of Taste* (1979; translation by Richard Nice 1984: Abingdon, 2005).

Bourdieu, P., *On Television and Journalism* (London, 1998).

Braybon, G., *Women Workers in the First World War* (London and New York, 1981).

Burleigh, M., *Death and Deliverance: 'Euthanasia' in Germany 1900–1945* (Cambridge, 1994).

Bury, M., 'Illness narratives: fact or fiction?', *Sociology of Health and Illness*, 23 (2001), 263–85.

Busfield, J., 'The female malady? Men, women and madness in nineteenth century Britain', *Sociology*, 28 (1994), 259–77.

Busfield, J., *Men, Women and Madness: Understanding Gender and Mental Disorder* (Houndmills, 1996).

Busfield, J., 'Restructuring mental health services in twentieth-century Britain', in M. Gijswijt-Hofstra and R. Porter (eds), *Cultures of Psychiatry and Mental Health Care in Postwar Britain and the Netherlands* (Amsterdam, 1998), pp. 9–28.

Butler, T., *Changing Mental Health Services: The Politics and Policy* (London, 1993).

Cantor, D., 'Representing "the public": medicine, charity and emotion in twentieth-century Britain', in S. Sturdy (ed.), *Medicine, Health and the Public Sphere in Britain, 1600–2000* (London, 2002), pp. 145–68.

Carpenter, M., 'Asylum nursing before 1914: a chapter in the history of labour', in C. Davies (ed.), *Rewriting Nursing History* (London, 1980), pp. 123–46.

Carpenter, M., *Working for Health: The History of the Confederation of Health Service Employees* (London, 1988).

Carpenter, M., *Normality Is Hard Work: Trade Unions and the Politics of Community Care* (London, 1994).

Carr, E. H., *What Is History?* (1961; Harmondsworth, 1990).

Cherry, S., *Mental Health Care in Modern England: The Norfolk Lunatic Asylum / St Andrew's Hospital c.1810–1998* (Woodbridge, 2003).

Chesler, P., *Women and Madness* (1972: New York, 1973).

Clark, M. J., 'Law, liberty and psychiatry in Victorian Britain: an historical survey and commentary, c. 1840–1890', in L. de Goei and J. Vijselaar (eds), *Proceedings of the First European Congress on the History of Psychiatry and Mental Health Care* (Amsterdam, 1993), pp. 187–93.

Clarke, L., 'Joshua Bierer: striving for power', *History of Psychiatry*, 8 (1997), 319–32.

Corrigan, P. W. (ed.), *On the Stigma of Mental Illness: Practical Strategies for Research and Social Change* (Washington, DC, 2005).

Cross, S., 'Visualizing madness: mental illness and public representation', *Television & New Media*, 5 (2004), 197–216.

Cross, S., *Mediating Madness: Mental Distress and Cultural Representation* (Houndmills, 2010).

Crossley, N., 'R. D. Laing and the British anti-psychiatry movement: a socio-historical analysis', *Social Science and Medicine*, 47 (1998), 877–89.

Crossley, N., 'Transforming the mental health field: the early history of the National Association of Mental Health', *Sociology of Health and Illness*, 20 (1998), 458–88.

Crossley, N., *Contesting Psychiatry: Social Movements in Mental Health* (Abingdon, 2006).

Curran, J. and Seaton, J., *Power Without Responsibility: The Press and Broadcasting in Britain* (London, 1997).

Delap, L., *Knowing Their Place: Domestic Service in Twentieth-Century Britain* (Oxford, 2011).

Dingwall, R., Rafferty, M. and Webster, C., *An Introduction to the Social History of Nursing* (London, 1988).

Eghigian, G., 'Deinstitutionalizing the history of contemporary psychiatry', *History of Psychiatry*, 22 (2011), 201–14.

Fennell, P., *Treatment without Consent: Law, Psychiatry and the Treatment of Mentally Disordered People since 1845* (London, 1996).

Finlayson, G., 'A moving frontier: voluntarism and the State in British social welfare 1911–1949', *Twentieth Century British History*, 1 (1990), 183–206.

Finlayson, G., *Citizen, State, and Social Welfare in Britain, 1830–1990* (Oxford, 1994).

Foucault, M., *Madness and Civilization: A History of Insanity in the Age of Reason* (London, 1967).

Fraser, N., 'Rethinking the public sphere: a contribution to the critique of actually existing democracy', in C. Calhoun (ed.), *Habermas and the Public Sphere* (1992; Cambridge, Mass., 1999), pp. 109–42.

Freeman, H., 'Psychiatry and the state in Britain', in M. Gijswijt-Hofstra, H. Oosterhuis, J. Vijselaar and H. Freeman (eds), *Psychiatric Cultures Compared: Psychiatry and Mental Health Care in the Twentieth Century* (Amsterdam, 2005), pp. 116–40.

Future Vision Coalition, *A Future Vision for Mental Health* (n.p., 2009).

Gilman, S. L., *The Face of Madness: Hugh W. Diamond and the Origin of Psychiatric Photography* (New York, 1977).

Gilman, S. L., *Disease and Representation: Images of Illness from Madness to AIDS* (Ithaca and London, 1988).

Gittins, D., *Madness in Its Place: Narratives of Severalls Hospital, 1913–1997* (London, 1998).

Goffman, E., *Stigma: Notes on the Management of a Spoiled Identity* (1963; Harmondsworth, 1968).

Griffiths, R., 'The bigger picture', *Mental Health Today* (January/February, 2012), 20.

Habermas, J., *The Structural Transformation of the Public Sphere*, trans. T. Burger (1962; Cambridge, 1999).

Hacking, I., *The Social Construction of What?* (1999; Cambridge, Mass., 2000).

Hall, L. A., 'Essay review: does madness have a gender?', *History of Psychiatry*, 20 (2009), 497–501.

Hallam, J., *Nursing the Image: Media, Culture and Professional Identity* (London, 2000).

Harding, T. W., '"Not worth powder and shot": a reappraisal of Montagu Lomax's contribution to mental health reform', *British Journal of Psychiatry*, 156 (1990), 180–7.

Harris, B., *The Origins of the Welfare State: Social Welfare in England and Wales, 1800–1945* (Basingstoke, 2004).

Harris, B., 'Voluntary action and the state in historical perspective', *Voluntary Sector Review*, 1 (2010), 25–40.

Henderson, L., 'Selling suffering: mental illness and media values', in G. Philo (ed.), *Media and Mental Distress* (Harlow, 1996), pp. 18–36.

Hess, V. and Majerus, B., 'Writing the history of psychiatry in the twentieth century', *History of Psychiatry*, 22 (2011), 139–45.

Hinshaw, S. P., *The Mark of Shame: Stigma of Mental Illness and an Agenda for Change* (Oxford, 2007).

Hornstein, G. A., *Agnes's Jacket: A Psychologist's Search for the Meanings of Madness* (2009; Ross-on-Wye, 2012).

Houston, R. A., '"Not simple boarding": care of the mentally incapacitated in Scotland during the long nineteenth century', in P. Bartlett and D. Wright (eds), *Outside the Walls of the Asylum: The History of Care in the Community 1750–2000* (London, 1999), pp. 19–44.

Hughes, K., *The Victorian Governess* (London, 1993).

Ingram, A. (ed.), *Voices of Madness: Four Pamphlets, 1683–1796* (Stroud, 1997).

Jackson, M., 'Images of deviance: visual representations of mental defectives in early twentieth-century medical texts', *British Journal for the History of Science*, 28 (1995), 319–37.

Jackson, M., *The Borderland of Imbecility: Medicine, Society and the Fabrication of the Feeble Mind in Late Victorian and Edwardian England* (Manchester, 2000).

Jenkins, K., *Rethinking History* (1991; Abingdon, 2009).

Joicey, N., 'A paperback guide to progress: Penguin books 1935 – c. 1951', *Twentieth Century British History*, 4 (1993), 25–56.

Jones, C., 'Raising the anti: Jan Foudraine, Ronald Laing and anti-psychiatry', in M. Gijswijt-Hofstra and R. Porter (eds), *Cultures of Psychiatry and Mental Health Care in Postwar Britain and the Netherlands* (Amsterdam, 1998), pp. 283–94.

Jones, K., *Asylums and After. A Revised History of the Mental Health Services: From the Early 18th Century to the 1990s* (London, 1993).

Karpf, A., *Doctoring the Media: The Reporting of Health and Medicine* (London, 1988).

Kitzinger, J., 'A sociology of media power: key issues in audience reception research', in G. Philo (ed.), *Message Received: Glasgow Media Group Research 1993–1998* (Harlow, 1999), pp. 3–20.

Larkin, G., 'Health workers', in R. Cooter and J. Pickstone (eds), *Companion to Medicine in the Twentieth Century* (London, 2003), pp. 531–42.

Lewis, J., *The Voluntary Sector, the State and Social Work in Britain: The Charity Organisation Society / Family Welfare Association Since 1869* (Aldershot, 1995).

Link, B. G. and Phelan, J. C., 'Conceptualizing stigma', *Annual Review of Sociology*, 27 (2001), 363–84.

Long, V., 'The Mental After Care Association: Public Representations of Mental Illness, 1879–1925' (MA thesis, University of Warwick, 2000).

Long, V., 'Changing Public Representations of Mental Illness in Britain, 1870–1970' (PhD dissertation, University of Warwick, 2004).

Long, V., '"A satisfactory job is the best psychotherapist": employment and mental health, 1939–60', in P. Dale and J. Melling (eds), *Mental Illness and Learning Disability since 1850: Finding a Place for Mental Disorder in the United Kingdom* (Abingdon, 2006), pp. 179–99.

Long, V., *The Rise and Fall of the Healthy Factory: The Politics of Industrial Health in Britain, 1914–60* (Basingstoke, 2011).

Long, V., '"Often there is a good deal to be done, but socially rather than medically": the psychiatric social worker as social therapist, 1945–1970', *Medical History*, 55 (2011), 223–39.

Long, V., 'Rethinking post-war mental healthcare: industrial therapy and the chronic mental patient in Britain', *Social History of Medicine*, advance access, published online, 10 March 2013.

Long, V., '"Surely a nice job for a girl?" Stories of nursing, gender, violence and mental illness in British asylums, 1914–1930', in P. Dale and A. Borsay (eds), *Nursing the Mentally Disordered: Struggles that Shaped the Working Lives of Paid Carers in Institutional and Community Settings from 1800 to the 1980s* (forthcoming).

Loughlin, K., '"Your Life in Their Hands": the context of a medical-media controversy', *Media History*, 6 (2000), 177–88.

Lunbeck, E., *The Psychiatric Persuasion: Knowledge, Gender and Power in Modern America* (Princeton, 1994).

MacDonald, D. F., *The State and the Trade Unions* (London, 1976).

MacDonald, M., *Mystical Bedlam: Madness, Anxiety, and Healing in Seventeenth-Century England* (Cambridge, 1981).

Maw, J., 'Revealing the Mind Bender General', BBC documentary, broadcast on Radio 4 on 17 March 2009.

McCandless, P., '"Build! build!" the controversy over the care of the chronically insane in England, 1855–1870', *Bulletin for the History of Medicine*, 53 (1979), 553–74.

McCandless, P., 'Liberty and lunacy: the Victorians and wrongful confinement', in A. Scull (ed.), *Madhouses, Mad-Doctors and Madmen: The Social History of Psychiatry in the Victorian Era* (Philadelphia, 1981), pp. 339–61.

McCarthy, H. and Thane, P., 'The politics of association in industrial life', *Twentieth-Century British History*, 22 (2011), 217–29.

McGann, S., Crowther, A. and Dougall, R., *A History of the Royal College of Nursing 1916–90: A Voice for Nurses* (Manchester, 2009).

Mehta, N., Kassam, A., Leese, M., Butler, G. and Thornicroft, G., 'Public attitudes towards people with mental illness in England and Scotland, 1994–2003', *British Journal of Psychiatry*, 194 (2009), 278–84.

Melling, J., 'Sex and sensibility in cultural history: the English governess and the lunatic asylum, 1845–1914', in J. Andrews and A. Digby (eds), *Sex and Seclusion, Class and Custody: Perspectives on Gender and Class in the History of British and Irish Psychiatry* (Amsterdam, 2004), pp. 177–219.

Melling, J., '"Buried alive by her friends": asylum narratives and the English governess, 1845–1914', in J. Melling and P. Dale (eds), *Mental Illness and Learning Disability since 1845: Finding a Place for Mental Disorder in the United Kingdom* (Abingdon, 2006), pp. 65–90.

Melling, J. and Forsythe, B., *The Politics of Madness: The State, Insanity and Society in England, 1845–1914* (Abingdon, 2006).

Mitchell, D., 'Parallel stigma? Nurses and people with learning disabilities', *British Journal of Learning Disabilities*, 28 (2000), 78–81.

Muijen, M., 'Scare in the community: Britain in moral panic', in T. Heller, J. Reynolds, R. Gomm, R. Muston and S. Pattison (eds), *Mental Health Matters: A Reader* (Houndmills, 1996), pp. 143–55.

Neve, M. and Turner, T., 'What the doctor thought and did: Sir James Crichton-Browne (1840–1938)', *Medical History*, 39 (1995), 399–432.

Nolan, P., *A History of Mental Health Nursing* (London, 1993).

Nolan, P., 'Annie Altschul's legacy to 20th century British mental health nursing', *Journal of Psychiatric and Mental Health Nursing*, 6 (1999), 267–72.

Nolan, P. and Hopper, B., 'Revisiting mental health nursing in the 1960s', *Journal of Mental Health*, 9 (2000), 563–73.

Norman, P., *In the Way of Understanding – Part of a Life: Lantern Slides in a Rough Time Sequence* (Godalming, 1982).

Nottingham, C., 'The rise of the insecure professionals', *International Review of Social History*, 52 (2007), 445–75.

Oakley, A., *A Critical Woman: Barbara Wootton, Social Science and Public Policy in the Twentieth Century* (London, 2011).

Parry-Jones, W., *The Trade in Lunacy: A Study of Private Madhouses in England in the Eighteenth and Nineteenth Centuries* (London, 1972)

Paterson, D., *A Mad People's History of Madness* (Pittsburgh, 1982).

Payne, S., 'Outside the walls of the asylum? Psychiatric treatment in the 1980s and 1990s', in P. Bartlett and D. Wright (eds), *Outside the Walls of the Asylum: The History of Care in the Community 1750–2000* (London, 1999), pp. 244–65.

Philo, G., (ed.), *Media and Mental Distress* (Harlow, 1996).

Philo, G., 'The media and public belief', in G. Philo (ed.), *Media and Mental Distress* (Harlow, 1996), pp. 82–104.

Philo, G., 'Users of services, carers and families', in G. Philo (ed.), *Media and Mental Distress* (Harlow, 1996), pp. 105–14.

Philo, G. (ed.), *Message Received: Glasgow Media Group Research 1993–1998* (Harlow, 1999).

Philo, G., McLaughlin, G. and Henderson, L., 'Media content', in G. Philo (ed.), *Media and Mental Distress* (London, 1996), pp. 45–813.

Pickstone, J. V., 'Psychiatry in general hospitals: history, contingency and local innovation in the early years of the National Health Service', in J. V. Pickstone (ed.), *Medical Innovations in Historical Perspective* (Houndmills, 1992), pp. 185–99.

Plumb, A., '. . . Distress or disability?' (1994), reproduced in J. Anderson, B. Sapey and H. Spandler (eds), *Distress or Disability? Proceedings of a Symposium Held at Lancaster University, 15–16 November 2011* (Bowland North, 2012), pp. 4–12.

Pols, H., '"Beyond the clinical frontiers": the American mental hygiene movement, 1910–1940', in V. Roelcke, P. Weindling and L. Westwood (eds), *International Relations in Psychiatry: Britain, Germany and the United States to World War II* (Rochester, 2010), pp. 111–33.

Porter, R., *Mind-Forg'd Manacles: A History of Madness in England from the Restoration to Regency* (Cambridge, Mass., 1987).

Porter, R. (ed.), *The Faber Book of Madness* (London, 1991).

Porter, R., 'Hearing the mad. Communication and excommunication', in L. de Goei and J. Vijselaar (eds), *Proceedings of the First European Congress on the History of Psychiatry and Mental Health Care* (Amsterdam, 1993), pp. 338–52.

Porter, R., 'Psychiatry and its history: Hunter and Macalpine', in L. de Goei and J. Vijselaar (eds), *Proceedings of the First European Congress on the History of Psychiatry and Mental Health Care* (Amsterdam, 1993), pp. 167–77.

Porter, R., *A Social History of Madness: Stories of the Insane* (London, 1999).

Porter, R., and Micale, M. S., 'Introduction: reflections on psychiatry and its histories', in M. S. Micale and R. Porter (eds), *Discovering the History of Psychiatry* (New York and Oxford, 1994), pp. 3–36.

Prior, L., *The Social Organization of Mental Illness* (London, 1993).

Prochaska, F. K., *Women and Philanthropy in Nineteenth-Century England* (Oxford, 1980).

Ramon, S., *Psychiatry in Britain: Meaning and Policy* (London, 1985).

Redfield Jamison, K., *Touched With Fire: Manic Depressive Illness and the Artistic Temperament* (New York, 1994).

Reid, F., 'Distinguishing between shell-shocked veterans and pauper lunatics: the Ex-Services' Welfare Society and mentally wounded veterans after the Great War', *War in History*, 14 (2007), 347–71.

Renvoize, E., 'The Association of Medical Officers of Asylums and Hospitals for the Insane, the Medico-Psychological Association, and their presidents', in G. E. Berrios and H. Freeman (eds), *150 Years of British Psychiatry, 1841–1991* (London, 1991), pp. 29–78.

Rollin, H. R., 'The Red Handbook: an historic centenary', Psychiatric Bulletin, 10 (1986), 279.

Rolph, S., Atkinson, D. and Warmsley, J., '"A pair of stout shoes and an umbrella": the role of the mental welfare officer in delivering community care in East Anglia: 1946–1970', British Journal of Social Work, 33 (2003), 339–59.

Rose, N., Governing the Soul: The Shaping of the Private Self (London, 1989).

Sartorius, N. and Schulze, H., Reducing the Stigma of Mental Illness: A Report from a Global Programme of the World Psychiatric Association (Cambridge, 2005).

Sayce, L., From Psychiatric Patient to Citizen: Overcoming Discrimination and Social Exclusion (Houndmills, 2000).

Scannell, P., 'Public service broadcasting: the history of a concept', in A. Goodwin and G. Whannel (eds), Understanding Television (London, 1990), pp. 11–29.

Scottish Government, Towards a Mentally Flourishing Scotland: Policy and Action Plan, 2009–2011 (Edinburgh, 2009).

Scull, A. T., Museums of Madness: The Social Organization of Insanity in Nineteenth-Century England (London, 1979).

Scull, A., (ed.), The Asylum as Utopia: W. A. F. Browne and the Mid-Nineteenth Century Consolidation of Psychiatry (London and New York, 1991).

Scull, A., The Most Solitary of Afflictions: Madness and Society in Britain, 1700–1900 (New Haven and London, 1993).

Scull, A., 'Somatic treatments and the historiography of psychiatry', History of Psychiatry, 5 (1994), 1–12.

Scull, A., Madhouse: A Tragic Tale of Megalomania and Modern Medicine (New Haven and London, 2005).

Scull, A., MacKenzie, C. and Hervey, N., Masters of Bedlam: The Transformation of the Mad-Doctoring Trade (Princeton, 1996).

Searle, G. R., Eugenics and Politics in Britain 1900–1914 (London, 1976).

Shakespeare, T. and Watson, N., 'The social model of disability: an outdated ideology?', Research in Social Science and Disability, 2 (2002), 9–28.

Shorter, E., A History of Psychiatry: From the Era of the Asylum to the Age of Prozac (New York, 1997).

Shortland, M., 'Screen memories: towards a history of psychiatry and psychoanalysis in the movies', British Journal for the History of Science, 20 (1987), 421–52.

Showalter, E., The Female Malady: Women, Madness and English Culture, 1830–1980 (1987; London, 2001).

Small, H., '"In the guise of science": literature and the rhetoric of nineteenth-century English psychiatry', History of the Human Sciences, 7 (1994), 27–55.

Smith, J., 'Forging the "missing link": the significance of the Mental After Care Association archive', History of Psychiatry, 8 (1997), 407–20.

Soanes, S., 'Reforming asylums, reforming public attitudes: J. R. Lord and Montagu Lomax's representations of mental hospitals and the community, 1921–1931', Family and Community History, 12 (2009), 117–29.

Soanes, S., 'Rest and Restitution: Mental Convalescence and the English Public Mental Hospital, 1919–1939' (PhD thesis, University of Warwick, 2011).

Spandler, H., *Asylum to Action: Paddington Day Hospital, Therapeutic Communities and Beyond* (London, 2006).

Spandler, H., 'From social exclusion to inclusion? A critique of the inclusion imperative in mental health', *Medical Sociology Online*, 2:2 (2007), 3–16.

Stedman Jones, G., *Outcast London: A Study in the Relationship between Classes in Victorian Society* (1971: Harmondsworth, 1992).

Stewart, J., 'Angels or aliens? Refugee nurses in Britain, 1938 to 1942', *Medical History*, 47 (2003), 149–72.

Stewart, J., 'Psychiatric social work in inter-war Britain: child guidance, American ideas, American philanthropy', *Michael Quarterly*, 3 (2006), 78–91.

Stewart, J., '"I thought you would want to come and see his home", child guidance and psychiatric social work in inter-war Britain', in M. Jackson (ed.), *Health and the Modern Home* (Abingdon, 2007), pp. 111–27.

Stewart, J., 'The scientific claims of British child guidance', *British Journal for the History of Science*, 42 (2009), 407–32.

Stewart, J., *Child Guidance in Britain, 1918–1955: The Dangerous Age of Childhood* (London, 2013).

Strong, S., *Community Care in the Making: A History of MACA 1879–2000* (London, 2000).

Sturdy, S., 'Hippocrates and state medicine: George Newman outlines the funding policy of the Ministry of Health', in C. Lawrence (ed.), *Greater than the Parts: Holism in Biomedicine, 1920–1950* (Oxford, 1998), pp. 112–34.

Sturdy, S., (ed.), *Medicine, Health and the Public Sphere in Britain, 1600–2000* (London, 2002).

Suzuki, A., *Madness at Home: The Psychiatrist, the Patient, and the Family in England, 1820–1860* (Berkley and Los Angeles, 2006).

Tansey, E. M., '"They used to call it psychiatry": aspects of the development and impact of psychopharmacology', in M. Gijswijt-Hofstra and R. Porter (eds), *Cultures of Psychiatry and Mental Health Care in Postwar Britain and the Netherlands* (Amsterdam, 1998), pp. 79–101.

Taylor, B., 'The demise of the asylum in late twentieth-century Britain: a personal history', *Transactions of the Royal Historical Society*, 21 (2011), 193–215.

Thom, B., *Dealing with Drink: Alcohol and Social Policy from Treatment to Management* (London, 1999), pp. 36–9.

Thom, D., 'Wishes, anxieties, play and gestures: child guidance in inter-war England', in R. Cooter (ed.), *In the Name of the Child: Health and Welfare, 1880–1940* (London, 1992), pp. 200–19.

Thomson, M., *The Problem of Mental Deficiency: Eugenics, Democracy, and Social Policy in Britain, c. 1870–1959* (Oxford, 1998).

Thomson, M., 'Status, manpower and mental fitness: mental deficiency in the First

World War', in R. Cooter, M. Harrison and S. Sturdy (eds), *War, Medicine and Society* (Stroud, 1998), pp. 149–66.

Thomson, M., *Psychological Subjects: Identity, Culture and Health in Twentieth-Century Britain* (Oxford, 2006).

Todd, S., *Young Women, Work, and Family in England 1918–1950* (Oxford, 2005).

Toms, J., 'Mental Hygiene to Civil Rights: MIND and the Problematic of Personhood, c.1900–c.1980' (PhD thesis, University of London, 2005).

Toon, E., '"Cancer as the general population knows it": knowledge, fear, and lay education in 1950s Britain', *Bulletin of the History of Medicine*, 81 (2007), 116–48.

Topp, L., Moran, J. and Andrews, J. (eds), *Madness, Architecture and the Built Environment: Psychiatric Spaces in Historical Context* (Abingdon, 2007).

Trent Jr, J. W., *Inventing the Feeble Mind: A History of Mental Retardation in the United States* (Berkeley and Los Angeles, 1994).

Tringo, J. L., 'The hierarchy of preference towards disability groups', *Journal of Special Education*, 4 (1970), 295–30.

Turner, T., '"Not worth powder and shot": the public profile of the Medico-Psychological Association, c. 1851–1914', in G. E. Berrios and H. Freeman (eds), *150 Years of British Psychiatry, 1841–1991* (London, 1991), pp. 3–16.

Ungerson, C., *Policy Is Political: Sex, Gender and Informal Care* (London, 1987).

Ussher, J., *Women's Madness: Misogyny or Mental Illness?* (London, 1991).

Vincent, A. W., 'The Poor Law reports of 1909 and the social theory of the Charity Organisation Society', *Victorian Studies*, 27 (1984), 343–63.

Webster, C., 'Healthy or hungry thirties?', *History Workshop Journal*, 13 (1982), 110–29.

Westwood, L., 'Avoiding the Asylum: Pioneering Work in Mental Health Care, 1890–1939' (DPhil thesis, Sussex University, 1999).

Westwood, L., 'A quiet revolution in Brighton: Dr Helen Boyle's pioneering approach to mental health care, 1899–1939', *Social History of Medicine*, 14 (2001), 439–57.

White, H., *The Content of the Form: Narrative Discourse and Historical Representation* (Baltimore and London, 1987).

Woodroofe, K., *From Charity to Social Work in the United States and England* (London, 1962).

Wright, D., 'The discharge of pauper lunatics from county asylums in mid-Victorian England: the case of Buckinghamshire', in J. Melling and B. Forsythe (eds), *Insanity, Institutions and Society 1800–1914: A Social History of Madness in Comparative Perspective* (Abingdon, 1999), pp. 93–112.

Yanni, C., *The Architecture of Madness: Insane Asylums in the United States* (Minneapolis and London, 2007).

Younghusband, E., *Social Work in Britain: 1950–197. A Follow-Up Study Vol. 2* (London, 1978).

Internet sources

Andrews, J., 'Savage, Sir George Henry (1842–1921)', *Oxford Dictionary of National Biography*, Oxford University Press, 2004; online edition, May 2007: www.oxforddnb.com/view/article/38635.

Beresford, P., 'Mental health discrimination is coming from the top, not the public', *The Guardian* (30 November 2011): www.guardian.co.uk/society/joepublic/2011/nov/30/mental-health-discrimination-campaign.

Corley, T. A. B., 'Wakefield, Charles Cheers, first Viscount Wakefield (1859–1941)', *Oxford Dictionary of National Biography*, Oxford University Press, 2004; online edition, January 2011: www.oxforddnb.com/view/article/36679.

Department of Health, '£20 million to knock down mental health stigma', 10 October 2011: http://mediacentre.dh.gov.uk/2011/10/10/20-million-to-knock-down-mental-health-stigma/.

Digby, A., 'Tuke, Daniel Hack (1827–1895)', *Oxford Dictionary of National Biography*, Oxford University Press, 2004: www.oxforddnb.com/view/article/27804, accessed 15 November 2011.

Firemonkee, 'Time to Change': www.mentalhealthforum.net/forum/thread4637.html, 10 May 2011.

Fisher, P., 'James Bickford', *Guardian*, 3 April 2009: www.guardian.co.uk/theguardian/2009/apr/03/obituary-james-bickford.

'Health: Dobson outlines Mental Health Plans', 29 July 1998: http://news.bbc.co.uk/1/hi/health/141651.stm.

Hornstein, G., 'Bibliography of first-person narratives of madness in English (5th edition)', last revised December 2011: www.gailhornstein.com/files/Bibliography_of_First_Person_Narratives_of_Madness_5th_edition.pdf.

Lentin, A., 'McCardie, Sir Henry Alfred (1869–1933)', *Oxford Dictionary of National Biography*, Oxford University Press, 2004: www.oxforddnb.com/view/article/34677, accessed 10 October 2011.

Lombard, P., 'Mental Health Act: demand for community orders swamps services', *Community Care*, 30 March 2009: www.communitycare.co.uk/articles/30/03/2009/111151/mental-health-act-demand-for-community-orders-swamps-services.htm.

http://mary-barnes.net/about.htm, consulted 17 February 2012.

Mental Health Foundation, 'What are mental health problems?': www.mentalhealth.org.uk/help-information/an-introduction-to-mental-health/what-are-mental-health-problems/?view=Standard, accessed 30 January 2012.

Mind: www.mind.org.uk/.

Powell, E., speech given to the National Association for Mental Health (1961): reproduced on the webpage http://studymore.org.uk/xpowell.htm.

Rethink Mental Illness: http://www.rethink.org/.

Roberts, A., 'Mental Health History Timeline': http://studymore.org.uk/.

Royal College of Psychiatrists: www.rcpsych.ac.uk.

Russell, K. F. 'Berry, Richard James Arthur (1867–1962)', *Australian Dictionary of*

Biography (1979): http://adb.anu.edu.au/biography/berry-richard-james-arthur-5220/text8703, accessed 8 February 2013.

See Me: www.seemescotland.org.

Springhall, J., 'Brabazon, Reginald, twelfth earl of Meath (1841–1929)', *Oxford Dictionary, of National Biography*, Oxford University Press, 2004; online edition, January 2011: www.oxforddnb.com/view/article/32019.

'This week in . . .', *Worcester News* (August 18 2008): www.worcesternews.co.uk/news/nostalgia/thisweekin/3601926.AUGUST_16_23/.

Time to Change: www.time-to-change.org.uk.

Together, 'Henry Hawkins: Founder of Together': www.together-uk.org/uploads/pdf/history/henryhawkins.pdf, accessed 8 November 2011.

http://topdocumentaryfilms.com/how-mad-are-you/, consulted 17 February 2013.

Willis, S., 'Shiny happy service users – is the TTC campaign about to become counter-productive?', 18 September 2010: www.dawnwillis.wordpress.com/2010/09/18/shiny-happy-service-users-%E2%80%93-is-the-ttc-campaign-about-to-become-counter-productive/.

Index